Evaluation of Acupuncture

Culture and Knowledge
Edited by Friedrich G. Wallner

Vol. 24

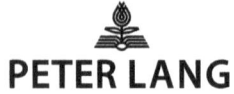

Friedrich G. Wallner /
Fengli Lan (eds.)

Evaluation of Acupuncture

An Intercultural and Interdisciplinary Approach

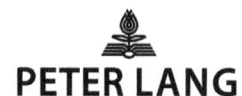

Bibliographic Information published by the Deutsche Nationalbibliothek
The Deutsche Nationalbibliothek lists this publication in the Deutsche Nationalbibliografie; detailed bibliographic data is available in the internet at http://dnb.d-nb.de.

Library of Congress Cataloging-in-Publication Data
A CIP catalog record for this book has been applied for at the Library of Congress.

Gefördert von der Kulturabteilung der Stadt Wien, Wissenschafts- und Forschungsförderung.

ISSN 1613-902X
ISBN 978-3-631-74709-4 (Print)
E-ISBN 978-3-631-76145-8 (E-Book)
E-ISBN 978-3-631-76146-5 (EPUB)
E-ISBN 978-3-631-76147-2 (MOBI)
DOI 10.3726/b14376

© Peter Lang GmbH
Internationaler Verlag der Wissenschaften
Berlin 2018
All rights reserved.

Peter Lang – Berlin · Bern · Bruxelles · New York · Oxford · Warszawa · Wien

All parts of this publication are protected by copyright. Any utilisation outside the strict limits of the copyright law, without the permission of the publisher, is forbidden and liable to prosecution. This applies in particular to reproductions, translations, microfilming, and storage and processing in electronic retrieval systems.

www.peterlang.com

Dedicated

to

my friend

Alfred Pritz

Contents

Friedrich Wallner and Fengli Lan
Introduction 9

About the Authors 11

Friedrich Wallner
Manifesto for a *Non-Competing Parallel Research Programme*
on Acupuncture 17

Lixing Lao and Mingxiao Yang
Evidence-Based Acupuncture and Mechanistic Studies of Acupuncture 37

Fengli Lan
Interpreting Literature: A Key to Transmit and Enrich Knowledge
System of Acupuncture 55

Ephraim Ferreira Medeiros, Lixing Lao, and Fengli Lan
An Overview of the Evolution of Acupuncture Treatment:
From Stone Needle to Laser Beam 67

Andrea-Mercedes Riegel
Translations of Chinese Medical Texts and Their Impact on the
Theories and Practice of Chinese Medicine 83

Lixing Lao and Mingxiao Yang
Difficulties and Challenges Clinical Acupuncture Trials Are Facing 103

Fengli Lan
Women's Health: Fundamentals, Lifestyles and Acupuncture Approach 117

Andrea-Mercedes Riegel
Acupuncture Treatment for Lifestyle Related Diseases 147

Kwon Jong Yoo
Acupuncture and Placebo Effect 169

Andrea-Mercedes Riegel
The Names of Acupoints in Chinese Medicine: A Mirror of
Chinese Culture Misunderstood in the Western World 185

Ephraim Ferreira Medeiros, Andrea-Mercedes Riegel,
Mildred Ferreira Medeiros and Fengli Lan
Understanding Baomai 胞脉 and Baoluo 胞絡: A Multidisciplinary
Approach 215

Andrea-Mercedes Riegel
Baomai and *Baoluo*: Two Vessels of Importance Not Only for
Female Health 239

Introduction

This book is the newest publication of the international research group "Theory, Methodology, and Structure of TCM" which has been working since 2008. It starts to outline a methodology which is adequate for research on Classical Chinese Medicine (CCM). Such a methodology must take care of the ontological and methodological structure of CCM, which is incompatible with the Western Medicine. After this we show in a detailed way and careful analysis of research procedures which are now common–Evidence-Based Acupuncture and Mechanistic-Based Acupuncture research–, and discuss the challenges and difficulties in clinical acupuncture trials that are still faced today. The results of these studies show that Chinese medicine offers serial and secured options for medical treatment and alternative for Western medicine – even though we subordinate with the Western methodology (a critical view on evidence-based medicine (EBM) and double-blind methodology offers a report of placebo theories.)

Besides the external critique on acupuncture we concentrate on the improvement of theoretical basis and exact understanding of acupuncture. This is done by analysis of classical texts and hermeneutical treatments. To this undertaking we also offer historical studies.

A fruitful way to solve misunderstandings and increase the theoretical understanding is a study on translations of Chinese medical texts.

The analysis of acupuncture in respect of concrete health problems also offers specific theoretical insights and possibilities. The discussions of lifestyle-related diseases and women's diseases open additional insights on the theoretical background of acupuncture.

Besides this you can see the broad and open basis of Chinese medicine in the research on *Baomai* and *Baoluo* by different members of our research group.

This book shows that our research group is on the way to general and explicit theories of Chinese medicine. It will demonstrate that Chinese medicine is a scientific system which is independent from modern Western medicine.

The editors

About the Authors

Fengli LAN

Prof. Dr. Lan Fengli (1972–), Currently a faculty member of the Five Branches University, Graduate School of Traditional Chinese Medicine (TCM); California Licensed Acupuncturist (Acupuncture and Chinese Herbal Medicine); Former Professor at the Shanghai University of TCM (SHUTCM, until 2015); Guest Professor at the University of Vienna in Austria in Winter Semester 2010–2011.

Studied Medicine, English Language and Literature, Applied Linguistics, Philosophy of Science, and Anthropology: Bachelor in Medicine (also known as MD), 1990–1995, Hebei Medical University; Master in Medicine, 1995–1998, SHUTCM; PhD in Medicine, 2002–2005, SHUTCM; B.A. in English Language and Literature, 2001–2003, Shanghai International Studies University; Postdoctoral Fellowship in Applied Linguistics, 2005–2008, Shanghai Jiao Tong University and China Postdoctoral Science Foundation; Visiting Faculty in Constructive Realism, 2007–2010, University of Vienna and OeAD in Austria; Visiting Faculty in Anthropology, 2014–2016, University of California Santa Cruz and San Diego, USA.

Has published 36 peer-reviewed journal papers; 38 book chapters, 27 conference papers, and 24 books. Fields of research: Philosophical and Intercultural Interpretation of Chinese Medicine, Acupuncture, Gynecology in Chinese Medicine, Ancient Chinese Medical Classics; Classical Chinese Language, Culture, and Philosophy; Cross-Cultural and Translation Studies of Chinese Medicine; Applied Linguistics; Constructive Realism; Medical, Psychological, Linguistic, and Cultural Anthropology. Favorite publications: *Culture, Philosophy, and Chinese Medicine: Viennese Lectures* (Peter Lang, 2012); *Metaphor: The Weaver of Chinese Medicine* (Bautz, 2015).

Lixing LAO

Prof. Dr. Lao Lixing (1954–), Vivian Taaam Wong Endowed Professor in Integrative Medicine, Professor and Director in the School of Chinese Medicine, The University of Hong Kong. Adjunct Professor of Family Medicine and the Director of Traditional Chinese Medicine Research Program in the Center for Integrative Medicine of the School of Medicine, University of Maryland, Baltimore (UMB), USA.

An elected vice president of the World Federation of Acupuncture and Moxibustion Societies (WFAS) and an appointed Secretary General of the Consortium for Globalization of Chinese Medicine (CGCM). Board member of the SAR and a co-president of the Society for 5 years 2003–2007.

Graduated from the Shanghai University of Traditional Chinese Medicine (TCM) in 1983 and completed his Ph.D. in physiology at UMB in 1992. Also, a licensed acupuncturist over 30 years and served as a Board member for 5 years on the Maryland State Board of Acupuncture.

Has led over 20 clinical trials and pre-clinical studies in acupuncture and Chinese herbal medicines funded by the National Institutes of Health (NIH) and Department of Defense, USA. Published over 230 peer-reviewed scientific papers and over 10 book chapters. Has also given over 300 presentations at national and international conferences/symposia. Serves on editorial boards in a number of journals including associate editor in the Journal of Alternative and Complementary Medicine and the Journal of Alternative Therapies in Health and Medicine, and co-Editor in Chief in the Journal of Integrative Medicine. Research focus on translational research that bridges basic science, clinical trials, and "real world" acupuncture/Chinese medicine clinical practice.

Ephraim Ferreira MEDEIROS

Director of the International Education and Research Department – CEATA (Center for Study of Acupuncture and Alternative Therapies) – Brazil/China (www.ceata.com.br).

He was born in 1973 in Rio de Janeiro. Bachelor of Science in Biomedicine – State University of Campinas – Brazil (1995).

Postgraduate specialization course in Acupuncture – Brazilian Association of Acupuncture – ABA (1997).

Created and developed the technique of Aromatic Acupuncture that combines the therapeutic effects of acupuncture with energetic functions of essential oils used in aromatherapy (1999).

Pioneer in the implementation of web platforms to the study of Chinese Medicine in Brazilian Portuguese language (since 1995).

Founder, webmaster, and Content Designer of the projects Acupunturabrasil. org – 1995 (previously Acupuntura.pro.br), Medicinachinesaclassica.org, Mei huanet.com, and Bencaobrasil.org.

Lives in China since October 2006, conducting advanced clinical studies in hospitals and clinics in Beijing and Sichuan (Gulou Hospital, Tongren Hospital, Beijing Hospital, Acupuncture Hospital of the China Academy of Chinese Medical

Sciences (CACMS), and Mianyang TCM Hospital) and training in Japanese acupuncture in Meiji University of Integrative Medicine (Kyoto, Japan). Currently researching Philosophy of Science in Traditional Chinese Medicine (Acupuncture).

Mildred MEDEIROS

Born in 1976 in Rio de Janeiro (Brazil). Bachelor in Biological Sciences from the Federal University of Rio de Janeiro (1999), Master in Morphology from the State University of Rio de Janeiro (2002). She holds a Ph.D. in Sciences from the State University of Rio de Janeiro (2014). In her scientific initiation and master's degree, she performed histochemical, immunocytochemical and stereological investigations on the pineal gland of rats, and published scientific articles on the subject. In her doctorate, she developed research on inflammatory infiltrates and some chemokines on biopsied nerves of patients with the pure neural form of leprosy, having published works in the area.

Currently, she teaches the following subjects at the Estácio de Sá University (RJ): Histology and Embryology, Cellular Biology, Morphology I and II in nursing, physiotherapy and dentistry courses. She is also conducting research on the following topics: fetal alcohol syndrome, Down's Syndrome, pregnancy gestation, the morning-after pill, congenital syphilis, bacterial endocarditis, health education and hematopoietic stem cell transplantation, involving undergraduate nursing and dentistry students in Estacio de Sá. She is a researcher with a scholarship at the Estácio de Sá University (Brazil). Since February 2016, she has been an assistant professor of Systems Anatomy, Parasitology, Epidemiology and Cellular and Molecular Biology at the University Center Augusto Motta (RJ – Brazil). Since July 2017, she also has been cooperated as an assistant professor of Histology and Embryology at Universidade Veiga de Almeida University – RJ.

Andrea-Mercedes RIEGEL

Born in 1957 in Rastatt, Germany; studied applied linguistics and science of translation (French, Spanish, and law) in Heidelberg (1976–1983). Afterwards studies in Chinese language (classic and modern) philosophy and culture, German linguistics and literature and medical history in Heidelberg and Munich. M.A: in 1992. Between 1989 and 1991 studies abroad in Taibei (Taiwan), classes in Western and Chinese Medicine, 6 months of clinical practice in a Taibei hospital.

Between 1993 and 1999 postgraduate studies in classical Chinese medical literature in Munich, doctorate (Dr. Phil.) in 1999. Since 1999 practitioner of Chinese medicine and interpreter in lessons for Chinese medicine in China. Since 2003 lecturer at the "Academy for holistic medicine" in Heidelberg. In 2005 she started her studies in medical sciences at the University of Witten/Herdecke and her second doctorate (Dr. rer. medic.) in 2010. During 2010 and 2015 several stays in Asia for studies in theories of Chinese medicine and acupuncture practice.

Main research areas are the *Yijing* and its influence on the theories and practice of Chinese medicine., the value of old medical theories for the treatment of modern diseases, the interpretation of Chinese medical terms in modern medicine and the translation of classical texts of Chinese medicine.

Numerous articles and lectures about Chinese medicine and 16 books about clinical practice and medical theories.

Friedrich WALLNER

Born in 1945 in Weiten, Lower Austria/Austria, University Professor for Philosophy and Philosophy of Science at the University of Vienna since 1987 (studied Philosophy, Psychology, Education, German and Classic Literature, etc.). His areas of expertise include the Vienna Circle, Ludwig Wittgenstein, Karl Popper, the Philosophy of Science of Psychotherapy, the Philosophy of Science of Traditional Chinese Medicine, as well as Epistemology, Applied Philosophy of Science, and Intercultural Philosophy.

Among professorships at the Institute of Theoretical Physics at the University of Vienna, Wallner worked on behalf of the Austrian Federal Ministry for Education, Arts and Culture in the field of pedagogy research. During 1985–1995 he developed a new Philosophy of Science, i.e. Constructive Realism, which makes the manifold scientific approaches understandable based on different cultures.

Since the 1990s, he has devoted his scientific and academic work especially to the research of TCM. His research activities are particularly focused on the complex relationship between the field of scientific practice and the 258 sociocultural contexts of presuppositions. More specifically, his research intensively concentrates on structural analytic studies of TCM and other local and indigenous systems of knowledge. Against the background of the cultural dependency of science, Wallner is intensively working on the argumentative structure of TCM with the aim to provide scientific fundament for the research of TCM as well as to refine the scientific research on the basis of theoretical concepts of Philosophy of Science.

Numerous visiting professorships in 14 countries; scientific guidance and presidencies of famous international conferences, congresses, workshops and seminars; numerous guest lectures all over Europe, Asia, Australia, New Zealand, Africa, Latin America, USA and Canada, Wallner advocates international, intercultural and interdisciplinary research projects and cooperation. Scientific Emphases: Theory, Methodology and Structure of Chinese Medicine; Cultural Dependency of Science; How to Research and Modernize Chinese Medicine; Applications of Constructive Realism in Developing an Integrative Medicine; Intercultural Philosophy and Chinese Medicine, etc.

Up to this date, he has published over 200 scientific essays, 20 monographs (Die Verwandlung der Wissenschaft, 2002; What Practitioners of TCM should know, 2006; Traditionelle Chinesische Medizin – Eine Alternative Denkwei-se, 2006; Five Lectures on the Foundations of Chinese Medicine, 2009; Systemanalyse als Wissenschaftstheorie I–III, 2008–2011, etc.) and 40 omnibus volumes. Since 2004 to 2010, Wallner was the chairman of the research unit "Interdisciplinarity and Interculturality" of the University of Vienna.

Wallner was listed 2014 in "The Encyclopedia Intelligentsia" and 2016 honored with the "Austrian Cross of Honor, First Class, for Science and Art".

Mingxiao YANG

Dr. Yang Mingxiao (1988–), Postdoctoral Fellow of the School of Chinese Medicine, The University of Hong Kong. Member of the China Association of Acupuncture and Moxibustion 2016–2022. Graduated from the Chengdu University of Traditional Chinese Medicine (CDTCM) in 2014 and completed his Ph.D. in Acupuncture and Massage at CDTCM in 2017. Also, a registered TCM doctor for over 3 years.

Has participated in 4 clinical trials and pre-clinical studies in acupuncture, including two National 973 programs. Published over 20 scientific papers in peer-reviewed journals including JAMA, Internal Medicine, PloS One, etc.

Serves as an associate editor of peer-reviewed journal TRIALS.

Directions of ongoing research: evidence-based medicine and randomized clinical trials in acupuncture and moxibustion for pain conditions, metabolomics in acupuncture and TCM, and gut microbiota research in acupuncture treating cardiovascular diseases.

Kwon Jong YOO

Born in 1959 in Goesan, Southern province in South Korea, University Professor of Philosophy at the Chung-Ang University since 1995 (studied Confucianism, Taoism, Buddhism, and cognitive Science, Systems Thinking, etc.). His areas of expertise include East Asian Confucianism, Taoism, Buddhism, Confucian Classics, Taoist Classics, Korean Traditional Philosophy, Korean history of Philosophy,

Comparative Studies of the Mind, Constructivism, Constructive Realism, Rituals and Lifestyle.

He has developed a constructivist framework to develop traditional Confucianism into modern self-organizational methodology, especially for sound lifestyle by applying traditional Confucian rituals in everyday life. Relating to this, he has been linking mind studies on Confucianism, Taoism, and Buddhism to the self-organizational/cultivational methodology. According to this study direction, he has paid attention to differences in understanding mind in every language, culture, and academic field and thus went further to comparative studies of mind understanding. From 2012 to 2016, as the Director of the Institute for Philosophical Studies at the Chung-Ang University, he has completed a three-year project supported by the National Research Foundation of Korea. The project was to make a dictionary of comparison of understanding mind.

Now he extends his research concern into how to establish and continue a sound lifestyle not only of an individual but of a society. Relating to this, he has joined in Professor Wallner's TCM project and is developing a philosophical refinement of meridian system with concepts and theories of systems view and cognitive science. In addition, he applied Professor Wallner's Constructive Realism to his comparative studies of the mind and human soundness.

He had studied about Constructive Realism and Constructivism as a visiting scholar at the University of Vienna for a year from 2005 to 2006 and at the same time as LG Yonam Research Professor. From 2014 to 2015, he visited the New York State University, Stony Brook and performed comparative studies of mind.

He has served as the President of Korean Society of Confucian Studies from 2015 to 2017, as the President of the Society of Mind Studies from 2011 to 2015, as the President of the International Association fo Bio-Cosmology from 2013 to 2016, and also as the Chair of the International Conference on Comparative Studies of Mind since 2010 until now. His Research Papers and Publications include:

2006 "Korean Culture and Korean Thought, Asian and African Studies", Journal of the Department of Asian and African Studies University of Ljubljana – Faculty of Arts.
2011 "Ecologism and Confucian Pro-life-ism", ACTA Koreana.
2013 "Dasan's Approach to the Ultimate Reality", Korean Journal, Vol. 53, No. 2, Korean National Commission for the UNESCO.
2013 "Ecology and Korea Confucianism", Kyemyeong University Press.
2014 "Ethical Activism with Consideration of the Routine of Food culture", entry of the Encyclopedia of Food and Agricultural Ethics, Springer Reference.
2017 "On a Harmony Principle of Body-Mind-Life", Lifestyle and Health.

Friedrich Wallner

Manifesto for a *Non-Competing Parallel Research Programme* on Acupuncture*

Abstract: The article's point of departure is the methodological shortcomings of researching Classical Chinese Acupuncture. Referring to Imre Lakatos's concept of *Parallel Research Programmes* and the epistemological stand of *Constructive Realism* it aims to lay the foundations for the development of a *Non-Competing Parallel Research Programme* on Acupuncture.

1 Introduction

To date the most complete studies into the effect and effectiveness of acupuncture have been the so-called German Acupuncture Trials (GERAC). Taking place between 2001 and 2017, more than 3500 patients with chronic conditions were treated with either standard methods of Western medicine, with acupuncture based on the traditional Chinese acupuncture points (*verum*), or with what has henceforth become known as *sham acupuncture* (setting the needles without regard for the traditional acupuncture points).[1]

Yet, the outcome of the studies has been puzzling—even foregoing any of themore or less valid critiques of the trials—and ultimately produced more questions than answers. While both *sham* and *verum* acupuncture outperformed the treatment with standard tools of Western medicine, their effects on patients seemed to be indifferent to whether the correct acupuncture points where needled or not.[2]

On a first view, this result allows to draw the conclusion that we can easily separate the question of scientificity of acupuncture as part of the whole system of Classical Chinese medicine (CCM) from the question of its healing effect. I have argued elsewhere that this would be a mistake. I also argued that the surprising outcome of the study can be explained (at least mostly) by what is essentially a categorical error: namely, trying to explain the inner workings of a scientific system

---

* I am very grateful to Dr. Jan Brousek for cooperating on this text.
1 Cf. Birch, Stephen: "Reflections on the German Acupuncture Studies". In: *Journal of Chinese Medicine* 83, February 2007, pp. 12–17.
2 Meanwhile, the official explanation is that the acupuncture points of sham acupuncture have been still in the segment of the traditional acupuncture points. But, this does not change the fact the study is built on a methodological mistake, as I will show within this article.

based on an utterly different ontology, like the CCM, by judging it according to the standards of a different (our modern) science.

On the other hand, if I'm correct about the CCM being a comprehensive scientific proposition system in its own right, this opens the question of how we are then to evaluate the claims of acupuncture, besides the immediate health merits of its practice, in such a way that our evaluation can still provide orientation for our modern world? In other words, how can we provide an assessment of the proposition system that guides the practice of acupuncture that is not doomed to fail from the start? In what follows I'm going to propose how the philosophy of science can contribute to this question by providing a proper theoretical framework that allows us to analyze and evaluate ontologically incommensurable proposition systems.

At this point I would like to point out that Western medicine is a very young discipline, only about 200 years young. It was fundamentally influenced by Western sciences, especially by Newton and the concept of mechanics. In turn, Newtonian mechanics builds on a descriptivist concept of reality whose basis is highly metaphysical. This traces back to Parmenides, whose formulation "noein kai einai tauton",[3] which means "thinking and being identical",[4] has become of axiomatic character for Western science. Its main idea was that knowledge should be the mirror of the world. This conviction survived up to the point when descriptivism died within the last century. Descriptivism just could not be managed and finally turned out to be a metaphysical fantasy. Until the 20th century the equation "science=truth" was believed by any intellectual in Europe, for example by the so-called Vienna Circle, which in the end showed that this is impossible: science is not a mirror of the world, science is a construct which replaces some aspects of the world by technical reasons.

If we now compare this axiom with one from the CCM we become aware of the fundamental difference between the two approaches. The axiom from the CCM has the formulation "Tian Ren He Yi", which we can translate as "heaven and men in harmony".[5] It does neither say, man and heaven "should be" in harmony, nor

---

3 Cf. Parmenides: *Sein und Welt:* Die Fragmente neu übersetzt und kommentiert von Helmuth Vetter. (Mit einem Anhang von Alfred Dunshirn über neue Literatur zu Parmenides). Verlag Karl Alber: Freiburg/München. 2016.
4 It actually does not say "is" identical or "should" be identical, rather just "thinking and being identical".
5 Cf. Lan, Fengli: "Metaphors in the Framework of Tian Ren He Yi: Aspects of Lifestyle Related Diseases." In: F. L. Lan/F.G. Wallner/G. Klünger (eds.): *Lifestyle and Health.* Traugott Bautz: Nordhausen. 2017. pp. 77–108.

does it say, "harmony is the condition"; both would already be metaphysical and follow a totally wrong line.

Therefore, we should start to change our approach, otherwise we will lose all that what CCM can offer and Western medicine does not offer.

In the following, I will lay out the origins of the central ideas of Lakatos's *Methodology of Scientific Research Programmes*, which in parts inspired this paper, and then explain why, as a theory of science, it ultimately failed. The next section explains the rough outlines of a theory of science called *Constructive Realism* (CR), whose major assumptions will then use to replace the problematic parts of the Lakato's theory. With all that as a proper theoretical background, I can then offer a more thorough motivation for why we *need* a *Non-Competing Parallel Research Programme* on acupuncture. The last section then ties all the former parts together and outlines the concrete tasks that flow from the theoretical framework provided.

2 Lakatos's Scientific Research Programmes

Both practice and public discourse of modern science are still guided by an understanding of science that, at best, is hopelessly idealistic or, at worst, inconsistent with and deluded about actual scientific work. The general picture here is one in which science is on an ever-expanding journey of progress toward complete and true knowledge concerning everything that there is to know about the universe. In this—let's call it the *naïve picture of science*—all things are, at least in theory, objectively knowable and statements about the world are either true or false.

These unreflected assumptions are mostly innocent and seldom damaging to the actual business of doing science. However, as we have already seen our question faces a set of unique challenges that make it necessary to understand how problematic some of these assumptions actually are. I will illustrate some of these problems by drawing on the seminal work in History of Science by Imre Lakatos (which I will later modify to make it more suitable to deal with our challenge here).

Imre Lakatos was a mathematician and philosopher from Hungary, who was concerned that philosophy of science had gotten caught up the pursuit of elegant and idealistic theory of science that had nothing to do with how science actually happened. In this regard, Lakatos agreed with Thomas Kuhn. The main opponent for Kuhn had been Karl Popper who held that science was a mix of making bold explanatory claims about the world, and then seeking out evidence that could *falsify* that theory, which in turn would give rise to new bold conjectures about the world. This process of *falsification*, he thought, would eventually lead to an ever-closer approximation of true knowledge about the world.[6] Popper's approach can somehow be described through the picture of going deeper and deeper into water: As soon as we realize a resistance, Popper would have said, now we have falsified this. Kuhn's investigations in the history of science showed clearly that this was not at all how scientific discoveries were made. Not only do scientists rarely seek actively for evidence to falsify their theories, they also don't treat empirical evidence that challenges the correctness of their theories, as falsifying. Instead such evidence is widely treated as an anomaly, which has to be explained as part of the original theory. It's not the theory that gets to be adapted to nature, but rather it's the mission of the scientist find a way of molding nature so that it fits the theory. Only in extraordinary times, when the pressure of the contradictory evidence gets too much, a theory will get replaced with a new one that is better equipped to explain the majority of the evidence. Kuhn famously coined the term "scientific revolution" for these transitions from one scientific paradigm into the next.[7]

Lakatos agreed with the general idea of Kuhn's history of science, but held that Kuhn didn't give Popper's ideas enough credit. He proposed that rather than being focused on isolated theories with a huge explanatory outreach, scientific paradigms consist of *sets of theories* around a hard core of unassailable assumptions that he called *research programme*. Within the research programme testable theories are generated that then become incorporated into the research programme and/or get modified to keep up with the new evidence. These theories, at the fringes of a research programme, are called *auxiliary hypotheses* and function as something like a protective belt for the sacred beliefs at the core.

Whenever an evidence surfaces which challenges or refutes the core of assumptions of a research programme, its disciples will modify the auxiliary hypotheses in such ways that the anomalies can be explained. This goes on and on until the generation of new auxiliary hypotheses has become purely defensive. Indeed, it is part of an implicit agreement of the adherents of a research programme that the core beliefs are accepted without further proof or debate. It needs to be said that this is not a *carte blanche* to create random theories. Instead the modification and generation of new theories has to be governed by principles also contained in the hardcore of the research programme.

For Lakatos, a research programme can be in either one of the two states. It can be progressing or it can be degenerating. The idea is that a research programme is

---

6   Compare Popper, Karl R.: *The Logic of Scientific Discovery*. Routledge: London. 2002 (1959).
7   See Kuhn, Thomas: *The Structure of Scientific Revolutions*. Fourth edition (with an introductory essay by Ian Hacking). The University of Chicago Press: Chicago. 2012 (1962).

progressing as long as the modifications and additions of further auxiliary hypotheses keep increasing the overall explanatory power of the research programme. Increasing the explanatory power here means that a theory is able to predict novel facts about so far unknown phenomena on the basis of the explained facts, and that these predictions can be independently confirmed.

On the other hand, if more and more auxiliary hypotheses are needed to keep up with new contra-indicating evidences, without increasing the explanatory power, then the research programme is degenerating and its disciples should start to look for a new research programme that promises more and deeper explanations than the old one.

Unlike Kuhn's *paradigms* of which only ever one could exist at the same time, for Lakatos research programmes can exist in parallel and they often do so, competing for an advantage in explanatory power. What Kuhn called a scientific revolution is in effect just a progressive research programme superseding a degenerative one.

3 Pseudo-Science and the Demarcation Criterion

What is interesting about Lakatos's *Methodology of Scientific Research Programmes* is that the scientificity of a program can be assessed without assessing the facts itself. For him a theory can be factually wrong and still be progressive, while another research program may be all factually correct but degenerating nonetheless.

All degenerating theories are pseudo-science in his eye. So, for instance, when the Ptolomean worldview was gradually overcome by the Copernican model of the cosmos, the old theory had automatically become a pseudo-science according to Lakatos. The geocentric model could explain fewer features of the world than the new heliocentric model; it had rightly been abandoned.

However, it might have already come to your mind that Lakatos's methodology of evaluating scientific programs doesn't bode well for our project: The CCM and the philosophy that guides it was never meant as theory or research programme with the aim to advance our understanding of the world in any sense that Lakatos would accept as progressive. It is not aimed at explaining new and surprising facts about the universe in terms of causal relations. So, if we had to take Lakatos by his word, we could end our endeavor right here and thereby proclaiming all CCM as pseudo-science and go on to more fruitful ventures.

Fortunately for our project, it is not at all clear that Lakatos's demarcation criterion for separating good science from pseudo-science can do the work it is supposed to do.

One major objection that the *Methodology of Research Programmes* faces is what we could call the "Too wide or too narrow" objection. This objection—though not under this name—had been famously forwarded by Paul Feyerabend. Feyerabend claimed that Lakatos's theory faced a dilemma: on the one hand it seemed that the theory, when taken strictly, would have to exclude a lot of what could reasonably held to be good science from the good science category because it wasn't progressing.[8] Among the theories that wouldn't constitute progressive research programmes according to the Method of Competing Scientific Research Programmes are for instance Darwin's Evolutionary Theory and Einstein's General Theory of Relativity (although Lakatos did later find a way to argue that indeed the General Theory articulated a progressive research programme). Furthermore, Lakatos held that its perfectly possible for a research programme to be degenerating for some time until, with another breakthrough among the auxiliary hypotheses, it becomes progressive again. Basically it is impossible to say whether or when any degenerating research programme might recover again. Moreover, periods of degeneration—in Lakatos's sense—are fairly common in even the most "progressive" sciences.

Sometimes, while there is wide agreement that a certain theory is inescapably degenerative, there isn't a viable progressive alternative; in which case the program will have to be kept until there is. Abandoning a degenerative research programme without a progressive alternative would mean essentially that we'd reduce our explanatory reach even further then by sticking with degenerative paradigm. That's why this isn't an option of Lakatos.

Taken together, all of these individual problems make the theory seem way too narrow to be pragmatic. What then, Feyerabend wondered, should the consequences for a research programme if it is found to be degenerating? Should it still receive grants for research and if yes, how long should it receive any kind of financial or other support? Can it still be taught in school and university?

Lakatos's answer to these questions immediately exposed him to the second horn of Feyerabend's dilemma. His methodology, he said, doesn't presume to tell anyone what to do or what not. It merely advises scientists to be honest and forward about the current state of their research programme. This is, of course, a rather curious position to take, and Feyerabend was fast point this out. What sense does a demarcation criterion have, he asked, if it can't prescribe any actions to take? Such a toothless criterion dispenses with all of the critical bite one

---

8   See Feyerabend, Paul: *Against Method. Outline of an Anarchistic Theory of Knowledge.* New Left Books: London. 1975.

would expect it to have. Much like a police force that merely advises people not to rob others, but can't arrest anyone, isn't really a police, this isn't a demarcation criterion. Lakatos passed away before he could reply to this objection and so far no satisfying way out of the dilemma has been suggested.[9]

My own quarrel with Lakatos's methodology comes from a different direction, although the consequences are similar: we have to abandon the idea that we could somehow "demarcate" science into progressive and degenerating research programmes by measuring and comparing the total sum of empirical explanations they offer.

While Lakatos already got rid of a lot of the metaphysical ballast that had been weighing down Western culture since its very inception in the Greek antique, the concept of science progressing toward an ever greater explanatory power is still very much rooted in that past. Obviously, he wasn't as naïve as to believe that science would actually discover the absolute and complete truth about the universe. Yet, one reason why his approach to evaluating competing scientific programs is so appealing to people from my cultural background is precisely that he managed to translate the idea of *progress towards to truth*, into the more metaphysically-innocent-sounding *progress towards greater explanatory power*.[10]

Besides the aforementioned challenges of this approach, many basic concepts of the methodology of *Competing Parallel Research Programmes*—like causal explanations or indeed the idea of a basic reality 'behind' our perceptions, that we approximate with ever-higher accuracy through our research programs—are *still* metaphysical artifacts of our culture.

In the end, after 2000 years, the failure of Western science is that it was loaded by metaphysics. A problem, which Western sciences could not solve and not even see. The Vienna Circle and its proponents had the standard to take away every metaphysics. However, so they got dependent upon metaphysics more than ever. A vivid example is their idea of an observer without subjectivity. Such a *machine* without any qualities cannot observe. In the end, it would just be a duplication of reality. This wrong track based on metaphysics led to the death of the philosophical concepts of the Vienna Circle, but also pathed the way for the emergence of CR.

There is nothing *per se* wrong with doing science based on these background presuppositions. As a matter of fact, I don't think it's even possible to completely

---

9 Ibid.
10 Compare Schulz, Andreas: "How can different medical systems be true at the sametime? – Popper, Feyerabedand Wallner on science and truth". In: F. Wallner/F. L. Lan (eds.): *The Concepts of Health and Disease from the Viewpoint of Four Cultures*. (Libri Nigri 46). Traugott Bautz: Nordhausen. 2014, pp. 120–133.

escape the ontological heritage of one's culture. These beliefs are ingrained too deep into our manner of thinking. However, in certain cases as in ours it is necessary to be aware of deep assumptions that govern one's worldview, and be able to set them aside methodologically in order to understand and make good use of those tools that were conceived outside the narrow horizon of one's own culture.

This is precisely what we are setting out to do here. We are going to use the central idea of Lakato's Methodology of *Parallel Research Programmes* yet without the metaphysically problematic parts. In order to do so, we have to think about how we are going to replace those parts of Lakatos's program. We need to say something about what we think actually is science and we need to become really clear about some of the other methodological assumptions we are going to make before we can tie it all back in with the concept of *Parallel Research Programmes*.

Fortunately for us I have already laid out those assumptions in other parts of my work: combined they are called *Constructive Realism*.

4 *Constructive Realism* (CR) and the Nature of Science

Constructive Realism is a pragmatic philosophy of science that aims to be metaphysics free. Obviously,—in virtue of the limits of the human existence—even the dedicated constructive realist doesn't get around making ontological assumptions either. In fact, the inevitability of working with metaphysical assumptions, might already be one of those assumptions. Unlike other Philosophies of Science, however, CR explicitly chooses and posits these assumptions *as assumptions*. That way, at least the most central assumptions of CR are chosen because of their pragmatic value for enhancing our understanding, rather than (just) being the unconscious expression of ancient cultural hopes and anxieties.

Those central assumptions are conceptualized in terms that sometimes make it hard for people to interpret them with the very metaphysical assumptions they are designed to avoid. Thus, the best way to present them is by explaining each central concept in concert with the most common misconception.

The first misconception refers to my concept of *Wirklichkeit*. Many people who start out reading my books are quickly convinced that what I must be talking about is really something like the Kantian *thing in itself*. But that was actually the first metaphysical fiction we threw right out of the window, right in the beginning. One reason so many people tend to fall into this trap is because they look up the German word *Wirklichkeit* in the dictionary and the closest translation to English they find is *reality*. Unfortunately, *reality* is a very metaphysically loaded term and it is also not an adequate translation. I don't think there is even an accurate translation.

Even if you had a more accurate translation or read it in German, if you have a Kantian background, which is very natural for many physicists, for instance, you will have a tendency to interpret *Wirklichkeit* as *thing in itself* regardless. This misconception will put an almost insurmountable blockage into your path to understanding CR. A good (or rather bad) example for this, is my good friend Herbert Pietschmann, a physicist among whose greatest influences was the Kantian physicist Wolfgang Pauli. Because of his inability to *not* understand *Wirklichkeit* in the sense of the *thing in itself*, Pietschmann would never comprehend CR.

The thing about the *thing in itself* is that it is completely unnecessary. It restricts the scientific research to specific area without giving clear reasons for what must be avoided or what can be done. It is also somewhat disturbing because no one *can* really believe that the world we experience is really completely unrelated, to what it (the world) *really* is, something allegedly unfathomable "behind" the world we see, the *real* reality. This is not the message of CR.

Now the second misunderstanding, once it is understood that *Wirklichkeit* does not refer to the *thing in itself*, is to believe that CR must be some sort of *Idealism*. Obviously, if there is no transcendental 'thing in itself', then what is left of transcendental idealism is the idealism. Thus, CR must be idealism. Yet, whoever truly believes this did not read carefully enough: our idea of how we, as human beings, relate to *Wirklichkeit* has little to do with idealism. Rather we hold that our relation to *Wirklichkeit* is realized by the living processes of human beings. *Wirklichkeit* is our destiny, but it is not something that we grapple with intellectually or that we even could investigate. Granted, *Wirklichkeit* does resemble a little bit the *thing in itself*, but, unlike Kant, we do not pretend that we could say anything about it. *That* would be engaging in metaphysical speculation. There is nothing we can say about it, nothing about whether it is pre-structured or not. And so we don't. We also don't need to. There is no need for us to say anything about the 'true nature' of *Wirklichkeit* because we never have to deal with it anyway. *Wirklichkeit* is just the necessarily presupposed world in which our *Lebenswelt* (*environment*) and the manifold *Realitäten* (realities) produced by different sciences are situated.

The good news (or the bad news, depending on whom you ask) is that because of our inability to say anything substantive about *Wirklichkeit* is that we will never solve all problems of science. And that is because science never deals with *Wirklichkeit* but rather 'only' with very limited aspects of our life-world (*Lebenswelt*). And, because *Lebenswelt* is constantly evolving and changing, not that we would even take note of that most of the times, the areas of possible scientific investigations are structurally unlimited. It is structurally impossible that we could ever give a coherent scientific explanation for every single aspect of the ever-evolving

Lebenswelt that we can investigate. Irrespective of any ideas one might have about the possibilities of uniting all of these explanations under the roof of just one science. We will never solve all problems of science, because that is structurally impossible. *Lebenswelt* is the constructive realist concept for the world we are embedded in our ordinary lives, the world we are familiar with. Or better, it is the wholeness of all the presuppositions that—mostly unquestioned and often unbeknownst to ourselves—govern our lives. It is the world we know without thinking about it. It is the way we relate to our environment before we even can engage in any scientific investigation. It is only from living inside *Lebenswelt* that we can pick certain highly specific aspects of it, for instance, the biological nature of my beating heart and shine the spotlight of scientific research onto it. Thus, *Lebenswelt* always precedes scientific *"reality"*. When I have developed CR, probably, I have read the book from Einstein, where he states that the life-world is the starting point of science and that all scientific theories are refinements of the life-world. My idea was also that we must look to the life-world of a culture, which is able to produce science.[11] The life-world is a system which has a set of convictions, what is real and not real; likewise, it has rules for arguing. All this is basic for scientific work.

Our *Lebenswelt* is constructed more or less randomly by our culture. And it is only inside the *Lebenswelt* that science finds the ideas for its research. This means that science, whether it wants to do so or not, is always investigating the structure of a construction which itself has no constructor.

While *Lebenswelt* has no constructor in the sense of an intentional entity, the scientific *micro-worlds* of what I called *Realität* (in contrast to *Wirklichkeit*) of course have constructors, namely the individual scientists. For example, if the scientist fails with respect to *Wirklichkeit*, he can learn successful actions. By successful actions he can build up so-called *micro-worlds*, which are replacing some aspects of the world by theoretical reasoning. The term *micro-world* does not mean that they are small but that they are not *real*. It is something which is working within the world but it is not real. A good example is the Newtonian physics. The classical mechanics is the *micro-world* of movement; but now no movement is going along the classical mechanics. Rather it is a system which explains movements but does not describe specific movements. Therefore, it is not *real*.

What we call *Realität* is the sum of all the scientifically structured aspects of our *Lebenswelt*. Any science produces *Realität*, whether it is physics or psychology,

---

11 Einstein, Albert: "Physik und Realität". In: ders. (Hg.): *Aus meinen späten Jahren*. Wunderkammer-Verlag: Neu-Isenburg. 2005, pp. 63–105.

whether it is biology or CCM. Although of course, in the case of CCM things are understood as processes, because it was sparked by a culture which has a very different understanding of *Realität*.

5 Motivating a *Parallel Research Programme* into Chinese Acupuncture

If we accept (at the very least for the sake of argument) the above concepts about our complicated relationship to the world around us, it should become immediately obvious why building a *Parallel Research Programme* on acupuncture is not an idle fancy but an urgency: without it we are going to miss out enormously!

Viewed from Latakos's paradigm of doing philosophy of science, not understanding CCM and the elaborate circular logics that guide it is not a big loss.[12] In the direct face-off between Western medicine and CCM the latter simply turned out to be less able to advance our explanatory power about the world. History has made its call—CCM is lost. From a constructive-realist background we discover that this is a little like simultaneously watching a Formula One driver driving laps and chess player making moves on a chessboard and then declaring the Formula One driver as the winner because he was faster. If this example seems ridiculous then that's because it is. It makes no sense at all to judge the skills of chess player according to the standards that apply to Formula One drivers. If anyone tried doing this in real life we would certainly shake our heads in utter disbelief proclaim that person to be insane.

And, yet when it comes to science and systems of belief we have no problem to judge a system that is built on non-causal, circular reasoning by the standards of a system that is built on causal reasoning and a strict dualist view of the world. And if we look just a little deeper we find out that the reason we think ourselves to be entitled to doing so is just—to stay with our analogy—that our Formula One driver is going so incredibly fast. In other words, because our sciences seem to have so much explanatory power, regarding certain *micro-worlds* that they constructed themselves, the idea is very convincing to us that, thus, all possible *micro-worlds* "must be" race tracks.[13]

---

12 Compare Lakatos, Imre: *The Methodology of Scientific Research Programmes*. (Philosophical Papers: Volume 1). J. Worrall/G. Currie (eds.), Cambridge University Press: Cambridge. 1978.
13 A dangerous misjudgement in my eyes that gets further intensified because of the erroneous but pervasive idea that our technological advancements are somehow the consequence of our science, while in fact it is rather the reverse.

I believe that the reason, so many incredibly smart people fall into this trap is that the very ontological presuppositions of Western culture inherently facilitate a view that has immense difficulty to transcend the narrow borders of its worldview. Luckily, with the ontological assumptions of CR in the background, we can zoom out of that narrow picture and see that there are other games out there worthy to be played, watched and understood. Just like the die-hard Formula One fan might realize one day that chess is really an interesting game to play and observe, or—better even—how the Formula One driver might realize that he can actually become a better race car driver through playing chess, our medical sciences can now realize that there are ways to profit *playing the game of classical Chinese acupuncture by its own rules.*

The case of acupuncture is, of course, way more dramatic because the loss we experience by trying to play it by our own rules, i.e. by the rules of modern science, is not that we are just having a little less or no fun, but that we are missing out on a majority of the health benefits, a lot of them in areas where Western medicine has little or no help to offer. That is a terrible price to pay.

At this point, we have to bring to mind that Western medicine is compared to other sciences at a very low level of reflection. It mainly focuses on the way of induction but it is not able to explain and understand its constructions. One important differentiation of Western science is the one between success and understanding: success alone does not make Western science. Rather, it would reduce Western science to a high degree. If we can see the way a medication is working, this is of course good for the doctor; no doubt. However, the programme of Western science is to understand because understanding is legitimation. As science is legitimated by understanding, we have to make a difference between success and understanding. Legitimation was always the biggest problem of philosophy of science. Regarding the history of Western science, the paths of legitimation have nearly always been metaphysical.

Due to the fact that classical China has no metaphysics, we are confronted with the question, which philosophy of science is structurally coming close to CCM in order to make the latter understandable. There are lots of books about Chinese medicine, which have these fantasies about the influence of meditation and holism on Chinese medicine. Although holism is right, the way of holism in CCM has nothing to do with holism, as it is grasped within Western thinking, namely metaphysically loaded holism. If you read classical Chinese texts as well as major classical Indian texts, like the Vedanta, our Western idea of a split between thinking and being is not at all understandable. This long Western list of questions about reality is simply not existing in classical Indian and classical

Chinese philosophy. This is a big difference, we must always be aware of, when approaching CCM.

In order to avoid paying that price of missing out on the valuable contribution of CCM we have to zoom out of our limited view of what rules healing systems have to follow. Rather, we have to search for ways to really understand Chinese acupuncture from within. This is the reason why we need a *Non-Competing Parallel Research Programme* on acupuncture that puts understanding first.

6 The Ingredients of a Parallel Research Programme

The initial question is: How could and how should a *Non-Competing Parallel Research Programme* on acupuncture look like in actual practice? Over the course of these pages we have already met most of the ingredients that will be necessary. First of all, we have a really strong motivation to start such a programme: namely the strong suspicion that acupuncture is a health system in his own right that will work much better if it were applied according to the philosophy it was conceived from. There is no lack of studies on the effectiveness of acupuncture, however, they all suffer from severe methodological flaws. They most certainly operate exclusively from a science paradigm that is categorically incapable to turn up genuine insights into the workings of acupuncture.

Second, by learning from the strengths and weaknesses of Lakatos's Methodology of Scientific Research Programmes we now know that successful[14] research programmes or paradigms are structured around a hard core of unassailable assumptions that are surrounded by a belt of auxiliary hypotheses. We also know that his competition-based demarcation criterion for what constitutes good science, does not hold fast against the scrutiny of modern philosophy of science. So, we will have to abandon it.[15]

Of course, the latter does not mean that we do not aim to gain greater explanatory power with our research programme because we do. Abandoning the principle of competition to sort good from bad or pseudo-science merely means, that this is not our criterion for what can be legitimately called science. Knowing all this allows us to free ourselves methodologically (at least to a certain extent) from the ontological constraints of our culture and consciously choose the kind

---

14 Please note, that I'm using 'successful' here in purely descriptive terms, i.e. as enduring historically, not in Lakatos's sense.
15 Compare Lakatos, Imre/Zahar, E.G.: "Why Did Copernicus's Programme Supersede Ptolemy's?" In: R. Westman (ed.): *The Copernican Achievement*. University of California Press: Los Angeles. 1976, pp. 354–383.

of unassailable assumptions that are supposed to make up the hard core of our research programme.

Third, we need to decide on the concrete areas we want to focus our research efforts on within the framework I laid out. Three large tasks come to mind:

The first of these tasks, already a part of our on-going research, is concerned with mitigating the translation problem. There are many wonderful translations of classical Chinese texts on acupuncture, however, even the best translations remain meaningless if their content lacks meaning in the context in which they are received. In the case of modern Western culture, in virtue of the many deep ontological differences we already recounted earlier, the context could probably not be less conducive to factor genuine understanding from even the best translations.

There is this saying that describes quite well the effect of getting lost in translation: I hear what you say but not what you mean. In the worst case our subsequent, hap-hazarded impromptu interpretations of the translated texts distorts their original meaning so badly that they can't guide effective treatment. To work against this effect we need to find ways to intertwine the source text's context and its manifold implicit presuppositions with the translation. This is something we can achieve through careful "strangification". We also need to develop understanding based criteria and standards for people who are qualified to be acupuncturist in a classical sense. Last, we need to find ways to conduct large-scale, long-time studies that compare the effectiveness of *sham* and *verum* acupuncture, and of westernized acupuncture with classical Chinese acupuncture. Such studies, especially the latter, if indeed they show a difference in the effectiveness of treatment depending on the background understanding the practitioner has, would without doubt be our most powerful to sway modernity to invest more resources and time into science, education and practice of acupuncture.

Fourth, we also know that the pragmatic choice for our hardcore assumptions is going to be a theory of science that does not force us to mistake chessboards for racetracks—metaphorically speaking. I hold that CR does all that while also offering us a further methodological tool to gain the painfully needed understanding of the scientific background of acupuncture. The method I am talking about here is called *strangification* and we already applied it with great success on this subject. Strangification is a method inspired by *Hermeneutics*. There have been various philosophers, especially in the phenomenological tradition of Heidegger, Husserl, Gadamer and others who have employed the German term for strangification, *Verfremdung*, long before the birth of CR. But this does not mean that strangification is the same as the hermeneutical methods. Only, that it is influenced by hermeneutics.[16] Strangification is the technique of intentionally taking an accepted proposition from one scientific system and putting in into a completely different context. Then, as the second step, one has to look at what happens to the sentence in the different context. This method will reveal all the presuppositions that govern the "truth" of the proposition in the original system. When strange ideas are coming together, interesting things happen. It allows us to gauge the limits of our proposition system, of our convictions, to glimpse the silent beliefs that run in the background. You can, for example, take propositions from psychology and put them into the context of physics or vice versa and you will learn a lot about what your own science presupposes and what the other science presupposes.

We have developed the methodology of strangification within interdisciplinary working groups during the 1980s. These seminars with members of various disciplines, like psychology, physics, musicology, literature and medicine were full of strangifications. We experienced that there are a lot of theories and opinions, contradicting to each other. While the university usually solves the problem of contradiction by having different disciplines, which are organised in different faculties, we actually tried to bring these contradictions to the fore. However, we also experienced that interdisciplinary cooperation only works when people really try to explain and explain their own concepts to people of other disciplines who do not have the specific disciplinary knowledge of the counterpart. Another important proposition is that the members are able to concede that their concepts might be wrong, respectively abridged in terms of not having reflected upon specific presuppositions of their own theories. In this regard, I had very good experiences with psychology and physics, but I remember one professor of physics who was totally unable to work interdisciplinary. He always told me that this was his discipline and therefore I was not allowed to judge about his discipline; respectively if I did not agree, I would be wrong. The experiences we have made with students and assistants of medicine have also been very interesting. The various ways of strangifications of Western medical concepts showed the high degree of naivity, in terms of lack of reflection about underlying presuppositions of Western medicine.[17]

When practising strangification, the result is mostly nonsense. But this is only the first step. If you are patient enough to find out why the other system becomes

---

16 See Wallner, Friedrich: "Language cannot be fathomed out". In: H. Hashi/F. Wallner (eds.): *Globalisierung des Denkens von Ost und West – Resultate des österreichisch-japanischen Dialogs*. (Libri Nigri 4). Traugott Bautz: Nordhausen. 2011, pp. 116–125.
17 Compare Lakatos, Imre: "Criticism and the Methodology of Scientific Research Programmes". In: *Proceedings of the Aristotelian Society* 69. Oxford University Press: Oxford. 1968, pp. 149–186.

nonsense, you have got insight into a system or into both systems. The best example for this is the strangification of classical Chinese thinking into Western thinking and vice versa; a work which mainly Prof. Lan and I have done within the last years. If you strangify ideas from Western ontology by probing them in the context of classical Chinese ontology, you will become very confused because nothing seems to fit. But this is a very productive confusion because, in the end, you will learn that much of the confusion was due to the fact that classical Chinese ontology doesn't make a difference between image and imagination. Image and imagination are one of them. In contrast, it is most natural for us Westerners to believe that there is a huge difference between image and imagination. That is why we always wonder what is behind the image, why we wonder how to get to the *Wirklichkeit*. For the Chinese on the other hand this makes no sense at all: There is no "behind the image" for them, so why look? This is quite a practical insight and Prof. Lan and I have published a very interesting paper on that topic.[18] The following scheme shows some of the outcomes of these cultural strangifications of Western and Chinese thinking.[19]

Table 1: Differences between European Thought and Chinese Thought

Type of Difference	European Thought	Chinese Thought
Ontology	Unchangeable basis of the changing things (Plato: Being)	Phenomena: unstable, emerging and disappearing
Methodology	Induction and Deduction	Governing Changes: Qu Xiang Bi Lei
Manner of Thought	Linear Reasoning: Cause and Effect	Circular Reasoning: One Point is Explained by All the Others
Theoretical Structure	Separation of Theory and Practice	Unity of Theory and Practice
Experience	A passive reception of information	A specific way of activity, an interaction

---

18 Wallner, Friedrich/Lan, Fengli: "Ontological Ambiguity and Methodological Circularity: QU-XIANG BI-LEI". In: F. Wallner/F. L. Lan/M. J. Jandl (eds.): *The Way of Thinking in Chinese Medicine. Theory, Methodology and Structure of Chinese Medicine.* (Culture and Knowledge: Vol. 13). Peter Lang: Frankfurt am Main. 2010, pp. 103–117.

19 For didactical reasons, we "compare", but be aware that the comparison of cultures is the biggest mistake of Western cultural sciences. Western sciences take other cultures under the theoretical framework of their culture. Therefore, the result is in the best case strangification.

If we take the example of ontology. The question "what is real?" is a good question. We are trained to make a clear division between real and unreal. Therefore, the ontology in the sense of the Western world is based on the idea of unchangeable things; of an unchangeable basis of the changeable things. This was already the idea of Plato and Democrit which remained up to quantum mechanics. All this science is working based upon the idea of the existence of an unchangeable basis of the changeable things. But, how is this in Chinese thinking? Chinese thinking is oriented on phenomena, as I have already shown by the Chinese axiom, which I have quoted above. Chinese thinking is aware of unstable, emerging and disappearing things. It has a total different idea about the real reality. For the Westerner the real reality is the one, which cannot be changed, what is eternal. This is clearly due to the combination of Plato with Christian belief. This has a lot of consequences for the methodology. The Western science is going the way of induction and deduction; going from the single case to the general and the more general one until the universal until you come to the *world formula*, a dream of physics in the 70es of the last century. A dream which was typical European.

The focus of methodology in Chinese thinking is totally different. Chinese thinking is concentrated in governing changes. Changes are more important than the reappearing of the same. The reappearing of the same makes the Westerner happy. The classical Chinese man would say this boring and not interesting. In this context, we have found the formula QU-XIANG BI-LEI ("governing changes"), which means not to go the way of induction and until you come to the most general—to the universal—but go the way to pick up something what is interesting, which is important.

Regarding the differences concerning the *Manner of Thought*, we realize that the thinking of the Westerner is linear: linear reasoning of cause and effect. If you look at the Chinese thinking, you see that it is circular. You can see that one point is explained by all the others. This style is richer in content but a little bit more unclear, than the western one of causality; apart from the fact that causality is a pure fiction. Of course, saying that there is no causality is again metaphysical, but at least there is no visible causality in the nature.

In Chinese thinking everything remains a little bit unclear but with every further step of circular reasoning it becomes clearer. Therefore, the collection of knowledge is richer in CCM. The Western medicine, which is focus on cause and effect, is a poor compared with CCM. On the other hand, CCM has some uncertainty, which clearly cannot be fixed like in the Western thinking.

Regarding the theoretical structure of Western thinking we a separation of theory and practice. Now, this separation has a little bit changed within the last 20 or 30 years, but it is basic for the Western thinking, that theory must go before the practice. In the Chinese thinking, there is the idea of a unity of theory and practice. In respect to experience, how to get to information, the Westerner beliefs in passive information reception. If you do not passively receive the information, the Westerner thinks that you are cheating the other one. If I have an interest that some result is coming, the other one would say, we must exclude him, because he is cheating us. Therefore, the observer must always be without any interest, what actually is impossible.

Experience in the Chinese thinking is a specific way of activity and interaction. The scheme shows the methodological mistake of the double-blind trials (GERAC). They make a split between imagination and *Wirklichkeit*, the reality. Imagination becomes dependent on reality. In the thinking of the Chinese classics reality does not play this role. In this point it is similar to the Indian Vedanta. There, nobody asks what is *real* real; not only what is real, but what is *real* real. This question is neither understandable in the classical Chinese context nor in the classical Indian one. The funny point about this is that we are so proud about this task which looks like nonsense in other cultures, like wasting time. The double-blind trials are based on this question. If you practice sham acupuncture and real acupuncture and the sham acupuncture has nearly the same result as the real one, you must say that acupuncture has no claim to reality. I know that the practitioner wants to know and it is good to know. I would also like to have a doctor who knows how to treat me; equal if he is practicing Chinese or Western medicine. But, we must be aware, that we—in this manner—exclude a lot of possible aspects of CCM, which are important for understanding it. At this level, we are only on the level of success, and this is reducing science. The main question must be, how can we understand what is going on here.

In the context of developing a *Parallel Research Programme* the philosopher is always like a signpost. You must be aware that philosophy can only show which direction is *good* in terms of for example epistemologically grasping CCM. However, the proposed direction then has to be followed by experts on CCM. Therefore, interdisciplinary working is indispensable in this regard. My task is to convince experts to realize a different way of researching CCM. This does not mean that I refute the classical way, the way of double-blind studies. Double-blind studies are important for many things. It is important to have a doctor who is able to recommend a certain way of acupuncture for example for arthritis, low back pain and so on. But this is only reducing science to the level of application of science. We want a full science and I am sure that, when we are able to make a framework for a research concept on CCM, we will get exciting results. But it will be a hard job. And according to my information, nobody did it so far.

References

Birch, Stephen: "Reflections on the German Acupuncture Studies". In: *Journal of Chinese Medicine* 83, February 2007, pp. 12–17.

Einstein, Albert: "Physik und Realität". In: ders. (Hg.): *Aus meinen späten Jahren*. Wunderkammer-Verlag: Neu-Isenburg. 2005, pp. 63–105.

Feyerabend, Paul: *Against Method. Outline of an Anarchistic Theory of Knowledge*. New Left Books: London. 1975.

Kuhn, Thomas: *The Structure of Scientific Revolutions*. Fourth edition (with an introductory essay by Ian Hacking). The University of Chicago Press: Chicago. 2012 (1962).

Lakatos, Imre: "Criticism and the Methodology of Scientific Research Programmes". In: *Proceedings of the Aristotelian Society* 69. Oxford University Press: Oxford. 1968, pp. 149–186.

Lakatos, Imre: *The Methodology of Scientific Research Programmes*. (Philosophical Papers: Volume 1). J. Worrall/G. Currie (eds.), Cambridge University Press: Cambridge. 1978.

Lakatos, Imre/Zahar, E.G.: "Why Did Copernicus's Programme Supersede Ptolemy's?" In: R. Westman (ed.): *The Copernican Achievement*. University of California Press: Los Angeles. 1976, pp. 354–383.

Lan, Fengli: "Metaphors in the Framework of Tian Ren He Yi: Aspects of Lifestyle Related Diseases." In: F. L. Lan/F. G. Wallner/G. Klünger (eds.): *Lifestyle and Health*. Traugott Bautz: Nordhausen. 2017. pp. 77–108.

Parmenides: *Sein und Welt: Die Fragmente neu übersetzt und kommentiert von Helmuth Vetter*. (Mit einem Anhang von Alfred Dunshirn über neue Literatur zu Parmenides). Verlag Karl Alber: Freiburg/München. 2016.

Popper, Karl R.: *The Logic of Scientific Discovery*. Routledge: London. 2002 (1959).

Schulz, Andreas: "How can different medical systems be true at the same time? – Popper, Feyerabed and Wallner on science and truth". In: F. Wallner/F. L. Lan (eds.): *The Concepts of Health and Disease from the Viewpoint of Four Cultures*. (Libri Nigri 46). Traugott Bautz: Nordhausen. 2014, pp. 120–133.

Wallner, Friedrich/Lan, Fengli: "Ontological Ambiguity and Methodological Circularity: QU-XIANG BI-LEI". In: F. Wallner/F. L. Lan/M. J. Jandl (eds.): *The Way of Thinking in Chinese Medicine. Theory, Methodology and Structure of Chinese Medicine*. (Culture and Knowledge: Vol. 13). Peter Lang: Frankfurt am Main. 2010, pp. 103–117.

Wallner, Friedrich: "Language cannot be fathomed out". In: H. Hashi/F. Wallner (eds.): *Globalisierung des Denkens von Ost und West – Resultate des österreichisch-japanischen Dialogs*. (Libri Nigri 4). Traugott Bautz: Nordhausen. 2011, pp. 116–125.

Lixing Lao and Mingxiao Yang

Evidence-Based Acupuncture and Mechanistic Studies of Acupuncture

Abstract: Nowadays, evidence-based acupuncture and mechanistic-based acupuncture research are two emerging concepts established upon evidence obtained from clinical trials and discoveries of mechanisms of action. This paper summarized recent advance in evidence-based acupuncture studies, as well as progress in mechanistic studies.

1 Introduction

Acupuncture is an archaic healing art which has been used in China and other East Asian countries for thousands of years. In history, this traditional therapy was only well documented in Chinese culture dating back to more than 2,000 years ago[1]. After thousands of years of development, this nonpharmacological intervention is now used in more than 183 countries in the world, according to the '*WHO traditional medicine strategy: 2014-2023*'[2]. Despite rapid dissemination of acupuncture in the world, the medical communities always question whether there is any scientific evidence supporting this ancient healing art. This paper will discuss the scientific evidence of acupuncture and its possible mechanisms of action in the following sections.

2 A Pyramid of Evidence for Acupuncture

In the 1990s, the evidence-based medicine (EBM) as an emerging field of medical research gained enormous attention. With the aim of improving healthcare, EBM has been explicitly defined as '*the conscientious, explicit, and judicious use of current best evidence in making decisions about the care of individual patients*'[3]. Such visions in some ways fitted in the rising demands of the public on credible

---

1   Chiu J-H. *History of Acupuncture [M]. Acupuncture for Pain Management.* Springer. 2014: 3-11.
2   Organization W.H.O. *WHO Traditional Medicine Strategy 2014-2023.* Geneva, 2013 [M]. 2014.
3   Sackett D L, Rosenberg W M C, Gray J a M, et al. Evidence Based Medicine: What it is and What it isn't [J]. *BMJ*, 1996, 312(7023): 71-2.

evidence in clinical settings[4]. By employing EBM approaches, modern medicine in recent years has generated a large body of evidence, which was used as a powerful tool to assist clinicians, patients and policymakers making healthcare decisions. Therefore, in the delivery of qualified medical care to patients, the importance of evidence is highlighted. EBM in a revolutionary manner changed the traditional way of medicine. Clinical decisions no longer merely rely on physicians' personal experience[5]. Moreover, EBM framework has contributed significantly to the recognition of acupuncture, for it provided a unified language that enables traditional medicine to communicate with western medicine.

Since 1990s numerous clinical trials of acupuncture have been published which significantly enriched the evidence foundations of acupuncture. In 1997, the National Institute of Health (NIH) of the United States held a consensus conference of acupuncture, which is regarded as a landmark in the history of acupuncture research[6]. This conference formally endorsed acupuncture for the treatment of many diseases, and stated that there was clear evidence showing the effect of acupuncture on postoperative pain, postoperative dental pain, and nausea and vomiting. It also stated that there were promising evidence showing that acupuncture was effective on arthritis, menstrual cramp, headache, low back pain, etc. It called further investigation on these conditions were needed.

According to a retrospective literature analysis on the global trend and performance of acupuncture research from 1991 to 2009, there was a dramatic increase of publications of acupuncture research since 1998[7]. Evidence-based research paradigm became a major tool for determining the effect of acupuncture. For example, in patients with chronic pains, an international group of acupuncture trialists conducted an individual patient data (IPD) meta-analysis to evaluate the benefits of acupuncture[8]. The pooled analysis of 29 randomized controlled trials (RCTs) with 17,992 patients demonstrated that patients receiving acupuncture experienced less pain in back/neck pain, osteoarthritis or headache, as compared with those receiving sham treatment. The authors found that the effect size of

---

4   Rosenberg W, Donald A. Evidence Based Medicine: An Approach to Clinical Problem-Solving [J]. *BMJ*, 1995, 310(6987): 1122-6.
5   Haynes R B. What Kind of Evidence is it that Evidence-Based Medicine Advocates want Health Care Providers and Consumers to Pay Attention to? [J]. *BMC Health Services Research*, 2002, 2(1): 3.
6   NIH Consensus Conference. Acupuncture [J]. *JAMA*, 1998, 280(17): 1518-24.
7   Han J-S, Ho Y-S. Global Trends and Performances of Acupuncture Research [J]. *Neuroscience & Biobehavioral Reviews*, 2011, 35(3): 680-7.
8   Vickers A J, Linde K. Acupuncture for Chronic Pain [J]. *JAMA*, 2014, 311(9): 955-6.

acupuncture in treating neck and back pain is 0.37 standard deviations (SDs) over the sham control; and 0.26 SDs for osteoarthritis and 0.15 and 0.62 SDs for treating chronic headache and shoulder pain, respectively. The results showed that acupuncture has substantial therapeutic effects for treating chronic pains. When compared to no-acupuncture treatments, the effect size of acupuncture was even bigger, indicating that acupuncture may be more effective than other interventions.

EBM highly values the quality of evidence and has built up a hierarchical pyramid to classify the level of evidence[9]. In those models, systematic reviews, meta-analysis, and RCT are ranked at the top of the evidence hierarchy, as they are the most reliable source of clinical evidence[10]. Randomized controlled trials as the golden standard of medicine are used to assess the clinical effect of medical interventions though diminishing potential biases caused by confounders commonly existed in non-randomized trials, or even non-controlled trials. Employing this approach in acupuncture research can minimize placebo/non-specific effect of acupuncture.

As a result, large numbers of RCTs were accordingly formulated and strictly conducted in a perspective manner for the generation of reliable clinical evidence for acupuncture. For example, Prof Berman and Prof Lao conducted a double-blind RCT to assess acupuncture's effect for knee osteoarthritis (KOA)[11]. The research recruited 570 eligible patients who were suffering from osteoarthritis of the knee, and randomly divided them into three groups, acupuncture group, sham control group and education group. After baseline assessment, the patients were treated by acupuncture twice per week for 8 weeks, and then tapered down to once a week, every other week, and once a month for up to 26 weeks. Patients in the sham control group received sham acupuncture (SA) treatment. Meanwhile, patients in the education group received 6 sessions of healthcare education and got no additional treatment. After the completion of treatment, a standard outcome known as Western Ontarian McMaster Osteoarthritis Index (WOMAC) was used at 8 and 26 weeks to assess the changes in pain intensity and joint function. The results showed that patients in acupuncture group experienced greater

---

9   Murad M H, Asi N, Alsawas M, et al. New Evidence Pyramid [J]. *Evidence Based Medicine*, 2016, 21(4): 125–7.
10 Rosner A L. Evidence-based Medicine: Revisiting the Pyramid of Priorities [J]. *Journal of Bodywork and Movement Therapies*, 2012, 16(1): 42–9.
11 Berman B M, Lao L, Langenberg P, et al. Effectiveness of Acupuncture as Adjunctive Therapy in Osteoarthritis of the Knee: A Randomized, Controlled Trial [J]. *Annals of Internal Medicine*, 2004, 141(12): 901–10.

improvement in WOMAC function scores (mean difference [MD]: −2.9) than sham control group at 8 weeks but not in pain scores, indicating that acupuncture is more effective in recovering knee joint function immediately after treatment. At 26 weeks, patients in acupuncture group experienced greater improvement in function scores (MD: −2.5) and pain scores (MD: −8.7). The clinical effect observed is very significant. It is even better than that of the conventional KOA treatment, the intra-articular injection of hyaluronic acid[12].

Clinical studies also have been carried out to assess the analgesic effect of acupuncture for acute pain. In a study by Shin et al., 58 eligible patients with acute low back pain (aLBP) have been recruited and randomly assigned in a 1:1 ratio to receive 1 session of either conventional diclofenac injection or motion style acupuncture treatment[13]. The investigators applied a treatment in which patients were required to passively or actively move their body during needle retention. The outcomes included improvement of pain intensity measured by a 10-point visual analog scale (VAS), and change in functional disability measured by the Oswestry Disability Index (ODI) at 30 minutes and at 2, 4, and 24 weeks after treatment. The results showed that 30 min after treatment acupuncture group had more pain relief (MD: 3.12, $P<0.0001$) and more functional improvement (MD: 32.95%; $P<0.0001$) than conventional diclofenac injection. Moreover, the therapeutic effect lasted for 4 weeks after treatment.

Despite the above-mentioned studies showing the effect of acupuncture for pain conditions, in recent years, more clinical trials started to investigate the effect of acupuncture on non-painful conditions. For example, in 2016 and 2017, several high influential journals such as *JAMA, Annals of Internal Medicine*, and *Journal of Clinical Oncology* published articles that demonstrate acupuncture is effective to treat visceral or functional diseases, including functional gastrointestinal disease[14], cancer therapy-related hot flashes[15], and stress urinary

---

12 Van Der Weegen W, Wullems J A, Bos E, et al. No Difference Between Intra-Articular Injection of Hyaluronic Acid and Placebo for Mild to Moderate Knee Osteoarthritis: A Randomized, Controlled, Double-Blind Trial [J]. *The Journal of Arthroplasty*, 2015, 30(5): 754–7.
13 Shin J-S, Ha I-H, Lee J, et al. Effects of Motion Style Acupuncture Treatment in Acute Low Back Pain Patients with Severe Disability: A Multicenter, Randomized, Controlled, Comparative Effectiveness Trial [J]. *PAIN®*, 2013, 154(7): 1030–7.
14 Liu Z, Yan S, Wu J, et al. Acupuncture for Chronic Severe Functional Constipation: A Randomized Trial [J]. *Annals of Internal Medicine*, 2016, 165(11): 761–9.
15 Lesi G, Razzini G, Musti M A, et al. Acupuncture as an Integrative Approach for the Treatment of Hot Flashes in Women with Breast Cancer: A Prospective Multicenter

incontinence[16]. A study by G. Lesi et al. (2016) found that 10 sessions of acupuncture treatment plus enhanced self-care was more effective in the management of hot flashes and improving quality of life of patients with breast cancer, as compared with enhanced self-care alone[15]. A trial (2016) evaluated the efficacy of electro acupuncture (EA) vs. sham EA (SA) in treating functional constipation[14]. Patients were randomly assigned to receive 28 sessions of either EA treatment or SA treatment in over 8 weeks. EA significantly increased spontaneous bowel movements during the treatment phase (week 1 to 8), and during follow-up period (week 9 to 20) ($P<0.001$). The effect sustained up to 6 months after treatment. In addition, Z. Liu et al. (2017) found that EA stimulation at the lumbosacral region was more effective to manage urinary leakage among women with stress urinary incontinence when compared with sham EA, providing a useful treatment for this common condition ($P<0.05$)[16]. A trial by Minchom A. et al. showed that all three treatment options, acupuncture, morphine, or acupuncture combined with morphine, could significantly alleviate dyspnoea in patients with advanced non-small cell lung cancer and mesothelioma (responder rate: 74% vs. 60% vs. 66%, respectively)[17]. Therefore, the authors concluded that acupuncture could be an alternative therapy for dyspnoea in patients with lung cancer. A trial from Japan found that the incidence of emergence agitation was significantly lower in transcutaneous electrical nerve stimulation (TENS) treatment (on acupuncture point H7) group compared with a sham TENS treatment group (31.7% vs. 56.7%, respectively; $P=0.010$)[18].

On the other side, clinical trials that yield negative results are not uncommon. However, most of these negative results were at least partially due to non-specific effect produced in sham control. For examples, a study by C. Ee et al. found that 8-week standard traditional Chinese medicine (TCM) acupuncture treatment was

---

Randomized Controlled Trial (AcCliMaT) [J]. *Journal of Clinical Oncology*, 2016, 34(15): 1795–802.

16 Liu Z, Liu Y, Xu H, et al. Effect of Electroacupuncture on Urinary Leakage Among Women with Stress Urinary Incontinence: A Randomized Clinical Trial [J]. *JAMA*, 2017, 317(24): 2493–501.

17 Minchom A, Punwani R, Filshie J, et al. A Randomised Study Comparing the Effectiveness of Acupuncture or Morphine Versus the Combination for the Relief of Dyspnoea in Patients with Advanced Non-Small Cell Lung Cancer and Mesothelioma [J]. *European Journal of Cancer*, 2016, 61(Supplement C): 102–10.

18 Hijikata T, Mihara T, Nakamura N, et al. Electrical Stimulation of the Heart 7 Acupuncture Site for Preventing Emergence Agitation in Children: A Randomised Controlled Trial [J]. *European Journal of Anaesthesiology (EJA)*, 2016, 33(7): 535–42.

not better in alleviating hot flashes in perimenopausal women than non-insertive SA (mean hot flash score: 15.36 vs. 15.04, $P=0.77$)[19]. Another study carried out by X. Wu and colleagues demonstrated that the use of acupuncture with or without clomiphene, did not increase live birth rate in women with polycystic ovarian syndrome, as compared with placebo acupuncture and placebo[20]. Their results show that the effect of placebo controls was too powerful to let acupuncture demonstrate its clinical effect. In Wu's study, the birth rate for both placebo controls were much higher (16.8%) than that assumed for sample size estimation (only 5%). This suggests that the sham controls used by this trial were not physiologically inert as it was supposed to be[21,22,23,24]. The methodological challenges will be discussed in the next paper.

Some researchers argue that classic RCT are predisposed with limitations that they may not reflect real-world condition. In order to produce 'real-world' evidence and to better inform clinical practice, the concepts of comparative effectiveness research need to be incorporated into current clinical research scheme[25,26]. A pragmatic RCT by Prof Macpherson et al. (2015) set a good example of using such methods to efficiently inform clinical decision making[27]. In their study, eligible

---

19 Ee C, Xue C, Chondros P, et al. Acupuncture for Menopausal Hot Flashes: A Randomized Trial [J]. *Annals of Internal Medicine*, 2016, 164(3): 146–54.
20 Wu X-K, Stener-Victorin E, Kuang H-Y, et al. Effect of Acupuncture and Clomiphene in Chinese Women with Polycystic Ovary Syndrome: A Randomized Clinical Trial [J]. *JAMA*, 2017, 317(24): 2502–14.
21 Lund I, Näslund J, Lundeberg T. Minimal Acupuncture is not a Valid Placebo Control in Randomised Controlled Trials of Acupuncture: A Physiologist's Perspective [J]. *Chinese Medicine*, 2009, 4(1): 1.
22 Paterson C, Dieppe P. Characteristic and Incidental (Placebo) Effects in Complex Interventions Such as Acupuncture [J]. *BMJ*, 2005, 330(7501): 1202–5.
23 Macpherson H, Vertosick E, Lewith G, et al. Influence of Control Group on Effect Size in Trials of Acupuncture for Chronic Pain: A Secondary Analysis of an Individual Patient Data Meta-Analysis [J]. *PLOS One*, 2014, 9(4): e93739.
24 Lund I, Lundeberg T. Are Minimal, Superficial or Sham Acupuncture Procedures Acceptable as Inert Placebo controls? [J]. *Acupuncture in Medicine*, 2006, 24(1): 13–5.
25 Witt C M, Manheimer E, Hammerschlag R, et al. How Well do Randomized Trials Inform Decision Making: Systematic Review Using Comparative Effectiveness Research Measures on Acupuncture for Back Pain [J]. *PLoS One*, 2012, 7(2): e32399.
26 Witt C M, Aickin M, Baca T, et al. Effectiveness Guidance Document (EGD) for Acupuncture Research-A Consensus Document for Conducting Trials [J]. *BMC Complementary and Alternative Medicine*, 2012, 12(1): 148.
27 Macpherson H, Tilbrook H, Richmond S, et al. Alexander Technique Lessons or Acupuncture Sessions for Persons with Chronic Neck Pain: A Randomized Trial [J]. *Annals of Internal Medicine*, 2015, 163(9): 653–62.

patients with chronic neck pain (average history over 6 years) were recruited and randomly assigned to receive one of the three pain management approaches: acupuncture plus usual care, Alexander techniques plus usual care, or usual care alone. They used the Northwick Park Questionnaire (NPQ) to assess the improvement in neck pain and its associated disability, and showed that at 12 months both acupuncture and Alexander techniques significantly ameliorated neck pain and improved its associated disability as compared with usual care. Moreover, both acupuncture and Alexander techniques exerted long-term therapeutic effects to patients with chronic neck pain. This study, therefore, showed that in clinical settings both therapies could be referred to patients to alleviate chronic neck pain. Similar research protocol used by other teams also found acupuncture was effective in 'real-world' settings for the treatment of chronic low back pain[28], chronic shoulder pain[29], chronic headache[30], allergic rhinitis[31], menopausal symptoms[32], postoperative nausea and vomiting in children after tonsillectomy and adenoidectomy[33], etc.

Based on previous clinical studies, a clear map of evidence of acupuncture therapy starts to emerge. In 2003, the World Health Organization systematically summarized the results of many clinical trials and divided 100 indications of acupuncture into four groups concerning the strength of existing evidence[34]. In this report, it stated that acupuncture has been proven to be an effective treatment for 28 conditions (mostly pain); 63 conditions are with promising evidence but

---

28 Witt C M, Jena S, Selim D, et al. Pragmatic Randomized Trial Evaluating the Clinical and Economic Effectiveness of Acupuncture for Chronic Low Back Pain [J]. *American Journal of Epidemiology*, 2006, 164(5): 487–96.
29 Molsberger A F, Schneider T, Gotthardt H, et al. German Randomized Acupuncture Trial for chronic shoulder pain (GRASP) – A Pragmatic, Controlled, Patient-Blinded, Multi-Centre Trial in an Outpatient Care Environment [J]. *PAIN*, 2010, 151(1): 146–54.
30 Vickers A J, Rees R W, Zollman C E, et al. Acupuncture for Chronic Headache in Primary Care: Large, Pragmatic, Randomised Trial [J]. *BMJ*, 2004, 328(7442): 744.
31 Brinkhaus B, Roll S, Jena S, et al. Acupuncture in Patients with Allergic Asthma: A Randomized Pragmatic Trial [J]. *The Journal of Alternative and Complementary Medicine*, 2017, 23(4): 268–77.
32 Avis N E, Coeytaux R R, Isom S, et al. Acupuncture in Menopause (AIM) Study: A Pragmatic, Randomized Controlled trial [J]. *Menopause*, 2016, 23(6): 626–37.
33 Liodden I, Sandvik L, Valeberg B T, et al. Acupuncture Versus Usual Care for Postoperative Nausea and Vomiting in Children After Tonsillectomy/Adenoidectomy: A Pragmatic, Multicentre, Double-Blinded, Randomised Trial [J]. *Acupuncture in Medicine*, 2015, 33(3): 196–203.
34 Chmielnicki B. *Evidence Based Acupuncture: WHO Official Position [M]*. 2016.

for which further proof is needed; 9 conditions are only reported by individual controlled trial; therefore, acupuncture is recommended to be tried because there is no satisfactory treatment till now for those conditions. For the rest 7 conditions, acupuncture was recommended to be performed by practitioners with special modern medical knowledge and adequate monitoring equipment. Furthermore, according to the '*Evidence Map of Acupuncture*' completed by the Department of Veteran Affairs of the United States in 2014, acupuncture has now been shown to have strong evidence in treating many painful conditions and mental disorders, as well as keeping wellness[35]. The 'Map' clearly illustrates the positive effect of acupuncture for headache, chronic pain and migraine. It also demonstrated that acupuncture has potential therapeutic effect on dysmenorrhea, labor pain, cancer pain, as well as many non-painful conditions such as insomnia, smoking, postoperative nausea/vomiting, restless legs, depression, schizophrenia, etc. However, for diseases like rheumatoid arthritis, shoulder pain, cancer adverse effect, and irritable bowel syndrome, there is still unclear evidence. For carpal tunnel syndrome and cocaine addiction, current evidence does not support the effect of acupuncture. "No evidence of effect" does not mean "evidence of no effect". Therefore, more rigorously and innovatively designed clinical trials are needed to determine the effect of acupuncture.

In conclusion, recently developed research methodology known as EBM played a major role to assess the clinical effect of acupuncture and has a big impact on the clinical implication worldwide. Currently, in the USA, over 42% of the hospitals provide outpatient and inpatient services of acupuncture and it is listed as the second most common alternative medicine treatment in these hospitals[36]. As the results of these evidences, at least 24 clinical guidelines in the West medical societies recommended acupuncture as one of the alternative treatment or integrative medicine treatment modality (From National Guideline Clearinghouse, https://www.guideline.gov/).

3 Mechanisms of Actions Revealed by Basic Studies in Acupuncture

Although acupuncture has been shown effective to many diseases, its mechanism of actions is still largely unknown. Therefore, many basic studies have been

---

35 West Los Angeles V, Hempel S, Shekelle P G, et al. Evidence Map of Acupuncture [J]. 2014.
36 Ananth S. *Complementary and Alternative Medicine Survey of Hospitals [J]*. Alexandria, VA: Samueli Institute, 2011.

conducted. The early stage of mechanistic studies mainly focused on acupuncture analgesia (AA), because at that time acupuncture was mainly used for pain conditions. Especially, in the late 1960s a Chinese research team led by Prof *Jisheng Han* initially started their research in investigating the anti-nociceptive mechanism of acupuncture by using neuropsychological methods. Their studies demonstrated that acupuncture increased the release of endogenous opioid peptides in the central nervous system, which played an essential role in AA. They further found that transfusion of cerebrospinal fluid (CSF) from acupuncture-treated donor rabbit to acupuncture-naïve recipient rabbit led to transplantation of AA effect[37]. Moreover, pain suppression induced by acupuncture was reversed by injecting opioid receptor antagonists, Naloxone[38]. Their studies also found an EA parameter-dependent phenomena of neuropeptides release. For example, EA with 2 Hz induced the release of encephalin, β-endorphin, and endomorphin; while 100 Hz EA selectively improved dynorphins release. A medium frequency of 15 Hz EA stimulation increased all kinds of endogenous opioid peptide aforementioned[39,40].

However, such studies using intact animal models to elucidate AA mechanism was frequently associated with methodological limitations. Because, those models were not corresponding to any pathological conditions and the modeled condition was transient which could only last for a couple of minutes. In addition to the contribution by the early studies about β-endorphin, recent years researchers use pathological animal models to explore the mechanism of AA. Various pain models, such as inflammatory pain models (e.g. Complete Freund's Adjuvant (CFA)-Induced Inflammatory Pain model)[41], neuropathic pain models (e.g. spinal/sciatic nerve ligation model)[42,43], cancer pain models (e.g. cancer-cell

---

37 Han J-S. Acupuncture and Stimulation Produced Analgesia [J]. *Opioids II*, 1993, 104: 105–25.
38 Mayer D J, Price D D, Rafii A. Antagonism of Acupuncture Analgesia in Man by the Narcotic Antagonist Naloxone [J]. *Brain Research*, 1977, 121(2): 368–72.
39 Han J-S. Acupuncture and Endorphins [J]. *Neuroscience Letters*, 2004, 361(1): 258–61.
40 Han J-S. Acupuncture: Neuropeptide Release Produced by Electrical Stimulation of Different Frequencies [J]. *Trends in Neurosciences*, 2003, 26(1): 17–22.
41 Wm L, Km C, Li N, et al. Analgesic Effect of Electroacupuncture on Complete Freund's Adjuvant-Induced Inflammatory Pain in Mice: A Model of Antipain Treatment by Acupuncture in Mice [J]. *The Japanese Journal of Physiology*, 2005, 55(6): 339–44.
42 Cidral-Filho F, Da Silva M, Moré A, et al. Manual Acupuncture Inhibits Mechanical Hypersensitivity Induced by Spinal Nerve Ligation in Rats [J]. *Neuroscience*, 2011, 193: 370–6.
43 Liou J-T, Liu F-C, Hsin S-T, et al. Inhibition of the Cyclic Adenosine Monophosphate Pathway Attenuates Neuropathic Pain and Reduces Phosphorylation of Cyclic

transplantation model)[44], and visceral hyperalgesia models (e.g. irritable bowel syndrome model)[45], have been used. It was demonstrated that on the behavioral level EA was able to alleviate both sensory and affective pain. Those studies also found an EA parameter-dependent effect, the traits of which, however, was quite different from Han's. It showed that EA with frequency of 2 Hz to 10 Hz exhibited more potent anti-inflammatory effect and anti-nociceptive effect for neuropathic pain model than that with frequency of 100 Hz[46]. While, higher frequency EA (100 Hz) can more rapidly induce pain relief as compared with low frequency in short term.

A review paper authored by Prof Lao's team summarized mechanisms of actions of acupuncture on pain. These mechanisms occur in all three levels in peripheral, spinal and supraspinal[47,48,49,50]. *At peripheral sites*, EA could increase opioid level by recruiting opioid-containing cell via activating sympathetic nerves, and by disrupting endocannabinoid metabolism through hypothalamus-pituitary-adrenal axis in inflammatory pain and neuropathic pain models. The accumulated opioids further inhibited the response of immune cells and the release of proinflammatory cytokines was diminished. Moreover, opioids secreted nearby injury site and endocannabinoid may inhibit the activities of peripheral sensory nerves. *At the*

Adenosine Monophosphate Response Element-Binding in the Spinal Cord After Partial Sciatic Nerve Ligation in Rats [J]. *Anesthesia & Analgesia*, 2007, 105(6): 1830–7.

44 Lee H-J, Lee J-H, Lee E-O, et al. Substance P and Beta Endorphin Mediate Electroacupuncture Induced Analgesic Activity in Mouse Cancer Pain Model [J]. *Acupuncture & Electro-Therapeutics Research*, 2009, 34(1–2): 27–40.

45 Wu J C, Ziea E T, Lao L, et al. Effect of Electroacupuncture on Visceral Hyperalgesia, Serotonin and Fos Expression in an Animal Model of Irritable Bowel Syndrome [J]. *Journal of Neurogastroenterology and Motility*, 2010, 16(3): 306.

46 Zhang R-X, Lao L, Wang X, et al. Electroacupuncture Attenuates Inflammation in a Rat Model [J]. *Journal of Alternative & Complementary Medicine*, 2005, 11(1): 135–42.

47 Zhang R, Lao L, Ren K, et al. Mechanisms of Acupuncture–Electroacupuncture on Persistent Pain [J]. *Anesthesiology: The Journal of the American Society of Anesthesiologists*, 2014, 120(2): 482–503.

48 Li A, Wang Y, Xin J, et al. Electroacupuncture Suppresses Hyperalgesia and Spinal Fos Expression by Activating the Descending Inhibitory System [J]. *Brain Research*, 2007, 1186:171–9.

49 Silva J R, Silva M L, Prado W A. Analgesia Induced by 2-or 100-Hz Electroacupuncture in the Rat Tail-Flick Test Depends on the Activation of Different Descending Pain Inhibitory Mechanisms [J]. *The Journal of Pain*, 2011, 12(1): 51–60.

50 Zhang R-X, Lao L, Wang L, et al. Involvement of Opioid Receptors in Electroacupuncture-Produced Anti-Hyperalgesia in Rats with Peripheral Inflammation [J]. *Brain Research*, 2004, 1020(1): 12–7.

spinal level, EA decreased prostaglandin E2 (PGE2) to alleviate pain through ameliorating cyclooxygenase-2 (COX-2). EA also may inhibit glutamate receptor, ionotropic, N-methyl D-aspartate 1 (GluN1) phosphorylation and pain by down regulating glutamate release in pre-synaptic level. Moreover, 5-hydroxytryptamine 1A receptor (5-HT1AR) in post-synaptic level was upregulated by EA to inhibit GluN1 phosphorylation. Moreover, opioids released in spinal cord modulated the release of pain-related substances which further inhibited immune response. Consequently, the release of IL-1β, IL-6, TNF-α, p-Akt, and P38 was suppressed[51]. Moreover, *at the supraspinal level*, EA may block N-Methyl-D-Aspartate-Receptor (NMDAR) function to inhibit affective pain mechanism in the anterior cingulate cortex (ACC).

Furthermore, more finding of mechanisms of AA has been reported in recent years, such as the role of adenosine in AA and the central mechanism of AA revealed by neuroimaging technology. Current studies demonstrated that acupuncture treatment released adenosine triphosphate/adenosine diphosphate (ATP/ADP) from keratinocytes and mast cells in the surrounding skin where needle was inserted[52]. The accumulation of adenosine, adenosine monophosphate (AMP), ADP and ATP may subsequently activate its receptors, P2 receptors (P2Rs) at fibroblast and P1/P2Rs at nerve endings in skin[53]. Because adenosine participates in the peripheral sensation of noxious stimuli and nociceptive signal transmission in the CNS, it is hypothesized that inhibitory signals produced by peripheral sensory nerve during acupuncture treatment might be transduced to the central pain centre via the spinoparabrachial and spinothalamic tracts[53,54,55,56]. Moreover, neuroimaging technologies are now available for researchers to use

---

51 Zhang R-X, Li A, Liu B, et al. Electroacupuncture Attenuates Bone Cancer Pain and Inhibits Spinal Interleukin-1β Expression in a Rat Model [J]. *Anesthesia & Analgesia*, 2007, 105(5): 1482–8.
52 Goldman N, Chen M, Fujita T, et al. Adenosine A1 Receptors Mediate Local Anti-Nociceptive Effects of Acupuncture [J]. *Nature Neuroscience*, 2010, 13(7): 883–8.
53 Zhang Q, Zhao Y, Guo Y, et al. Activation and Sensitization of C and Aδ Afferent Fibers Mediated by P2X Receptors in Rat Dorsal Skin [J]. *Brain Research*, 2006, 1102(1): 78–85.
54 Burnstock G. Purinergic P2 Receptors as Targets for Novel Analgesics [J]. *Pharmacology & Therapeutics*, 2006, 110(3): 433–54.
55 Burnstock G. Purinergic Receptors and Pain [J]. *Current Pharmaceutical Design*, 2009, 15(15): 1717–35.
56 Burnstock G. Chapter Four-Purinergic Mechanisms and Pain [J]. *Advances in Pharmacology*, 2016, 75: 91–137.

for the exploration of the central mechanism of acupuncture in human[57]. Studies found that acupuncture with *Deqi* sensation could evoke comprehensive deactivation of the limbic system and activation of the somatosensory brain regions, functions of which are responsible to process affective and sensory pain signals[58,59]. They also demonstrated that in chronic pain patients (carpel tunnel syndrome), acupuncture elicited response in a coordinated limbic network including hypothalamus and amygdala[60].

4 Conclusion

In recent decades, many clinical trials of acupuncture have been conducted. Those trials demonstrated that acupuncture is effective to treat not only painful conditions but also many non-painful disorders, which formed a solid evidence for acupuncture. Meanwhile, the understanding of mechanisms of acupuncture's analgesia has greatly advanced our knowledge. However, further studies are still warranted to elucidate its actions, particularly for non-painful conditions.

References

Amunts K, Ebell C, Muller J, et al. The Human Brain Project: Creating a European Research Infrastructure to Decode the Human Brain [J]. *Neuron*, 2016, 92(3): 574–81.

Ananth S. *Complementary and Alternative Medicine Survey of Hospitals [J]*. Alexandria, VA: Samueli Institute, 2011, http://www.samueliinstitute.org/File%20Library/Our%20Research/OHE/CAM_Survey_2010_oct6.pdf.

Avis N E, Coeytaux R R, Isom S, et al. Acupuncture in Menopause (AIM) Study: A Pragmatic, Randomized Controlled Trial [J]. *Menopause*, 2016, 23(6): 626–37.

---

57 Amunts K, Ebell C, Muller J, et al. The Human Brain Project: Creating a European Research Infrastructure to Decode the Human Brain [J]. *Neuron*, 2016, 92(3): 574–81.
58 Hui K K S, Liu J, Marina O, et al. The Integrated Response of the Human Cerebro-Cerebellar and Limbic Systems to Acupuncture Stimulation at ST 36 as Evidenced by fMRI [J]. *NeuroImage*, 2005, 27(3): 479–96.
59 Hui K K S, Liu J, Makris N, et al. Acupuncture Modulates the Limbic System and Subcortical Gray Structures of the Human Brain: Evidence from fMRI Studies in Normal Subjects [J]. *Human Brain Mapping*, 2000, 9(1): 13–25.
60 Napadow V, Kettner N, Liu J, et al. Hypothalamus and Amygdala Response to Acupuncture Stimuli in Carpal Tunnel Syndrome [J]. *PAIN*, 2007, 130(3): 254–66.

Berman B M, Lao L, Langenberg P, et al. Effectiveness of Acupuncture as Adjunctive Therapy in Osteoarthritis of the Knee: A Randomized, Controlled Trial [J]. *Annals of Internal Medicine*, 2004, 141(12): 901-10.

Brinkhaus B, Roll S, Jena S, et al. Acupuncture in Patients with Allergic Asthma: A Randomized Pragmatic Trial [J]. *The Journal of Alternative and Complementary Medicine*, 2017, 23(4): 268-77.

Burnstock G. Chapter Four-Purinergic Mechanisms and Pain [J]. *Advances in Pharmacology*, 2016, 75: 91-137.

Burnstock G. Purinergic P2 Receptors as Targets for Novel Analgesics [J]. *Pharmacology & Therapeutics*, 2006, 110(3): 433-54.

Burnstock G. Purinergic Receptors and Pain [J]. *Current Pharmaceutical Design*, 2009, 15(15): 1717-35.

Chiu J-H. *History of Acupuncture [M]. Acupuncture for Pain Management.* New York, NY: Springer. 2014: 3-11.

Chmielnicki B. *Evidence Based Acupuncture: WHO Official Position [M].* 2016.

Cidral-Filho F, Da Silva M, Moré A, et al. Manual Acupuncture Inhibits Mechanical Hypersensitivity Induced by Spinal Nerve Ligation in Rats [J]. *Neuroscience*, 2011, 193: 370-6.

Ee C, Xue C, Chondros P, et al. Acupuncture for Menopausal Hot Flashes: A Randomized trial [J]. *Annals of Internal Medicine*, 2016, 164(3): 146-54.

Han J-S. Acupuncture and Stimulation Produced Analgesia [J]. *Opioids II*, 1993, 104: 105-25.

Han J-S. Acupuncture and Endorphins [J]. *Neuroscience Letters*, 2004, 361(1): 258-61.

Han J-S. Acupuncture: Neuropeptide Release Produced by Electrical Stimulation of Different Frequencies [J]. *Trends in Neurosciences*, 2003, 26(1): 17-22.

Han J-S, Ho Y-S. Global Trends and Performances of Acupuncture Research [J]. *Neuroscience & Biobehavioral Reviews*, 2011, 35(3): 680-7.

Haynes R B. What Kind of Evidence is it that Evidence-Based Medicine Advocates want Health Care Providers and Consumers to Pay Attention to? [J]. *BMC Health Services Research*, 2002, 2(1): 3.

Hempel S, Taylor S L, et al. Evidence Map of Acupuncture [J]. Los Angeles, CA: Evidence-based Synthesis Program (ESP) Center. 2013.

Hijikata T, Mihara T, Nakamura N, et al. Electrical Stimulation of the Heart 7 Acupuncture Site for Preventing Emergence Agitation in Children: A Randomised Controlled Trial [J]. *European Journal of Anaesthesiology (EJA)*, 2016, 33(7): 535-42.

Hui K K S, Liu J, Marina O, et al. The Integrated Response of the Human Cerebro-Cerebellar and Limbic Systems to Acupuncture Stimulation at ST 36 as Evidenced by fMRI [J]. *NeuroImage*, 2005, 27(3): 479–96.

Hui K K S, Liu J, Makris N, et al. Acupuncture Modulates the Limbic System and Subcortical Gray Structures of the Human Brain: Evidence from fMRI Studies in Normal Subjects [J]. *Human Brain Mapping*, 2000, 9(1): 13–25.

Goldman N, Chen M, Fujita T, et al. Adenosine A1 Receptors Mediate Local Anti-Nociceptive Effects of Acupuncture [J]. *Nature Neuroscience*, 2010, 13(7): 883–8.

Lee H-J, Lee J-H, Lee E-O, et al. Substance P and Beta Endorphin Mediate Electroacupuncture Induced Analgesic Activity in Mouse Cancer Pain model [J]. *Acupuncture & Electro-Therapeutics Research*, 2009, 34(1–2): 27–40.

Lesi G, Razzini G, Musti M A, et al. Acupuncture as an Integrative Approach for the Treatment of Hot Flashes in Women with Breast Cancer: A Prospective Multicenter Randomized Controlled Trial (AcCliMaT) [J]. *Journal of Clinical Oncology*, 2016, 34(15): 1795–802.

Li A, Wang Y, Xin J, et al. Electroacupuncture Suppresses Hyperalgesia and Spinal Fos Expression by Activating the Descending Inhibitory System [J]. *Brain Research*, 2007, 1186: 171–9.

Liodden I, Sandvik L, Valeberg B T, et al. Acupuncture Versus Usual Care for Postoperative Nausea and Vomiting in Children After Aonsillectomy/Adenoidectomy: A Pragmatic, Multicentre, Double-blinded, Randomised Trial [J]. *Acupuncture in Medicine*, 2015, 33(3): 196–203.

Liou J-T, Liu F-C, Hsin S-T, et al. Inhibition of the Cyclic Adenosine Monophosphate Pathway Attenuates Neuropathic Pain and Reduces Phosphorylation of Cyclic Adenosine Monophosphate Response Element-Binding in the Spinal Cord After Partial Sciatic Nerve Ligation in Rats [J]. *Anesthesia & Analgesia*, 2007, 105(6): 1830–7.

Liu Z, Liu Y, Xu H, et al. Effect of Electroacupuncture on Urinary Leakage Among Women with Stress Urinary Incontinence: A Randomized Clinical trial [J]. *JAMA*, 2017, 317(24): 2493–501.

Liu Z, Yan S, Wu J, et al. Acupuncture for Chronic Severe Functional Constipation: A Randomized Trial [J]. *Annals of Internal Medicine*, 2016, 165(11): 761–9.

Lund I, Näslund J, Lundeberg T. Minimal Acupuncture is not a Valid Placebo Control in Randomised Controlled Trials of Acupuncture: A Physiologist's Perspective [J]. *Chinese Medicine*, 2009, 4(1): 1.

Lund I, Lundeberg T. Are Minimal, Superficial or Sham Acupuncture Procedures Acceptable as Inert Placebo Controls? [J]. *Acupuncture in Medicine*, 2006, 24(1): 13–5.

Macpherson H, Tilbrook H, Richmond S, et al. Alexander Technique Lessons or Acupuncture Sessions for Persons with Chronic Neck Pain: A Randomized Trial [J]. *Annals of Internal Medicine*, 2015, 163(9): 653-62.

Macpherson H, Vertosick E, Lewith G, et al. Influence of Control Group on Effect Size in Trials of Acupuncture for Chronic Pain: A Secondary Analysis of an Individual Patient Data Meta-Analysis [J]. *PLOS One*, 2014, 9(4): e93739.

Mayer D J, Price D D, Rafii A. Antagonism of Acupuncture Analgesia in Man by the Narcotic Antagonist Naloxone [J]. *Brain Research*, 1977, 121(2): 368-72.

Minchom A, Punwani R, Filshie J, et al. A Randomised Study Comparing the Effectiveness of Acupuncture or Morphine Versus the Combination for the Relief of Dyspnoea in Patients with Advanced Non-Small Cell Lung Cancer and Mesothelioma [J]. *European Journal of Cancer*, 2016, 61(Supplement C): 102-10.

Molsberger A F, Schneider T, Gotthardt H, et al. German Randomized Acupuncture Trial for Chronic Shoulder Pain (GRASP) - A Pragmatic, Controlled, Patient-Blinded, Multi-Centre Trial in an Outpatient Care Environment [J]. *Pain*, 2010, 151(1): 146-54.

Murad M H, Asi N, Alsawas M, et al. New Evidence Pyramid [J]. *Evidence Based Medicine*, 2016, 21(4): 125-7.

Napadow V, Kettner N, Liu J, et al. Hypothalamus and Amygdala Response to Acupuncture Stimuli in Carpal Tunnel Syndrome [J]. *Pain*, 2007, 130(3): 254-66.

NIH Consensus Conference. Acupuncture [J]. *JAMA*, 1998, 280(17): 1518-24.

Organization W H O. *WHO Traditional Medicine Strategy 2014-2023*. Geneva, 2013 [M]. 2014.

Paterson C, Dieppe P. Characteristic and Incidental (Placebo) Effects in Complex Interventions Such as Acupuncture [J]. *BMJ*, 2005, 330(7501): 1202-5.

Rosenberg W, Donald A. Evidence Based Medicine: An Approach to Clinical Problem-Solving [J]. *BMJ*, 1995, 310(6987): 1122-6.

Rosner A L. Evidence-Based Medicine: Revisiting the Pyramid of Priorities [J]. *Journal of Bodywork and Movement Therapies*, 2012, 16(1): 42-9.

Sackett D L, Rosenberg W M C, Gray J a M, et al. Evidence Based Medicine: What it is and What it isn't [J]. *BMJ*, 1996, 312(7023): 71-2.

Shin J-S, Ha I-H, Lee J, et al. Effects of Motion Style Acupuncture Treatment in Acute Low Back Pain Patients with Severe Disability: A Multicenter, Randomized, Controlled, Comparative Effectiveness Trial [J]. *PAIN®*, 2013, 154(7): 1030-7.

Silva J R, Silva M L, Prado W A. Analgesia Induced by 2-or 100-Hz Electroacupuncture in the Rat Tail-Flick Test Depends on the Activation of Different

Descending Pain Inhibitory Mechanisms [J]. *The Journal of Pain*, 2011, 12(1): 51–60.

Van Der Weegen W, Wullems J A, Bos E, et al. No Difference Between Intra-Articular Injection of Hyaluronic Acid and Placebo for Mild to Moderate Knee Osteoarthritis: A Randomized, Controlled, Double-Blind Trial [J]. *The Journal of Arthroplasty*, 2015, 30(5): 754–7.

Vickers A J, Linde K. Acupuncture for Chronic Pain [J]. *JAMA*, 2014, 311(9): 955–6.

Vickers A J, Rees R W, Zollman C E, et al. Acupuncture for Chronic Headache in Primary Care: Large, Pragmatic, Randomised Trial [J]. *BMJ*, 2004, 328(7442): 744.

Witt C M, Manheimer E, Hammerschlag R, et al. How Well do Randomized Trials Inform Decision Making: Systematic Review Using Comparative Effectiveness Research Measures on Acupuncture for Back Pain [J]. *PLoS One*, 2012, 7(2): e32399.

Witt C M, Aickin M, Baca T, et al. Effectiveness Guidance Document (EGD) for Acupuncture Research-A Consensus Document for Conducting Trials [J]. *BMC Complementary and Alternative Medicine*, 2012, 12(1): 148.

Witt C M, Jena S, Selim D, et al. Pragmatic Randomized Trial Evaluating the Clinical and Economic Effectiveness of Acupuncture for Chronic Low Back Pain [J]. *American Journal of Epidemiology*, 2006, 164(5): 487–96.

Wm L, Km C, Li N, et al. Analgesic Effect of Electroacupuncture on Complete Freund's Adjuvant-Induced Inflammatory Pain in Mice: A Model of Antipain Treatment by Acupuncture in Mice [J]. *The Japanese Journal of Physiology*, 2005, 55(6): 339–44.

Wu X-K, Stener-Victorin E, Kuang H-Y, et al. Effect of Acupuncture and Clomiphene in Chinese Women with Polycystic Ovary Syndrome: A Randomized Clinical Trial [J]. *JAMA*, 2017, 317(24): 2502–14.

Wu J C, Ziea E T, Lao L, et al. Effect of Electroacupuncture on Visceral Hyperalgesia, Serotonin and Fos Expression in an Animal Model of Irritable Bowel Syndrome [J]. *Journal of Neurogastroenterology and Motility*, 2010, 16(3): 306.

Zhang Q, Zhao Y, Guo Y, et al. Activation and Sensitization of C and Aδ Afferent Fibers Mediated by P2X Receptors in Rat Dorsal Skin [J]. *Brain Research*, 2006, 1102(1): 78–85.

Zhang R, Lao L, Ren K, et al. Mechanisms of Acupuncture–Electroacupuncture on Persistent Pain [J]. *Anesthesiology: The Journal of the American Society of Anesthesiologists*, 2014, 120(2): 482–503.

Zhang R-X, Lao L, Wang L, et al. Involvement of Opioid Receptors in Electroacupuncture-Produced Anti-Hyperalgesia in Rats with Peripheral Inflammation [J]. *Brain Research*, 2004, 1020(1): 12–7.

Zhang R-X, Lao L, Wang X, et al. Electroacupuncture Attenuates Inflammation in a Rat Model [J]. *Journal of Alternative & Complementary Medicine*, 2005, 11(1): 135-42.

Zhang R-X, Li A, Liu B, et al. Electroacupuncture Attenuates Bone Cancer Pain and Inhibits Spinal Interleukin-1β Expression in a Rat Model [J]. *Anesthesia & Analgesia*, 2007, 105(5): 1482-8.

Fengli Lan

Interpreting Literature: A Key to Transmit and Enrich Knowledge System of Acupuncture

Abstract: Literature research, classical and/or modern, has been of the first significance before proceeding research of any kind. Interpreting classical and modern literature in modern clinical settings is a key to transmit and enrich the knowledge system of acupuncture.

1 Significance of Literature Research: Standing on Predecessors' Shoulders

1.1 Research and Science

As the word suggests, research is based on "search" of the related literature. *Oxford Dictionary of English* defines "research" as "the systematic investigation into and study of materials and sources in order to establish facts and reach new conclusions."[1]

The original meaning of "Science" is "knowledge of any kind."[2]

Britain's Science Council finally worked out a new definition of "science" as "the pursuit and application of knowledge and understanding of the natural and social world following a *systematic* methodology based on *evidence*."[3]

The philosopher AC Grayling thinks the Council has done a good job: "Because 'science' denotes such a very wide range of activities a definition of it needs to be general; it certainly needs to cover investigation of the social as well as natural worlds; it needs the words "systematic" and "evidence"; and it needs to be simple and short. The definition succeeds in all these respects admirably, and I applaud it therefore."[4]

---

1 *Oxford Dictionary of English*. 2nd Ed. Oxford University Press. 1998, 1999, 2001, 2003, 2005.
2 *Oxford Dictionary of English*. 2nd Ed. Oxford University Press. 1998, 1999, 2001, 2003, 2005.
3 http://sciencecouncil.org/about-science/our-definition-of-science/. Date of last access: April 27, 2018.
4 *Commending the definition in the Guardian*, March 2009 https://www.theguardian.com/science/blog/2009/mar/03/science-definition-council-francis-bacon. Date of last access: April 27, 2018.

According to Science Council, scientific methodology includes the following: Objective observation: Measurement and data (possibly although not necessarily using mathematics as a tool); Evidence; Experiment and/or observation as benchmarks for testing hypotheses; Induction: reasoning to establish general rules or conclusions drawn from facts or examples; Repetition; Critical analysis; and Verification and testing: critical exposure to scrutiny, peer review and assessment.[5]

1.2 Is Acupuncture Scientific?

Can acupuncture be mentioned in the same breath with "science?" According to the definition of science by Britain's Science Council, the answer is surely "Yes."

Acupuncture is a branch knowledge system of Chinese medicine, not just a technique or a skill. It is generally very safe without toxic or major side effects except for some minor events like minor bleeding or local bruise if practiced by qualified or licensed professionals, and it proves to be effective for many conditions (if not all). It produces favorable holistic changes to the live beings including humans and other animals in double direction – known as regulatory effects, which can be measured by objective indicators, and evaluated by patient-centered outcomes and practitioner-centered reports.[6] For example, Tianshu (ST25) for bowel movement – diarrhea, dysentery, or constipation, and Neiguan (PC6) for abnormal blood pressure (high or low) and abnormal heart rhythm (fast or low or irregular) are adequately proved to be true with numerous repeatable clinical trials and experimental studies.

Acupuncture takes its root in classical Chinese culture, and it is a live carrier of the pearl of Chinese wisdom.

In the framework of the new definition of science by Britain's Science Council, I explain the "Scienticity of Acupuncture" in three layers: cultural, theoretical, and practical.

Culturally, the Chinese understanding of life, health, disease, and treatment presupposes *Tian Ren He Yi* 天人合一 or Unity of Heaven and Humankind as its ontology, *Qu Xiang Bi Lei* 取象比类 or Taking Image and Analogizing as its methodology, and *He* 和 or Harmony as its ultimate aim. What Chinese medicine studies is the living being, the life process, not the dead body. The live being

---

5   http://sciencecouncil.org/about-science/our-definition-of-science/. Date of last access: April 27, 2018.
6   MacPherson, Hugh, Hammerschlag, Richard, Lewith, George, Schner, Rosa. *Acupuncture Research: Strategies for Establishing an Evidence Base*. Edinburgh: Elsevier Churchill Livingstone, 2007, p. 77.

A Key to Transmit and Enrich Knowledge System of Acupuncture 57

is constantly influenced by its outside environment, natural and social. The live being needs to keep in a balanced and harmonious state for mental and physical health; if one fails in maintaining such a balance and harmony in oneself as well as in between one and the universe, the one will be in a diseased state. Acupuncture is supposed to bring the balance and harmony back through its double-direction regulating effect.

Theoretically, yin-yang, five elemental phases, visceral manifestation, *Jing-Luo*, and acupoints, etc. weave all the knowledge together by following the systematic methodology *Qu Xiang Bi Lei* 取象比类 or Taking Image and Analogizing[7,8] thus making acupuncture, a part of Chinese medicine, as a member of "science" which is defined as "the pursuit and application of knowledge and understanding of the natural and social world following a ***systematic*** methodology based on ***evidence***."[9]

Practically, acupuncture has been practiced for thousands of years, and the effect and efficacy of acupuncture for many conditions have been proved, manipulated, repeated, and evidenced.

Dry needling, which was evolved from wet needling pioneered by Janet Travell and David Simons in the 1940s,[10] may be somehow a new invention in the Western medicine, but is not new at all for Chinese medicine. It is a part of classical Chinese acupuncture – Ashi Point Acupuncture, which has been practiced for thousands of years. Yeh searched "dry needle," "dry needling," "ashi point," "ashi point acupuncture," or "myofascial pain needling" in Google Scholar Database and PubMed Database in February 2016, and got 749,365 manuscripts,[11] which shows the rich evidence of dry needling for pain, known as ashi point acupuncture in Chinese medicine.

Research of any kind should be established on the research outcomes of the former researchers. Literature review of a certain topic, systematic review or meta-analysis, is a must to go further. Working behind closed doors without knowing the research progress of a certain topic or the current hot issues, or taking a

---

7   Lan, Fengli. *Metaphor: The Weaver of Chinese Medicine*. Nordhausen: Traugott Bautz, 2015.
8   Lan, Fengli, Wallner, Friedrich. Taking Image and Analogizing: The Metaphorizing Process and the Way of Forming Metaphors in Chinese Medicine. *Journal of Dialectics of Nature*, 2014, 36(2): 98–104.
9   http://sciencecouncil.org/about-science/our-definition-of-science/. Date of last access: April 27, 2018.
10 Lewit, K. The Needle Effect in the Relief of Myofascial Pain. *Pain*, 1979, 6(1): 83–90.
11 Yeh, Tse M. Dry Needling for Musculoskeletal Pain Management: A Survey of Current Literature. Capstone Project. Five Branches University, 2017, p. 4.

biased approach by only referring to the literature which supports the biased and predetermined viewpoint, should be avoided by serious scholars.

2 Research on Classical Acupuncture Literature: Tracing to Its Source and Root

Research on classical Chinese literature is of prime significance for the theoretical and cultural interpretation of effectiveness and efficacy of acupuncture. Interpretation of acupuncture classics, especially the parts on Jing-Luo system, acupoints, acupuncture treatment for various diseases of *Huang Di Nei Jing Su Wen* and *Ling Shu Jing* is extremely important since these parts involve the construction of the knowledge system of acupuncture.

Systematizing the ancient literature on acupuncture treatment of certain diseases chronologically, analyzing the evolution of treatment methods, selection of acupoints, diseases appropriate for acupuncture, etc. are needed to establish the possible best treatment protocols for better practices and clinical trials.

The parts of the ancient literature on the relationship of the arrival of Qi and effectiveness and efficacy of acupuncture, interactions and relationships between patient and practitioner need to be further investigated in order to clarify the backgrounds and rationality of taking sham acupuncture as placebo in clinical trials.

Here I give an example of my research on *Jing-Luo* system: from rivers in the nature to vessels in humans.[12]

What is *Jing-Luo* system? Several translations are available for "*Jing-Luo* system 經絡系統:"

a. "Meridian System," the standard translation approved by World Health Organization,[13] but the word "Meridian" only indicates a two-dimensional grid while *Jing Luo* system is supposed to carry *qi* and blood, and thus must be a three-dimensional system;

b. "Channel System," the most popular translation in the English literature on Chinese medicine, for example, in the textbooks by Giovanni Maciocia,[14] but the word "Channel" is polysemous, indicating something not so important or

---

12 Lan, Fengli. *Metaphor: The Weaver of Chinese Medicine*. Nordhausen: Traugott Bautz, 2015, p. 188.
13 *WHO International Standard Terminologies on Traditional Medicine in the Western Pacific Region*. Geneva: WHO, 2007, p. 28.
14 Maciocia, Giovanni. *The Foundations of Chinese Medicine: A Comprehensive Text*. 3rd ed. Edinburgh: Elsevier, 2015, p. 793.

essential while the *Jing-Luo* system is a most important theoretical foundation for acupuncture, moxibustion, *tuina* or Chinese massage, *Qi Gong* or breathing exercise and herbal prescriptions;

c. "Vessel System", a translation in an introduction book on *Huang Di Nei Jing Su Wen*,[15] can be taken as the best translation if we take into account the origin and development of the concepts of *Mai* (脈, vessel) and *Jing-Luo* (經絡).

Based on some anatomical knowledge on *Mai* (脈, vessel) and medical practice, especially the application of acupuncture, moxibustion, *tuina* or Chinese massage, and *qigong* or breathing exercise, the concepts of *Jing-Luo* (經絡) are actually metaphors formed in the way of observing, taking images of and analogizing the water flow in the rivers in the nature and the longitudinal lines of the textiles, which are embodied in their writing forms. The chapter *Water & Earth* of *Guan Tzu* states that "Water is the *qi* and blood of the earth, running on (under) the earth just like *qi* and blood flowing in the vessels."

The simplified form of "*mai* 脉" has 4 variant original complex forms.

脈 and 衇 are its common original complex forms. Its lesser seal script is 衇. This sinogram is a signific-phonetic compound: the left part is its signific component 月 (flesh moon) or 血 (blood), indicating that *mai* 脈 functions to carry and move blood and is a part of the human body; And the right part is its phonetic, indicating both pronunciation and meaning at the same time. In medical books unearthed from Mawangdui Han Tomb, most writing forms of "*mai* 脈" were written as "溫". "水" is the variant form of " 氵", "目" the variant form of "月 (flesh moon)", "皿" the variant form of "blood 血". The structure of the sinogram has clearly illustrated that ancient Chinese analogized or metaphorized water flow with blood flow.[16] It is thus clear that "*mai*" of the early days referred to blood vessel, so "*mai* 脉" is also known as "blood vessel 血脈", as stated in *Huang Di Nei Jing Su Wen · Mai Yao Jing Wei Lun* 脉要精微论 or *Huang Di's Inner Classic · Basic Questions ·Discourse on Subtleties and Essentials of Vessels* "The vessels 脈 are the residence of the blood. 脉者，血之府也。" Be aware, *Qi* does not show up in this quotation. Figure 1 shows original complex writing forms of "Mai 脉."

---

15 Unschuld, Paul U. *Huang Di Nei Jing Su Wen: Nature, Knowledge, Imagery in an Ancient Chinese Medical Text*. 1st ed. Berkeley, CA: University of California Press, 2003, contents.
16 Li, Ding. *Interpretation of Difficult Issues on Acupuncture*. Shanghai: Shanghai University of Traditional Chinese Medicine Press, 1998, pp. 2–3.

Fig. 1: Variant Original Complex Forms of "Mai 脉".[17]

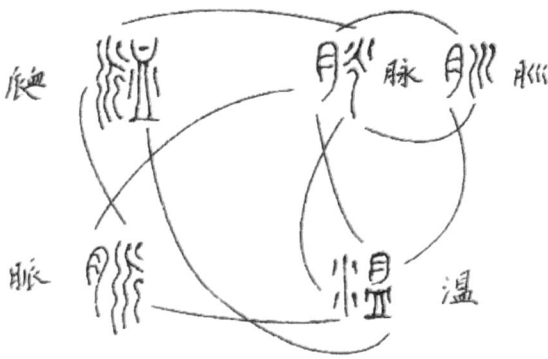

The concepts "*jing*" and "*luo*" appeared later than "*mai* or vessel". *Jing* and *luo* are further divisions of "*mai* or vessel", i.e. "*jing*" vessel and "*luo*" vessel, which was first recorded in the *Huang Di Nei Jing Ling Shu. Mai Du* 脉度 or *Huang Di's Inner Classic · Miraculous Pivot · On Vessels* "*Jing* vessels reside in the interior; their branches running transversely are known as *luo* vessels; the branches of *luo* vessels are known as grandchild vessels. 经脉为里，支而横者为络，络之别者为孙。"

The sinograms "經 *jing*" and "絡 *luo*" share the same radical – the silk part "糸", which is originally used in the textiles.

The concept "*jingmai* 經脈" is a metaphor formed in the way of *Qu Xiang Bi Lei* or taking images and analogizing. The right part of "經" is "巠", indicating both pronunciation and meaning, which is interpreted in *Shuo Wen Jie Zi* or *The Origin of Chinese Characters* as "water vessels, following (川, pictographic, indicating rivers), under the 一; 一, refers to the earth 水脉也，从巜 (川) 在一下；一，地也", that is to say, "巠" refers to the water vessels running under the earth. *Jing* 經 is explained in *Shuo Wen Jie Zi* or *The Origin of Chinese Characters* as "the longitudinal lines of the textiles or the warps 织纵丝也." The reason that "*Jing* 經" is used to name the main stems of the vessels is closely related to the origin of the sinogram "*jing* 經", which contains two images and reflects the similarities between the longitudinal lines of the textiles, the rivers running under the earth and the running routes of the main stems of the vessels.

---

17 Li, D. "Rationality of Acupuncture: The Origin and Development of Theories of Vessels and Acupoints". In: Lan, F.L./Wallner, F.G./Wobovnik, C. (eds.): *Shen, Psychotherapy, and Acupuncture: Theory, Methodology and Structure of Chinese Medicine*. Frankfurt a. M.: Peter Lang, 2011, p. 191.

Another part of "luo 絡" is "各", indicating both pronunciation and meaning, which is interpreted in *Shuo Wen Jie Zi* or *The Origin of Chinese Characters* as "divergent views being different 异辞也." Another interpretation of *Luo* 絡 is that "It originally meant unreeled silk, hemp, or cotton fiber, and from its association with stringy fibers came to be used in Chinese medicine as a noun that means network and as a verb that means to net."[18] Anyway, *Luo* 絡 is used to name divergent branches of the vessels.

Huang Di Nei Jing Ling Shu. Ben Zang 本藏 or *Huang Di's Inner Classic · Miraculous Pivot · On Viscera* states that "*Jing* vessels 經脈 function to move *qi* and blood, nourish yin and yang, moisten tendons and bones, and lubricate joints. 经脉者，所以行血气而营阴阳，濡筋骨，利关节者也." Compared to the statement that "The vessels 脈 are the residence of the blood", quite a lot new contents were supplemented to *jing* vessels, among which the most remarkable point is that the function of moving *blood* was extended to moving *qi and blood*.

"*Xue mai* 血脈", "*jing* 經" and "*luo* 絡" appeared together in the *Han Shu·Yi Wen Zhi* or *Treatise on Literature* of *The History of The Former Han Dynasty* 汉书·艺文志, "Medical classics explore the origins of *blood vessels* 血脈, *jing-luo* 經絡, bone marrow, yin-yang, exterior and interior in order to treat various diseases from the root," where blood vessels were differentiated from *jing-luo*.

Jing-luo 經絡 functions to carry and move *qi* and blood in the body. *Guan Tzu · Water & Earth* states that "Water is the *qi* and blood of the earth, running on the earth which is just like *qi* and blood flowing in the vessels." Judged from the cognizing order, the flow of *qi* and blood in man is analogized and inferred from the natural phenomenon of water flow in the rivers under the earth. The extensions from "vessel 脈" to "*jing-luo* 經絡" and from "blood" to "*qi* and blood" are also closely related to the application of acupuncture, moxibustion, *tuina*, *qigong*, etc., which explore the phenomenon of *qi* and blood flowing in the body, thus enriching the understanding on the "vessels".

Seeing that "*jing* 經" and "*luo* 絡" are subdivisions of "*Mai* 脉" or Vessel, i.e. *Jing* Vessel and *Luo* Vessel, *Jing-Luo* system is surely the "Vessel system" – being mainly composed of *Jing* Vessels and *Luo* Vessels.

To sum up, the concepts and theory of *jing-luo* were formed first on the basis of some anatomical knowledge on "vessel 脈"; then by the way of *Qu Xiang Bi Lei*, i.e. observing and taking images of the water flow in the rivers on/under the earth and the longitudinal lines of textiles, then analogizing, enlightened by the idea

---

18 Wiseman, Nigel, Zhang, Yuhuan. *Chinese Medical Characters, Volume One: Basic Vocabulary*. Brookline, MA and Taos, NM: Paradigm Publications, 2003, p. 174.

of *Tian Ren He Yi* or Unity of Heaven and Humans; and then have been proved and modified in the medical practice, especially the application of acupuncture, moxibustion, *tuina*, and *qigong*. That is to say, *jing-luo* or the vessels are metaphors, referring to the circular round pathways of the living system.

Jing-luo 經絡 system or the vessel system is a functional concept reflecting a certain image, which is embodied in their writing forms. As stated in the *Huang Di's Inner Classic · Basic Questions · Discourse on Leaving and Uniting of True Qi and Evil Qi* (*Huang Di Nei Jing Su Wen·Li He Zhen Xie Lun*) that "The sages formulated principles, which must conform to the heaven and earth. Therefore, the heaven has 365 degrees and 28 constellations, the earth has 12 *jing* rivers, and man has 12 *jing* vessels. 夫圣人之起度数，必应于天地，故天有宿度，地有经水，人有经脉。"

Is it possible to discover the physical substrate of this vessel system? It is well known that this vessel system is neither blood vessel system nor nervous system or lymph system. Recent studies show evidences about the anatomical basis for the Jing-Luo/vessel system in Chinese medicine – the fascia network. Specifically, this hypothesis is supported by anatomical observations of body scan data which demonstrates that the fascia network resembles the Jing-Luo system in salient ways, as well as physiological, histological, and clinical observations. This view represents a theoretical basis and means for applying modern biomedical research to examining Chinese medical principles and therapies in a holistic approach to diagnosis and treatment.[19]

3 Critical Review of Peer-Reviewed Journal Papers on Acupuncture

Randomized clinical trials have been considered as the gold standard for the efficacy of medical intervention. Acupuncture is no exception. It is imperative for the researchers who are going to apply for funding to sponsor their research proposals to do systematic critical reviews or meta-analysis of a certain topic in order to ensure the research question is in the frontier using methods of the most advanced and meeting the healthcare needs of patients, etc.

Most researchers and practitioners have no problem of accepting negative results about acupuncture from well-designed clinical trials. But papers published

---

19 Bai Yu, Wang Jun, Wu Jin-peng, et al. Review of Evidence Suggesting that the Fascia Network Could be the Anatomical Basis for Acupoints and Meridians in the Human Body. *Evidence-Based Complimentary and Alternative Medicine*, 2011. Article ID 260510. Available at: http://dx.doi.org/10.1155/2011/260510.

in top peer-reviewed medical journals are not guaranteed to be papers from well-designed researches. Readers, researchers in particular, always need to keep critical when reading peer-reviewed journal papers, and improve research designs by borrowing experiences, negative and positive, from others.

For example, an Australian clinical trial, published in the *Journal of the American Medical Association* (*JAMA*) in 2014 by Rana Hinman et al. evaluating the effectiveness of both needle and laser acupuncture for chronic knee pain, concluded that

"In patients older than 50 years with moderate or severe chronic knee pain, neither laser nor needle acupuncture conferred benefit over sham for pain or function. Our findings do not support acupuncture for these patients."[20]

Obviously, this statement does not reflect the clinical experiences of most practitioners. *JAMA* (Impact Factor: 44.4) has been one of the most influential peer-reviewed medical journals for years. How should we interpret the research outcome of this journal paper?

Dr. Hongjian He, AP, MD, PhD; Lixing Lao, PhD, MB; Wing-Fai Yeung, BCM, PhD; and Yong Ming Li, MD, PhD "poked" so many "holes" in this study after further investigation, including design flaws; violating ethics; the sample size being too small; the research outcome contradicting with that of larger scale clinical trials; ignoring intervention from non-steroidal anti-inflammatory drugs (NSAIDs); biased approach by ignoring the evidence of acupuncture efficacy in improving patients' overall pain score, and functional improvement (both $p<0.05$); the acupuncture intervention (including needle acupuncture and laser acupuncture) being far away from an optimal treatment in the terms of dosage and frequency; no licensed acupuncturist participated in that study, instead they used physician practitioners; and so and so forth.[21]

More critical reviews of such peer-reviewed journal papers on acupuncture with negative results need to be done in order to save acupuncture as a science in the future.

---

20 Hinman RS, McCrory P, Pirotta M, et al. Acupuncture for Chronic Knee Pain: A Randomized Clinical Trial. *JAMA*. 2014, 312(13): 1313–22.
21 Reddy, B. Chinese Doctors Poke Holes in Australian Study. *Acupuncture Today*. 2015, 16(7). Available at: http://www.acupuncturetoday.com/mpacms/at/article.php?id=33043. Date of last access: May 1, 2018.

4 Conclusion

Annotation and interpretation of classical texts alone or in combination with personal experiences has been a major method to develop acupuncture and Chinese medicine in the last thousands of years. Nowadays, literature research, classical and/or modern, has been of the first significance before proceeding research of any kind. Interpreting classical and modern literature in modern clinical settings is a key to transmit and enrich the knowledge system of acupuncture.

References

Hinman RS, McCrory P, Pirotta M, et al. Acupuncture for Chronic Knee Pain: A Randomized Clinical Trial. *JAMA*, 2014, 312(13): 1313–22.

Lan, F.L.. *Metaphor: The Weave r of Chinese Medicine*. Nordhausen: Traugott Bautz, 2015.

Lan, F. L., Wallner, F. Taking Image and Analogizing: The Metaphorizing Process and the Way of Forming Metaphors in Chinese Medicine. *Journal of Dialectics of Nature*, 2014, 36(2): 98–104.

Lan, F. L., Wallner, F. G., Wobovnik, C. (eds.). *Shen, Psychotherapy, and Acupuncture: Theory, Methodology and Structure of Chinese Medicine*. Frankfurt a. M.: Peter Lang, 2011.

Lewit, K. The Needle Effect in the Relief of Myofascial Pain. *Pain*, 1979, 6(1): 83–90.

Li, D. *Interpretation of Difficult Issues on Acupuncture*. Shanghai: Shanghai University of Traditional Chinese Medicine Press, 1998.

Maciocia, G. *The Foundations of Chinese Medicine: A Comprehensive Text*. 3rd ed. Edinburgh: Elsevier, 2015.

MacPherson, H., Hammerschlag, R., Lewith, G., Schner, R. *Acupuncture Research: Strategies for Establishing an Evidence Base*. Edinburgh: Elsevier Churchill Livingstone, 2007.

Reddy, B. Chinese Doctors Poke Holes in Australian Study. *Acupuncture Today*, 2015, 16(7). Available at: http://www.acupuncturetoday.com/mpacms/at/article.php?id=33043. Date of last access: May 1, 2018.

Unschuld, P. U. *Huang Di Nei Jing Su Wen: Nature, Knowledge, Imagery in an Ancient Chinese Medical Text*. 1st ed. Berkeley, CA: University of California Press, 2003.

WHO. *WHO International Standard Terminologies on Traditional Medicine in the Western Pacific Region*. Geneva: WHO. 2007.

Wiseman, Nigel, Yuhuan, Zhang. *Chinese Medical Characters, Volume One: Basic Vocabulary.* Brookline, MA and Taos, NM: Paradigm Publications. 2003.

Yeh, T. M.. Dry Needling for Musculoskeletal Pain Management: A Survey of Current Literature. Capstone Project or Dissertation for Doctor of Acupuncture Oriental Medicine. Santa Cruz and San Jose, California: Five Branches University, 2017, p. 4.

Ephraim Ferreira Medeiros, Lixing Lao, and Fengli Lan

An Overview of the Evolution of Acupuncture Treatment: From Stone Needle to Laser Beam

Abstract: Drawing from acupuncture's history, we analyze how globalization, data science, and cross-disciplinarity transformed the study and practice of Chinese Medicine. We argue that a thorough understanding of foundational acupuncture theories and metaphors could guide a harmonized way forward: reconstructing lost knowledge and incorporating discoveries.

1 Developing the "Zhen" 针 (Acupuncture Needles)

1.1 Zhen's First Shapes and Materials

We begin by recalling that Zhenjiu is the Chinese name for acupuncture where Zhen stands for the acupuncture's needling objects and techniques and Jiu stands for the moxibustion ones. It is important to notice that archeological evidence places moxibustion as being practiced for longer than acupuncture. Chinese medical texts found in the tomb of Ma Wangdui in Hunan only describe moxibustion channels. Ancient Chinese texts describe the use of sharp stone tools – called Bian – in practices such as bleeding and the draining of abscesses and carbuncles. Sharp bones, pointed crystals, and bamboo also were used for needle manufacture.

Remember: the character 针 Zhen (needle) is etymologically related to 箴, itself related to bamboo. Needles (sewing and acupuncture both) have the same root, both connecting to bamboo.[1]

Of note is that some needles displayed in museums as acupuncture ones have eyes on them. Their existence shows that the technology for producing metallic sharp objects was already well refined but on the other hand, it raises questions about its therapeutic uses, at least the ones found in tombs. There is no evidence of needles being used simultaneously as sewing and medicinal instruments.

---

1 The same bamboo that was important for the Japanese Acupuncture's development of shinkan, the needle guide by the blind acupuncturist Waichi Sugiyama during the Edo Period (1603–1867). Kobayashi, Akiko/Uefuji, Miwa/Yasumo, Washiro: "History and Progress of Japanese Acupuncture". *Evidence-Based Complementary and Alternative Medicine*, 7(3), 2010, pp. 359–365.

1.2 The Early Systematization of Acupuncture and Moxibustion

The emergence of the monumental works *Huangdi Neijing* at the Spring and Autumn Period (770–476 BCE)/Warring States Period (475–221 BCE) and *Nanjing* at the Han Dynasty (206–220 CE) were key moments for acupuncture's evolution and can be considered the starting point for the systematic practice of acupuncture and moxibustion in China.

Another milestone was the classic *Zhenjiu JiaYijing* by Huang-fu Mi (215–282 CE), a famous acupuncturist during the Wei (220–264 CE) and Jin (265–420 CE) Dynasties. This classic contains a summary of achievements in the field of acupuncture and moxibustion from the Qin (221–207 BCE) to the Han Dynasty (206–220 CE) and his own clinical experiences.

Before these systematization efforts (and even after it),[2] acupuncture practice was linked to Shamanic healing practices. The appearance of these texts sets the beginning of a clear separation between orthodox and heterodox practices in Chinese medicine in general, each group claiming the discourse and vying for practices, traditions, and lineages.

2 Acupuncture's First Epoch of Decline and Disuse

After these efforts, acupuncture all but disappears until the Song Dynasty. Chinese physicians became extremely cautious of using acupuncture in clinical practice, preferring moxibustion instead, being a safer therapy. Possible reasons are pointed by Mathias Vigouroux:

> After the disintegration of the Han Empire (206 bce–220 ce), the acupuncture classics circulation was limited to a very small number of physicians in China. Only a few diagrams were available to help practitioners visualize the acupuncture points in the body. Also, over time, discrepancies appeared between treatises.
> Immediate risks inherent to the practice of moxibustion were mostly limited to burns and blisters, whereas a needle wrongly inserted could cause bleeding, damage the tissues or the organs, and have even more dramatic consequences.[3]

In our opinion, we also must remind the high risks of cross infections from neglecting or lack of adequate methods to properly sterilize needles.

---

2 Strickmann, Michel/Faure, Bernard: *Chinese Magical Medicine*. Stanford University Press: Stanford (CA), 2005.

3 Burns, Susan L./Elman, Benjamin A.: *Antiquarianism, Language, and Medical Philology: From Early Modern to Modern Sino-Japanese Medical Discourses*. Brill: Leiden, 2015.

Keiji Yamada proposes that the development of the treatments begins with moxibustion practices, evolves to fire-needles and finally reaches filiform needles.[4] When studying practitioners after the classics *Huangdi Neijing*, *Nan Jing* and *Zhenjiu Jiayi Jing*, we notice that moxibustion was almost exclusively the only technique used. This is particularly clear in the works of Ge Hong (葛洪, 284–364 CE), Tao Hong-jing (陶弘景, 456–536 CE), Xu Zhi-cai (492–572 CE), and Chao Yuanfeng (徐之才). But the biography of Dr. Liu Juanzi (刘涓子), practicing during the Song dynasty, describes an acupuncture technique using fire-needles. This gives strength to Prof. Yamada's theory of gradual transition: moxibustion-fire needle-filiform needle. Fire needling is also hygienically safer, possibly removing one risk factor mentioned above needle contamination and cross-infection.

3 The Beginning of a Restructured Acupuncture Practice

Acupuncture was still being studied by scholars – even if rarely practiced – and always present in varying degree on almost every academic text. That allowed its continued acceptance as an orthodox therapeutic practice over the centuries.

4 Sui (581–618 CE) And Tang (618–907 CE) Dynasties

Acupuncture and moxibustion developed rapidly along with the increasingly prosperous economy and culture of the time.

Sun Simiao, known for Qianjin Yaofang (Prescriptions Worth a Thousand Gold for Emergencies or Precious Prescriptions for Emergencies) and the QianjinYifang (A Supplement to the Essential Prescriptions Worth a Thousand Gold or Supplement to Precious Prescriptions), develops the first known colored maps of channels and points and provides the first description of the Ashi points.

Wang Tao (670–755 CE). Wang Tao wrote an important reference book for moxibustion, *Waitai Miyao* (Essential Secrets from the Imperial Library), in which recorded a host of **moxibustion** applications of various schools.

---

4 See Yamada, Keiji: *The Origins of Acupuncture, Moxibustion, and Decoction: The Two Phases of the Formation of Ancient Medicine: The Origins of Acupuncture and Moxibustion, The Origins of Decoction*. International Research Center for Japanese Studies: Kyoto, 1998, also, Yamada, Keiji: "Formation of Prototype for Chinese Medicine". *Japan Review*, 2, 1991, pp. 203–207.

5 Song Dynasty (960–1279 CE): Standardizing the Teaching of Acupuncture and the Popularization of its Practice

During the Song dynasty (960–1279 CE) a renewed interest in the study of acupuncture and moxibustion, improvements in printing technology and governmental support were important factors in facilitating the creation and dissemination of study materials.

Wang Wei-yi (987–1067 CE) – *Tongren Shuxue Zhen Jiu Tujing* (Illustrated Manual of the Bronze Man Showing Acupuncture and Moxibustion Points). One of the most important work in acupuncture's history, it documents the location of acupuncture points and channels in a way that allowed the transmission of such knowledge to happen in a standardized way.

He also designed two life-size male bronze statues. The bronze statues were considered exquisite teaching models at that time and an advance in medical education and with the help of the models, meridian theory became more popular.

Neo-Confucianism, analyses regarding the nature of Qi (especially by the philosophers Zhangzai and Chen Brothers) and careful studies of The Book of Changes (Yijing) are defining moments of the Song dynasty. Also, neo-Confucianism philosophy provided for an ethics where the study and practice of medicine were highly prized and even some emperors became students and practitioners of medicine.[5]

6 Jin (1115–1234) and Yuan (1271–1368) Dynasties

With standardized teaching came a safer practice and more detailed clinical observations thus making acupuncture a fertile ground for new proposals. The influence of the philosophies in Zhou Yi and the concept of "Changes with Current Situation" has become an important theoretical foundation for guiding Chinese medicine to understand the physiological function and pathological changes of the human body as well as developing the treatment methods like the "chronobiological" use of acupuncture points by techniques such as, Zi Wu Liu Zhu 子午流注 and Lin Gui Ba Fa 灵龟八法.[6] Acupuncture practice became even

---

5　See Goldschmidt, Asaf: *The Evolution of Chinese Medicine: Song Dynasty, 960–1200*. Routledge: London, 2011, pp. 19–42.

6　See Lo, Kwaiching/Li, Lei: "Tao of Changes and Tao of Medicine – The Influence of the Philosophy of the Concepts of Time and Space in Zhou Yi on the Academic Development of Chinese Medicine". *Journal of Beijing University of Chemical Technology (Social Sciences Edition)*, 1, 2014 (In Chinese).

more personalized – e.g. taking into consideration the time of day. These methods allow the practitioner to select a time of day that would be best for acupuncture and choose points that resonate with it, i.e. have the best clinical while the consultation is happening. These are methods still employed today.[7]

Yuan dynasty Hua Boren's 《十四经发挥》 (*Exposition of the Fourteen Meridians*) studies the relationship between meridians and points, making important contributions to its understanding, including Ren Mai and Du Mai [and/with] the 12 regular meridians. The book had a significant influence on the science of acupuncture.

7 Ming Dynasty (1368–1644)

Arguably, the golden age of acupuncture practice began during the Imperial period. All previous dynasties developments – especially post-Song – bear fruit and both the practice and academic research of acupuncture bloom.

Xu Feng 徐凤 discussed needling techniques for supplementation and drainage as well as techniques for massaging channels to direct qi in his book (Zhēn Jiŭ Dà Quán, 针灸大全).

Gao Wu 高武 wrote 《针灸聚英》 Zhenjiu Juying (An Exemplary Collection of Acupuncture, Moxibustion and their Essentials) around 1529.[8]

Yang Jizhou 杨继洲 (1522–1620) published the most significant text of the period on acupuncture, *Zhengjiu Dacheng* (The Great Compendium of Acupuncture and Moxibustion).

8 Qing Dynasty (1644–1912 CE): Decline of Acupuncture and Moxibustion Usage

With the rise of Western medicine presence, acupuncture uses steadily declines while phytotherapy manages to still be in widespread use.[9] Politically, this was a troubled period: Opium War, unequal treaties, Taiping Rebellion (1850–1864), and Dungan Revolt (1862–1877).

---

7   The Mianyang TCM Hospital (Sichuan Province People's Republic of China) has a section solely devoted to using these methods to treat patients.
8   This book influenced deeply the foundations of Korean Acupuncture. See "Characteristic of Korean Medicine – In Clinic; Saam Acupuncture". *All That Korean Medicine*. Seoul, 2011, retrieved on April 28, 2017 from http://tkmedicine.blogspot.sg/2011/07/3-characteristic-of-korean-medicine-in.html.
9   Cheng, XN: *Chinese Acupuncture and Moxibustion*. Foreign Languages Press: Beijing, 1987.

9 Republic of China (1912–1949 CE): Redefining Chinese Medicine and the Emergence of a New Professional Class

The Western medicine influence completely reshapes the medical landscape in China and drastic measures such as banning the practice of Chinese medicine and replacing it with its western counterpart. As an act of resistance to this hostile encroachment, the practitioners of Chinese medicine rise as a professional class, struggling to survive and define a properly independent identity.

This becomes one of the most fascinating (and problematic) periods of the history of Chinese medicine: the coalescing of a fragmented collection of practitioners into an organized group, using its influence and abilities to urge politicians against banning Chinese medicine and ensuring its survival.[10]

In 1935, a resolution backed by a petition from traditional medicine societies demanding equal status for Chinese and Western medicine passed.[11]

Also in the early 1930s, Cheng Danan, a Chinese scholar-physician, used Euroamerican anatomy to rehabilitate acupuncture as a respectable skill and insisted that acupuncture must be an effective medical therapy because its mechanism of action was the stimulation of the nerves described in European medical theory.[12]

10 People's Republic of China (PRC) 1949 – Present Days

Traditional Chinese Medicine (TCM) becomes then grounded on Chinese classics but guided by scientific methods and the need to integrate western medicine. This fusion is what Mao Zedong envisioned as "The new medicine".[13]

The TCM practiced today is based on standardization efforts that took place in China in the 1950s with the creation of TCM colleges and hygiene schools,

---

10 See Taylor, Kim: *Chinese Medicine in Early Communist China, 1945-63*. Routledge: London, 2005 and Scheid, Volker: *Chinese Medicine in Contemporary China*. Duke University Press: Durham (NC), 2002, pp. 66–106. (Unschuld, *op. cit.* pp. 229–260), and Andrews, Bridie: *The Making of Modern Chinese Medicine, 1850-1960*. University of Hawaii Press: Honolulu, 2015, pp. 207–217.

11 Hillier, S.: *Health Care and Traditional Medicine in China 1800-1982*. Routledge, 2013, p. 311.

12 Cheng's new scientific acupuncture was a great success in China. In the 1950s, however, Cheng abandoned his own earlier insistence that acupuncture must work through the nerves alone. Instead, he attributed its efficacy to the power of qi and the doctor-patient relationship, in addition to the physical stimulation of the nerves. See Andrews, BJ: "Acupuncture and the Reinvention of Chinese Medicine". *APS Bulletin*, 9(3), 1999.

13 Taylor, *op. cit.*

hospitals, and clinics. The Communist state-building project mandated that TCM institutions be built in every provincial capital. From 1956 to 1963, TCM textbooks were written and TCM institutions were created.[14]

The China Academy of TCM was established in 1955[15] and in 1958, the first successful surgical operation with acupuncture anesthesia aroused great attention in the West.[16]

From 1966 until 1976, the Cultural Revolution movement affected China politically and produced a huge negative impact on the country's economy and society.

The Cultural Revolution had a tremendous impact in the practice of acupuncture and its aftershocks are still felt today, especially with regards to human resources as many of the practicing acupuncturists of the time were either persecuted or even killed by the regime or committed suicide, and many a book was obliterated.[17]

In 1975 entrusted by the World Health Organization (WHO) International training centers for acupuncture and moxibustion were set up in Beijing, Shanghai and Nanjing aiming to train physicians and acupuncturists from various countries and regions.[18]

With the 80s came the Chinese economic reform, and a resurgence of scientific publication. It also marks the appearance of new acupuncture techniques, for economic opening also meant information exchange between the then closed China and the world. Some of these are readily assimilated back into Chinese practice while others had more acceptance outside China, e.g.: classical electroacupuncture vs. Voll's electroacupuncture; traditional moxibustion vs. TDP mineral Lamp (Teding Diancibo Pu); Nogier's auriculotherapy vs. Chinese auriculotherapy; and different approaches to laser acupuncture (Chinese, Japanese, and Western).

---

14 Hsu, Elizabeth: "The History of Chinese Medicine in the People's Republic of China and its Globalization". *East Asian Science, Technology and Society: An International Journal*.
15 See Wiseman, Nigel: *Education and Practice of Chinese Medicine in Taiwan*. The speech was given at the 31st TCM Congress, Rothenburg, June 2000. Retrieved on April 28, 2017 from http://www.paradigm-pubs.com/sites/www.paradigm-pubs.com/files/files/TAIWAN.pdf.
16 Zhang, Ji/Zhao, Bai-xiao/Lao, Lixing: *Acupuncture and Moxibustion*. People's Medical Publishing House: Beijing, 2014, p. 4.
17 Scheid, *op. cit.*, pp. 76–81.
18 Zhang/Zhao/Lao, *op. cit. loc. cit.*

11 Globalization of Acupuncture/TCM

The 1980s saw the complete rehabilitation of Chinese medicine from the destructive forces of the Cultural Revolution and reinforcing of its presence within state structures. By 1984, there were twenty-nine academies of TCM in China, eleven medical schools with specialist departments of TCM, and over 26,000 students engaged in its study.[19] In 1987, the World Federation of Acupuncture-Moxibustion Societies (WFAS) was established and the first International Conference on Acupuncture and Moxibustion was held in Beijing. Composed of fifty-live acupuncture associations worldwide WFAS is headquartered in Beijing.[20]

In the 1990s, TCM was commodified as semi-private industries promoted TCM in global health markets. In China, TCM colleges became "Universities of Chinese medicine and pharmacotherapy"[21] and TCM truly enters the global stage, providing innovative (or at least new) services, products and research and development opportunities, to any those who pay.

Some of those new techniques include auricular, scalp, abdominal, feet, tongue and hand acupuncture in addition to the traditional body acupuncture. Other developments that enjoy large popularity are filiform and intradermal needling, electrical stimulation, warm needling, ultrasound stimulation, laser acupuncture, magnetic therapy and acupoint injection, catgut, small knife needle, and others.

11.1 Therapeutic Fusions: Creating Synergies beyond the Realm of TCM

With the advances in research, electro acupuncture virtually became the top choice technique when researching acupuncture effects and mechanisms both in China and outside.[22]

The use of laser beams in acupuncture has a tremendous boost in research and gain immense popularity during these years.[23]

---

19 Taylor, *op. cit.* p. 151.
20 Zhang/Zhao/Lao, *op. cit. loc. cit.*
21 "The Globalization of Chinese Medicine". *The Levin Institute – State University of New York*, 2012, last modified 2017, retrieved on April 28, 2017 from http://www.globaliza tion101.org/the-globalization-of-chinese-medicine/.
22 See Mayor, David F. et al.: *Electroacupuncture: A Practical Manual and Resource*. Churchill Livingstone/Elsevier Health Sciences: Edinburgh, 2007.
23 See Naeser, Margaret A./Wei, Xiu-Bing: *Laser Acupuncture: An Introductory Textbook for Treatment of Pain, Paralysis, Spasticity and Other Disorders: Clinical and Research Uses of Laser Acupuncture from Around the World*. Boston Chinese Medicine: Boston

In addition to these milestones in the late 1990s and early 2000s, acupuncture began being paired with different therapeutical approaches as homeopathy, aromatherapy, flower remedies and non-Chinese phytotherapy. All these initiatives follow the reasoning that, if western medicine can be integrated into Chinese medicine, the same could be attempted with Chinese medicine and other medical systems. Some remarkable examples follow.

12 Revival of Homeopuncture

In the 1950s, Dr. Roger de la Fuye (French Homeopath and Acupuncturist) researched and concluded that homeopathy can be used with acupuncture to treat patients. He was also able to utilize the points to confirm if the remedy was the proper one. With the popularization of acupuncture in West, his approach saw a revival and gained boost during 1990s.

Example[24]:

Homeopucture Protocol to Vascular Disorders	
Hypotension	Hypertension
Ren6 Qihai- Gelsemium St36 Zusanli- Sempervirens Sp6 Sanyinjiao	Du20 Baihui LI11 Quchi - Aurum metallicum 30C St36 Zusanli- or Sp6 Sanyinjiao- Phosphorus 30C Liv3 Taichong

---

(MA), 1994. And Naeser, Margaret A./Wei, Xiu-Bing: *Laser Acupuncture: An Introductory Textbook.* Boston Chinese Medicine: Boston (MA), 1994, pp. 197–203.

24 Morais, Justin: "Acupuncture + Homeopathy = Homeopuncture". Retrieved on April 27, 2017 from http://www.acupuncture.org.sg/cos/o.x?c=/wbn/pagetree&func=view&rid=35321.

13 Aromatic Acupuncture

Prof. Ephraim Ferreira Medeiros developed the use of essential oils with acupuncture to optimize treatments in 1999,[25] based on works of La Fuye,[26] Peter Holmes[27] and Gabriel Mojay.[28]

14 Phyto Acupuncture

The use of seeds, originally from Brazilian traditional medicinal, on acupuncture (or auriculo acupuncture) points was developed by the Brazilian acupuncturist Dr. Sérgio Franceschini Filho.[29]

Many other techniques increase in popularity: magneto-acupuncture and bioresonance therapy became popular in West and especially in Japan.

15 Effects of Globalization

During this period, niches and specializations were created, defining knowledge borders and ascribing them to different professionals. Those efforts also try to distance the study of acupuncture from traditional concepts like Yin and Yang, Wu Xing, and Qi (considered too ambiguous) instead of replacing them with neuro-physiological/anatomical terminology.

Resulting from this distancing and separation are therapies that appropriate practices from acupuncture but remove them from any cultural/foundational aspects. One example of such practice is the creation of the "Dry Needling" technique by Janet G. Travell[30] in the late 90s.

---

25 Medeiros, Ephraim F: "Acupuntura Aromatica". Retrieved on April 27, 2017 from http://www.zangfu.com.br/biblioteca/acupuntura-aromatica.pdf. It is important to note that in 1990s it was very hard to find Chinese herbs to work in Brazil but in another hand high-quality aromatherapy essential oils abounded and this was one of the main reasons that motivated this combination and research.
26 See Jayasuriya, Anton: *Clinical Homeopathy*. Kuldeep Jain for Health Harmony: New Delhi, 2002, p. 718.
27 Holmes, Peter: *The Energetics of Western Herbs: A Materiamedica Integrating Western and Chinese Herbal Therapeutics*. Snow Lotus Press: Cotati, 2007.
28 Mojay, Gabriel: *Aromatherapy for Healing the Spirit: A Guide to Restoring Emotional and Mental Balance Through Essential Oils*. Gaia: London, 2005.
29 Franceschini Filho, Sérgio: *Fitoacupuntura: A Simplicidade E a Força Das Plantas Como Facilitadoras Da Saúde*, Editora Roca Ltda., 2000.
30 Simons, David G./Travell, Janet G./Simons, Lois S.: *Travell & Simons' Myofascial Pain and Dysfunction: The Trigger Point Manual*. Williams & Wilkins: Baltimore (MD), 1999.

Specializing, even more, are practices like Mikio Sankei's Esoteric Acupuncture, removing themselves from both classical acupuncture and western medicine, targeting instead practitioners of western esoteric/mystic traditions.[31]

Finally, an effort to standardize terms and procedure names in acupuncture (and TCM in general) took place, looking for improvements in teaching and practice of Chinese medicine around the world. While definitely not problem-free, this effort did heavily contribute to the current global reach – and development – of Chinese medicine.[32]

16 The IT, High Tech and Post Needle Era

With internet's explosive popularization in the early 2000s, forums and social networks enabled professionals from across the world to exchange knowledge, removing entry barriers and fostering the creation of new materials and approaches to the teaching of acupuncture. Following the Big Data innovations, these platforms also became a prime source for data-mining opportunities and post-2010 the majority of TCM hospitals in China have electronic data collection and management systems, streamlining everything from inventory management to epidemiologic analysis initiatives.

Research in computer science relevant to TCM[33] and the design of wearable sensors and devices[34] are opening promising avenues for diagnosing and acupuncture treatment.

Many new techniques have been developed concurrent to these, further removing themselves from classical acupuncture views using these concepts on a surface level and appropriating only a few classes of points and channels. These techniques are also different from other recent *technological* advances in that they eschew altogether the use of needles. Despite positioning themselves far from the classical body of theories and practices to define an identity of their own, techniques like Dry Needling and Esoteric Acupuncture still use needling as their

---

31 Sankey, Mikio: *Esoteric Acupuncture*. Mountain Castle Pub.: Los Angeles (CA), 1999.
32 *WHO standard acupuncture point locations in the Western Pacific Region*. World Health Organization, Western Pacific Region: Manila, 2008.
33 Wu, Zhaohui/Chen, Huajun/Jiang, Xiaohong: *Modern Computational Approaches to Traditional Chinese Medicine*. Elsevier: London, 2012. And Poon, Josiah/Poon, Simon K.: *Data Analytics for Traditional Chinese Medicine Research*. Springer: Cham, 2014.
34 Lei, H. et al: "A Pilot Clinical Trial to Objectively Assess the Efficacy of Electroacupuncture on Gait in Patients with Parkinson's Disease Using Body Worn Sensors". *PLOS One*, 11(5), 2016 e0155613, https://doi.org/10.1371/journal.pone.0155613.

central practice. Laser beams, which were being used in acupuncture before this period, can be employed with or without needles. This suggests a gradual trend toward substituting needles (Zhen) for other different kinds of stimuli leading to the emergence of a myriad of new approaches that do not employ needles or moxibustion.[35]

In a counter-parallel movement, there is rising interest in research that studies the importance of the classical forms of Chinese acupuncture, and texts like Liu Lihong's *Sikao Zhongyi* (《思考中医》)[36] are voicing concerns about – and suggesting ways out of – the extended crisis that Chinese Medicine is going through.[37]

17 Final Remarks

We have shown how the practice and study of acupuncture have changed over the millennia, especially after western theories of medicine began being incorporated into the Chinese medicine practices. Currently, there is renewed interest in acupuncture as providing preventive measures (an ancient focus but neglected over the years) in addition to its efficacy when treating a host of maladies is of particular importance.

Globalization has steadily increased the reach of TCM and acupuncture: more patients, practitioners and researchers and an ever-expanding body of academic work.

Another facet of it, working perhaps via obfuscation or redirection, resulted on "new therapies": niche practices and a discourse that uses (or better, appropriates) only to select concepts from the foundational acupuncture theories in a bid to further their own agenda (e.g. Medical or Esoteric acupuncture). By positioning themselves far away from the practices and discourse of acupuncture in China (or eastern Asia) and claiming to hold "new truths" about it, they end up reinforcing stereotypes and building resistance to the understanding of philosophical concepts as Yin/Yang and the five movements. Perhaps this is the largest challenge for

---

35 Some examples are Crystal Acupuncture – use of stones and crystals in acupoints; Chromo Acupuncture – LED light and optic fibers to stimulate acupoints with specific colors; and Radionic Acupuncture – radionics and radiesthesia (dowsing) combined with acupuncture theories for the remote treatment of maladies.

36 *Sikao Zhongyi* [Contemplating Chinese medicine] 刘力红.思考中医.广西师范大学出版社.

37 See *Chinese Medicine in Crisis: Science, Politics, and the Making of "TCM"*. Classical-ChineseMedicine.org, Hai Shan Center, Inc. Retrieved on September 1, 2017 from https://classicalchinesemedicine.org/gpa/chinese-medicine-in-crisis-science-politics-and-the-making-of-tcm/.

academic research on acupuncture. Globalization created a new set of challenges to the survival of acupuncture and Chinese medicine, after the arrival of western remedies, technology, and therapies.

To be able to survive, acupuncture had to concede, removing from the discourse concepts like Li and Yi and instead focusing only on its practical and descriptive aspects, a focus imported from Western medicine.[38] This resulted in a fractured transmission and comprehension of the knowledge historically associated with Chinese medicine, and we have shown that these gaps are being filled not only by concepts originated from western medicine but from areas far removed from both. For a notable example of these movements, a cursory glance over the curriculum of a typical TCM post-secondary program finds about half of the curriculum filled by western science and medicine disciplines and courses. Another example, in clinical practice, is auriculotherapy.

Auriculotherapy is a practice originated in France, that was (rapidly) assimilated to such a degree in China that it has its maps and prescriptive practices differing considerably from the French ones, and for some maladies like Myopia (especially pediatric Myopia) it is the primary treatment choice. Contemporary Chinese medicine does look outside and forward.

While supported by the government the "export" of acupuncture professionals is not without its problems, mostly stemming from the excessive simplification necessary to make it fit into western paradigms. A possible way to reconstruct – or at least mend some of – these fractures might be to combine the philosophy of Constructive Realism[39] with a program of study centered on the understanding of the foundational metaphors of Chinese Medicine and acupuncture theories.

This could herald a new cycle of transformation for acupuncture, interested in the *reconstruction* of the missing spaces, not simply be forgoing all modern advances and trying to restore the "golden age" of acupuncture. Such transformation would leave Chinese medicine and acupuncture in a place where it would be able to better withstand future upheavals, for its metaphorical reasoning is as important for the foundational identity of acupuncture as the needles (Zhen) themselves.

---

38 See Scheid, Volker: "Remodeling the Arsenal of Chinese Medicine: Shared Pasts, Alternative Futures." *The Annals of the American Academy of Political and Social Science* 583(1), 2002, pp. 136–59.
39 See Slunecko, Thomas/Wallner, Fritz G.: *The Movement of Constructive Realism*. Braumüller: Wien, 1997.

Acknowledgments

I would like to acknowledge Fernando Girotto (MSc in Physics and currently working toward MA in English Literature at the University of Calgary) for help editing the English text and footnotes.

References

Andrews, Bridie: "Acupuncture and the Reinvention of Chinese Medicine". *APS Bulletin*, 9(3), 1999.

Andrews, Bridie: *The Making of Modern Chinese Medicine, 1850–1960*. University of Hawaii Press: Honolulu, 2015.

Burns, Susan L./Elman, Benjamin A.: *Antiquarianism, Language, and Medical Philology: From Early Modern to Modern Sino-Japanese Medical Discourses*. Brill: Leiden, 2015.

"Characteristic of Korean Medicine – In Clinic; Saam Acupuncture". *All That Korean Medicine*. Seoul, 2011, retrieved on April 28, 2017 from http://tkmedi cine.blogspot.sg/2011/07/3-characteristic-of-korean-medicine-in.html.

Fruehauf, Heiner: "Chinese Medicine in Crisis: Science, Politics, and the Making of 'TCM'". ClassicalChineseMedicine.org, Hai Shan Center, Inc. Retrieved on September 1, 2017 from https://classicalchinesemedicine.org/gpa/chinese-medicine-in-crisis-science-politics-and-the-making-of-tcm/.

Cheng, Xinnong: *Chinese Acupuncture and Moxibustion*. Foreign Languages Press: Beijing, 1987.

Franceschini Filho, Sérgio: *Fitoacupuntura: A Simplicidade E a Força Das Plantas Como Facilitadoras Da Saúde*, Editora Roca Ltda: Rio De Janeiro, 2000.

Goldschmidt, Asaf: *The Evolution of Chinese Medicine: Song Dynasty, 960–1200*. Routledge: London, 2011.

Hillier, Sheila: *Health Care and Traditional Medicine in China 1800–1982*. Routledge: London, 2013, p. 311.

Holmes, Peter: *The Energetics of Western Herbs: A Materiamedica Integrating Western and Chinese Herbal Therapeutics*. Snow Lotus Press: Cotati (CA), 2007.

Hsu, Elizabeth: "The History of Chinese Medicine in the People's Republic of China and its Globalization". *East Asian Science, Technology and Society: An International Journal*, 2, 2008, pp. 465–84.

Jayasuriya, Anton: *Clinical Homoeopathy*. Kuldeep Jain for Health Harmony: New Delhi, 2002.

Kobayashi, Akiko/Uefuji, Miwa/Yasumo, Washiro: "History and Progress of Japanese Acupuncture". *Evidence-Based Complementary and Alternative Medicine*, 7(3), 2010, pp. 359–365.

Lei, Hong et al.: "A Pilot Clinical Trial to Objectively Assess the Efficacy of Electroacupuncture on Gait in Patients with Parkinson's Disease Using Body Worn Sensors". *PLOS One*, 11(5), 2016, e0155613, https://doi.org/10.1371/journal.pone.0155613.

Lo, Kwaiching/Li, Lei: "Tao of Changes and Tao of Medicine: The Influence of the Philosophy of the Concepts of Time and Space in Zhou Yi on the Academic Development of Chinese Medicine". *Journal of Beijing University of Chemical Technology (Social Sciences Edition)*, 1, 2014, pp. 58–63 (In Chinese).

Mayor, David F. et al.: *Electroacupuncture: A Practical Manual and Resource*. Churchill Livingstone/Elsevier Health Sciences: Edinburgh, 2007.

Medeiros, Ephraim F: "Acupuntura Aromatica". Retrieved on April 27, 2017 from http://www.acupunturabrasil.org/acupuntura-aromatica.pdf (In Portuguese).

Mojay, Gabriel: *Aromatherapy for Healing the Spirit: A Guide to Restoring Emotional and Mental Balance through Essential Oils*. Gaia: London, 2005.

Morais, Justin: "Acupuncture + Homeopathy = Homeopuncture". Retrieved on April 27, 2017 from http://www.acupuncture.org.sg/cos/o.x?c=/wbn/pagetree&func=view&rid=35321.

Naeser, Margaret A./Wei, Xiu-Bing: *Laser Acupuncture: An Introductory Textbook*. Boston Chinese Medicine: Boston, 1994.

Poon, Josiah/Poon, Simon K.: *Data Analytics for Traditional Chinese Medicine Research*. Springer: Cham, 2014.

Sankey, Mikio: *Esoteric Acupuncture*. Mountain Castle Pub.: Los Angeles (CA), 1999.

Scheid, Volker: "Remodeling the Arsenal of Chinese Medicine: Shared Pasts, Alternative Futures". *The Annals of the American Academy of Political and Social Science*, 583(1), 2002, pp. 136–159.

Scheid, Volker: *Chinese Medicine in Contemporary China*. Duke University Press: Durham (NC), 2002.

Simons, David G./Travell, Janet G./Simons, Lois S.: *Travell & Simons' Myofascial Pain and Dysfunction: The Trigger Point Manual*. Williams & Wilkins: Baltimore (MD), 1999.

Slunecko, Thomas/Wallner, Fritz G.: *The Movement of Constructive Realism*. Braumüller: Wien, 1997.

Strickmann, Michel/Faure, Bernard: *Chinese Magical Medicine*. Stanford University Press: Stanford (CA), 2005.

Taylor, Kim: *Chinese Medicine in Early Communist China 1945–63.* Routledge: London, 2005.

"The Globalization of Chinese Medicine". *The Levin Institute – State University of New York*, 2012, last modified 2017, retrieved on April 28, 2017 from http://www.globalization101.org/the-globalization-of-chinese-medicine/.

Unschuld, Paul U.: *Medicine in China: A History of Ideas.* University of California Press: Berkeley (CA), 1985.

Wiseman, Nigel: *Education and Practice of Chinese Medicine in Taiwan.* The speech was given at the 31st TCM Congress, Rothenburg, June 2000. Retrieved on April 28, 2017 from http://www.paradigm-pubs.com/sites/www.paradigm-pubs.com/files/files/TAIWAN.pdf.

WHO Regional Office for the Western Pacific, *WHO standard acupuncture point locations in the Western Pacific Region.* World Health Organization, Western Pacific Region: Manila, 2008.

Wu, Zhaohui/Chen, Huajun/Jiang, Xiaohong: *Modern Computational Approaches to Traditional Chinese Medicine.* Elsevier: London, 2012.

Yamada, Keiji: "Formation of Prototype for Chinese Medicine". *Japan Review*, 2, 1991, pp. 203–207.

Yamada, Keiji: *The Origins of Acupuncture, Moxibustion, and Decoction: The Two Phases of the Formation of Ancient Medicine: The Origins of Acupuncture and Moxibustion, The Origins of Decoction.* International Research Center for Japanese Studies: Kyoto, 1998.

Zhang, Ji/Zhao, Bai-xiao/Lao, Lixing: *Acupuncture and Moxibustion.* People's Medical Publishing House: Beijing, 2014.

Andrea-Mercedes Riegel
Translations of Chinese Medical Texts and Their Impact on the Theories and Practice of Chinese Medicine

Abstract: The alienation of modern Chinese Medicine from the original ideas may have its origin in the transmission of Chinese medical ideas via translations of classical texts in western languages. It seems that the restoration of the original Chinese Medicine requires a retranslation of all classical texts as a collaboration work between experts of different disciplines.

1 Introduction

It is a matter of fact that Chinese medical theories are often misunderstood in the Western world and even in China, the origin of medical theories and their correct application, according to the classics have fallen into oblivion due to the cleansings which took place during the Cultural Revolution. The first expert to bring translations of Chinese medical terms or acupoint names to Europe was Soulié de Morant (1878–1955).[1] His career in China and his connections to medical doctors in China are hotly debated in the Western hemisphere: Some Western experts accuse him of having introduced false theories in the West and of imposture.[2] But many of his translations were nevertheless adopted, so p.ex. the name "méridiens" for the channels and networks (*jingluo*) or "enveloppe de coeur et de sexualité"

---

1 Born in Paris and educated by the Jesuits, he had the chance to learn the Chinese language in his youth. He was sent to China when he was 23 years old in 1901. Because of his knowledge of Chinese and his "Chinese" behavior he was well accepted in the upper classes in Beijing where he worked as an interpreter. It was his own experience with Chinese acupuncture which made him curious about this art of healing. From the beginning of the 1930s until his death in 1955 he dedicated himself to Chinese acupuncture. His first book had been about Mongolian grammar but in 1934 and in 1938 he published two special works on Chinese acupuncture. In 1950 he was nominated for the Nobel Prize in medicine for his book "Real Chinese Acupuncture". See Jacquemin, Jeannine: "George Soulié de Morant, sa vie et son oeuvre d'écrivain et de Sinologue". *SRevue française d'Acuponcture 42*, 1985, pp. 9–31.
2 See p. ex. Lehmann, Hanjo: "Am Anfang war ein Scharlatan". *Deutsches Ärzteblatt* 107(30), 2010, pp. A1454–A1457.

(circulation-sexus) for the pericardium *xinbao* 心包 as well as many translations of the acupoint names.

Interest in this healing art has been constantly growing since the 1970s and several practitioners of Western medicine have published introductions to Chinese Medicine or to acupuncture. For example, in 1975 the pioneering Johannes Bischko published an introduction to Chinese acupuncture which he expanded in 1997 (Praxis der Akupunktur). In recent years some practitioners of acupuncture who learnt some Chinese have even tried to translate certain chapters of the classics in order to propagate Chinese medical ideas in the West.

As a first example we may introduce the translations of the first sentences of the *Lingshu* (8). A comparison will be made between an author who is relatively well known in Western Europe and who also is involved in training medical practitioners in acupuncture, Franz Jost, and the renowned sinologist and translator of Chinese medical texts Paul Unschuld.

Franz Jost is a Swiss medical doctor who practices in Lugano.[3] In the *Journal for Acupuncture and Auriculoacupuncture (ZAA)* 3/2012, he published a translation of the first sentences of the *Lingshu* (8). His intention was to make the theories of Chinese medicine understandable for Western medical doctors and to propagate the practice of Chinese acupuncture. Paul Unschuld on the other side has never studied Chinese medicine and has not even experienced acupuncture treatment. His intention is to translate classical medical texts in a philologically correct way. He and his assistant Tessenow translated the whole *Huangdi neijing* including the *Suwen* and the *Lingshu*; the translation of the *Lingshu* being published in 2016.

Jost chose the first sentences of the *Lingshu* (8) because of the importance of this chapter for acupuncture therapy. In his introduction he makes some revealing statements demonstrating his ideas about Chinese medical theories and their relationship to Western medicine. He states that Chinese medical theories have to fit to theories and facts in Western medicine and all depends on the correct translation. He says, "the statements in a Chinese manuscript are principally not contradictory to Western medical knowledge, if they are translated in the right way; otherwise they are not understandable."[4] And "The interpretation of an antic (sic!) Chinese text (…) must not be influenced by speculation, but follow rational laws. The text should be even comprehensive for a natural scientist."[5]

---

3   The list of his numerous publications is published on his website.
4   Jost, Franz: "Der Ursprung des Shen". *Zeitschrift für Akupunktur und Aurikulomedizin* 03, 2012, pp. 2–6.
5   Ibid., p. 2. In the end he interprets the chapter in a moral sense and thinks it is about immoral behavior and its consequences for the psyche.

There were already some mistakes and misunderstandings in Morant's publications, but experience teaches us that the new translations made by Western practitioners may be even worse if they are done without the help of at least one native speaker.[6] As these publications are widespread and the authors are well-known experts, the contents and the ideas in these works are largely accepted and may become standard teachings.

The second topic in this chapter will be the birth of a theory concerning the responsibilities of the lung. In many books on Chinese medicine we read "The lung regulates the waterways". This theory is far from being reliably classic, but it definitely influences medical practice.

2 Huangdi Neijing Lingshu (8) – An Important Chapter Misunderstood

Lingshu (8) is entitled *"Ben shen"*. It is about the *shen* (spirit) and its different manifestations in the immaterial aspects which are stored in the Yin organs such as the two souls *po* 魄 and *hun* 魂 thought *yi* 意, the will *zhi* 志, deliberation *lü* 慮 and the consequences of emotional excitement for the body and the spirit in case of alterations or excesses. The most important aspect of this chapter is the very first statement which is the idea that in the needling practice, the therapy must be based on the *shen*. The very first sentence reads "The method of needling must first be based on *shen*".[7] That is why the chapter is called *"ben shen"*. Knowing this we might translate the title as Unschuld does, "To consider the spirit as the Foundation". But right here we might also begin discussion. We may see *"ben"* as a transitive verb related to the noun *shen*. The translation might also be "to root *shen*", the root being a symbol for stability and reflecting best the symbolism of the character *ben* 本. This would also be adequate because this first sentence of *Lingshu* (8) is one of the most basic statements concerning acupuncture theory because it demonstrates that Chinese acupuncture allows and even requires the therapist's stable *shen* and its input into the therapy for a good result.[8]

---

6   One example could be C. Schnorrenberger's translation of the *Huangdi neijing Lingshu* which in large parts does not seem to be a translation of the Chinese original text, but of another text in a Western language. Schnorrenberger, Claus: *Lehrbuch der Akupunktur*. Area Verlag: Erftstadt, 2008.
7   *Lingshuyishi*. Shanghai kexuechubanshe: Shanghai, 1997, p. 75.
8   Acupuncture therapy is a subjective art of healing which not only leaves space for spirituality but is even based on it. This short statement may also be a first indication

Translations of selected sentences of Lingshu (8)
本神
Translation I[9]
To root the Shen

Explanation: *Ben* is translated as a verb, *shen* being the object. The image of the root was chosen because it best reflects the symbolism of the character *ben* 本. (see above) *Shen* could be translated with "spirit" or with "consciousness" but as it is the key notion in this chapter it was just adopted as Chinese character in the title.

Jost:
The Origin of Shen

Jost reverses the relation between the two characters. His translation would be correct if the title was *Shen zhi ben* 神之本. The idea of the whole chapter is already lost in the translation of the title.

Unschuld:
To Consider the Spirit as the Foundation[10]

黄帝问于崎伯曰:
凡刺之法，先必本于神。血，脉，营，气，精，神，此五藏之所藏也。至其淫泆离藏则精失，魂魄飞扬，志意恍乱，智虑去身者，何因而然呼?

Translation I:
Huangdi asked Qibo:
The method of needling must first be rooted in the spirit. Blood, vessels, Ying, Qi essence and *shen* they are stored in the five depots. If it comes about that by excessive [emotions] (*yinyi*) they become detached from the depots, then the essence gets lost, the [souls] *hun* and *po* are flying about, the will and thought get confused, wisdom and deliberation leave the body, what is the reason for this?

Explanation: *Yinyi* 淫泆 here means an excess of the seven emotions. In classical medical texts the character *yin* 淫 may refer to excessive climate influences which might harm the body.[11] *Yi* 泆 means "overflowing, excessive". As it is question of emotions here, the term is introduced in brackets. *Zhi* 至 as a verb means "to arrive" and as a noun it denotes an extreme, the highest level. So in this context

---

for the fact that the methods of Western medicine might not be valuable for the proof of the efficiency of acupuncture.
9   Translation I has been made by the author of this article.
10 Unschuld, Paul: *Huang Di Nei Jing Ling Shu* (*The Ancient Classic on Needle Therapy*). University of California Press: Oakland, 2016, p. 147.
11 In this sense the climatic influences are called the "*liu yin*" (六淫), the "six excessive climatic influences".

it may be seen in relation to *yinyi*, the highest level of emotional excess. *Li* 离, "to leave" or "to get detached" is an image here for the detachment from the *zang*-organs; the second sentence is not clear here, the subject being either the above mentioned substances or the "excessive emotions". The following character *zang* 藏 may be interpreted as storage or as the depots. In the following the text makes pairs, It combines the two souls *po* 魄 and *hun* 魂, *zhi* 志 and *yi* 意 and *zhi* 智 and *lü* 虑. And this is not at random but because of the interrelationship between the words forming a pair. *Po* and *hun* are the two souls of man, the body soul and the wandering soul. *Zhi*, the will is the directed intention *yi* and *zhi*, the wisdom unites experience, intuition, knowledge and deliberation.

> Jost:
> Each needling therapy must first be rooted in the natural laws. Xue (blood), mai (blood-vessels), ying (the nourishing energy), Qi (Odem), jing (the fines) and shen – these five are native in the five viscera.
> Excesses in licentiousness[12] destroy the (function of) storage and normally one loses the fines, hun and povanish quickly, the ratio and the will are confused and rebel, wisdom and deliberation leave the body. What is the reason for this? [...]

Jost translates *shen* with "the natural laws" which means the physical laws of nature; but *shen* is what makes the human being a human being,[13] it is his consciousness. Here one might ask what kind of influence the physical laws of nature may have on the needling therapy?

The five elements mentioned in this paragraph are not native in the five viscera, they are stored there. Jost interprets *yinyi* as "excesses in licentiousness" which does not seem to be the right interpretation here (see above). "Ratio" for *zhi* is a Latin expression which gives the reader the impression that this is a modern text written by a physician of the Western world. Moreover ratio does not reflect the aspects of wisdom.

> Unschuld:
> All norms of piercing [require one] top firstof all consider the spirit as the foundation. Blood, vessels, camp [qi, guard], qi, essence and spirit, they are stored in the five long-term depots. When someone leads an excessive life and [these contents] leave the long-term depots, then [this person's] essence will be lost. His hun and po will rise into the air, his

---

12 Translations to discuss are indicated in bold.
13 *Suwen* (26) states: "Qi and blood are man's shen, one must nourish them." Yang Weijie: *Huangdi neijing Suwenshijie*. Wenhuashuyegongsi: Taibei, 1990, p. 226; and *Lingshu* (54) states clearly "When blood and Qi are united, Ying and Wei-Qi have contact, the five depots are complete, *shen*-Qi dwells in the heart, *hun* and *po* are mature then the human being is accomplished." *Lingshuyishi*, p. 335.

mind and intentions will be utterly confused. His knowledge and his considerations leave his body, why is that so?[14]

In the second sentence Unschuld introduces a new subject "someone" which is not necessary. Though Unschuld explains in his annotations that *yinyi* in this case means an "excess" in the seven emotions he translates with "to lead an excessive life". As already mentioned above it is not very probable that here it should be an issue about an excessive licentious life because the chapteraddresses to medical practitioners and physicians always had high ethical standards. As for the *zang*-organs it would be adequate to call them "the depots" instead of "long-term depots". This expression suggests there are also short-term depots. The translation "knowledge" for *zhi* 智 seems an inadequate translation because emotional excesses do have an impact on the different aspects of *shen* not on the knowledge which one once acquired. Camp (qi, guard) as a translation for the nourishing energy (Ying-Qi) in man seems unconvincing because the expression is somewhat meaningless.

(歧伯答曰):
天之在我者德也，地之在我者氣也，德流氣薄而生者也。故生之来谓之精。

Translation I
Qibo answered:
What is in me of Heaven is the virtue, what is in me of Earth is the Qi. The virtue [of Heaven] flowing [down] and the Qiextending [upward] brings about new life. For this the origin of life is called *jing*.

Explanation: Here the terms *De* 德 and *Qi* 气 are of particular interest. *De* 德 here means the virtue of Heaven as it is stated in the Great Appendix: 天地之大德曰生 "The Great virtue[15] of Heaven and Earth is to create life."[16] And the sentence of *Lingshu* (8) here is an allusion to this statement.[17] From the point of view of grammar, 德流 and 氣薄 must both be noun and verb, the particle *er* 而 makes an adverbial subordination. *Sheng zhe ye* 生者也 "life begins" is the result of the action mentioned before. *De liu* and *Qi bo* being an allusion to the *Yijing*'s main idea of

---

14 Ibid.
15 In the German language we might translate *De* with "Wirkkraft".
16 *Zhouyizhezhong*. Jiuzhouchubanshe: Beijing, 2003, p. 912.
17 In the *Zhuangzi* we find similar statements concerning the virtue of Heaven. In the chapter *Tiande* (Heaven and Earth) we find the statement "The capacity of things to create new life this is called virtue". Chan Guying: *Zhuangzi jinzhujinshi*. Taiwan shang-wuyinshu guan: Taibei, 1992, p. 341. The *Zhuangzi Tiandao* states: "To understand the virtue of Heaven and Earth this means that the extraordinary great ancestors were in harmony with Heaven." Ibid., p. 374.

the creation of new life by Heaven and Earth in permanent communication – and man and woman on the human level – the expression may be seen as an image: Heaven's virtue flowing downward and the Qi of Earth extending upward; the two may unite and bring about new life. The virtue of Heaven in man is his procreativeness; the Qi of Earth may be interpreted as the vital and metabolic force of man and the ability to bear new life; this is because according to the Great Appendix, the Earth completes the things by change (*hua* 化).

> Jost:
> Qibo answers:
> What is in me (*in man*) from Heaven is the elementary force de 德 (*Yin and Yang*). What is in me from the Earth is the odem 氣 Qi. The elementary force of nature flows to the scarce Qi and develops it. For this one calls what comes into existence and comes about the fines 精 Jing (*life*).

Jost interprets Qi here as ovum and sperm[18] and *De* 德, virtue, as the "natural laws" of Yin and Yang. He interprets *De* in a moral sense when he explains: "The elementary forces of the cosmos make man virtuous"; that means Yin and Yang make man's character straight.[19] Jost does not see that *bo* must be a verb here, so he has to introduce another verb for the sentence. He chose the verb "to develop". And the object is "the scarce Qi" which would be *bo* Qi 薄气. He completely ignores the fact that the character *sheng* 生 means "to bring about new life" and it is the main subject of the Great Appendix. It has nothing to do with "development". The main problem here seems to be the fact that Jost does not know the meaning of the particle *er* 而.

> Unschuld:
> Heaven manifests itself in me as virtue.
> The earth manifests itself in me as qi.
> When the virtue flows and the qi have joined, life begins.
> The fact is:
> The origin of life is called essence.[20]

Unschuld interprets the *De* of Heaven in the right way, referring to the *Zhuangzi*-chapter *Tiandao*. But it may be a source of misinterpretation in a moral sense when he says "Heaven manifests itself within me as virtue".

---

18 Jost, p. 3.
19 Ibid. He also sees *De* as a medical term when he complains that in a newly published nomenclature he didn't find the term *De*.
20 Unschuld, p. 148.

In the following sentence he translates *gu* 故 which indicates a reason with "The fact is" and by this he demonstrates that he did not understand the text. The origin of life necessarily is called "essence" being the result of the union of the essences of father and mother.

兩精相搏謂之神。
隨神往來者謂之魂;
並精而出入者謂之魄;
所以任物者謂之心;

Translation I
When the two essences [of male and female] unite this is called *shen*.
What goes to and fro following the *shen* is called *hun*,
What leaves and enters [the body] by being united with the essence is called *po*;
So what is responsible for the [human] affairs is called the heart.

Explanation: Here we find the next allusion to the Great Appendix in the statement *liang jing xiang bo* 兩精相搏, "the two essences seize one another"[21] The Great Appendix states: *nan nü gou jing* (…) 男女搆精, "man and woman unite their essences".[22]

Bing 并 is often used as an emphasizing particle or in the sense of "together with, joint"; but here it should be a verb because of the parallel construction of the two sentences concerning the *po* and *hun* soul and the particle *er* 而 which normally requires that the character preceding and the character following the particle *er* 而 be a verb.

Jost:
The elementary force of nature De and the odem Qi which both together are pulsing as fines are called *shen* 神[…].
Respectively, when *shen* comes and goes this is called the spiritual soul.
What unites with the fines during coming and going this is called *po*.
For this what is responsible for the fines is called the heart.

Jost overlooks the allusion to the Great Appendix. Unfortunately ignoring grammar he even denies that *liang* "two" might refer to "*jing*" because in his opinion "there is only one *jing*".[23] As an act of desperation he interprets *liang* as referring to Heaven and Earth and tries to make a sentence which seems somewhat plausible. It is the same problem for the next sentence: he ignores that *sui* 隨 here may be a verb and translates according to his knowledge: the *hun*-soul is

---

21 This means they unite.
22 *Zhouyizhezhong*, p. 932.
23 Jost, p. 5; here he makes his own idea into the standard for the translation.

the wandering soul. It is not clear why he translates *hun* with "spiritual soul" whereas he does not translate *po*. As he doesn't know the particle *er* 而 as a particle which makes an adverbial subordination, his translation remains far away from the original text. In the last sentence he interprets *wu* 物 as a synonym to *jing* 精. The basis for this might be the idea that the heart stores the *shen* and here it is question about the relation between essence and *shen*.

> Unschuld:
> The fact is:
> The origin of life is called essence.
> When two essences clash that is called spirit.
> That which comes and goes following the spirit is called the *hun* soul.
> That which enters and leaves together with the essence, that is called *po* soul.
> That which is responsible for all affairs, that is called the heart.

Unschuld also ignores the allusion to the *Yijing*, translating *liang jing xiang bo* with "two essences clash". It is not question of the clashing of two – indifferent – essences but of the unification of the essences of Heaven and Earth or father and mother. The introduction of the article "the" would have made the meaning somewhat clearer. For *sui* 随 and *bing* 并 he offers a solution which also preserves the parallel construction of the two sentences.

> (…)
> (故智者之养生也)
> 必顺四时而适寒暑,
> 和喜怒而安居处
> 节阴阳而调刚柔。
> 如是则僻邪不至, 长生久视。

> Translation I
> So as for the [method of] nourishing the life of the wise men,
> They had to live according tothe four seasons, to adapt themselves to cold and heat, to live in peace by harmonizing the emotions of joy and anger and to regulate hard and soft by balancing Yin and Yang. By this the pathogens [of climate] could not reach [the body] and one could enjoy a long life.

Explanation: The last two parts of the first sentence are constructed in a parallel way, *he* 和 (to harmonize) and *jie* 节 (to restrain) being the corresponding verbs. Yang and Yin and the hard *gang* 刚 and the soft *rou* 柔 seem to be synonymous as well as *jie* 节 and *tiao* 调. On the other hand the balance between hard and soft may be seen as the result of the restrain of Yin and Yang whereas the concrete meaning of Yin and Yang in this context is not very clear. The Hard and the Soft are manifestations of Yang and Yin and in the text here there may even be an allusion to the older commentaries of the *Yijing*, where there is not yet question about Yin and Yang.

As for *pi xie* 僻邪 one may interpret the two characters as single characters or as a compound. *Xie* 邪 may just refer to harmful influences, to pathogens like excessive climatic factors. In this sense it is the counterpart to the *zheng* Qi 正气, the "straight Qi", the defense strength. *Pi* 僻 may mean "low, mean". Read as single characters *pi* 僻 is the attribute to *xie* 邪, the two characters meaning "the mean pathogens". As a compound *xiepi* 邪僻 means "depraved, mean" and the compound *pixie* 辟邪 (pi 辟 written without the radical *ren* 人) means "to ward off evil influences" and it also denotes a fabled animal with two horns placed at the grave of feudal princes in order to prevent evil influences from penetrating it.[24]

Changsheng jiushi 长生久视 "to enjoy a long life" is a citation of the *Laozi* (59) and makes clear the Daoist background of these statements. It may be divided into two separate parts, *chang sheng* and *jiu shi*, "a long life" and "long vision" or be interpreted as an entity, the second part *jiu shi* in this case just being a synonym for a long life.[25]

> Jost:
> Surely one has to live according to the four seasons and to adapt to cold and heat.
> Joy, anger and peace live together.
> Under certain circumstances Yang and Yin change from hard to soft.
> If one lives like this the decadency seldom becomes the standard in the organism.
> And one may look forward to a continuous development of life.[26]

Here Jost makes three sentences out of one. And once more he ignores the meaning of the particle *er* 而. He interprets *pi* as "depraved" and once more he insists on his idea that it was a question about the moral decay of man here. In the last sentence he overlooks the allusion to the *Laozi*.

> Unschuld:
> The fact is:
> When those who are knowledgeable nourish their life, the following is for sure:
> They act in accordance with the four seasons and adapt themselves to cold and summer heat.
> They harmonize joy and anger, and they maintain calmness in their home.

---

24 See also *Zhongwendacidian*. Zhongguowenhuadaxuechubanbu: Taibei, 1982, vol. 8, p. 1787.
25 The *Laozi* (59) says, "*Chang sheng jiushizhidao* 长生久视之道". Ren Farong: *Daodejingshiyi*. Santaichubanshe: Xian, 1988, p. 137.
26 Jost, p. 6. Jost omits the first part of the sentence.

They are moderate in regard to [making use of] their yin and yang [qi] and they seek to find a balance between hard and soft.
This way they keep the evil away from them. They achieve longevity, and their vision lasts long.[27]

Unschuld interprets *bi* 必 as "a matter of fact". In the following sentences the particle *er* 而 is translated with "and" which is legitimate. The introduction of the word *qi* in respect to Yin and Yang does not clarify the meaning of Yin and Yang here.

The subject in the last sentence may be seen in the evils *xie* 邪; they cannot reach and penetrate the body of the wise men. Unschuld prefers to preserve the subject of the sentences above, which is "the wise". This decision doesn't alter the sense of the statement.

These few sentences may demonstrate that practitioners with little knowledge of the Chinese language and Chinese culture may ignore the Chinese original text. Stickingto their own ideas they may easily be tempted to translate a classical text in the seemingly most plausible sense. By these practices, the culture of Chinese medicine gets more and more lost and misunderstandings are transported and spread all over the Western hemisphere.

Unschuld on the other side is a translator who is rich in knowledge of the classical Chinese language but who never studied Chinese Medicine. On the one hand he tends to translate the Chinese text literally, sticking closely to the Chinese characters. On the other hand he tends to make clear statements where the Chinese original remains ambiguous by introducing elements[28] in sentences according to his understanding. This might in some cases be helpful for the reader's understanding but this method bears the danger of making mistakes by makinga wrong decision. Sometimes preserving ambiguity helps to avoid misunderstandings more than making a clear decision. Unfortunately Unschuld ignores – just as Jost does – the fundamental role of the *Yijing* and especially of the Great Appendix for medical theories and so he overlooks allusions to this work in the classical medical texts which sometimes may result in incomprehensible translations.

3 The Lung and Its Responsibilities

Another example of the transmission of misunderstandings due to translation problems is the idea that the lung "regulates the waterways". In many Western

---

27 Unschuld, p. 149.
28 Subjects, objects, verbs or even half-sentences.

textbooks[29] about Chinese medicine one finds the statement "the lung regulates the waterways."

What are the responsibilities of the lung according to the Chinese classics?

First the lung covers all the other organs, it is closely related to the heart and it is the organ which directly establishes man's contact to the cosmos by absorbing the cosmic Qi (*kong* Qi 空气). It is the first minister of the heart and together with the heart its Qi sends the blood into the periphery. As for the trigrams, the lung is associated with Qian 乾, which represents the Heaven and metal and in the body also the head.[30]

The graph *fei* 肺 is composed of the radical *rou* 肉 (flesh) and *shi* 市 (the marketplace). *Shi* 市, which also might be read *po*, is synonym to *bu* 布, to distribute, and to disperse widely and broadly.[31] From the point of view of its outer appearance this character may be seen as a symbol for the anatomic appearance of the lung in lobes and for its function of dispersing the Qi in the body. An important statement concerning the lung's position in the organism may be found in *Suwen* (8), which states: "肺者，　相傅之官，　治节出焉." "The lung is the organ of the prime minister, administration and rhythm[32] start here".[33] The heart is the ruler organ (*jun zhu* 君主), the lung is its prime minister.

> *Suwen* (5) gives a brief summary of the correspondences of the lung. It states:
> The west brings about dryness,
> Dryness brings about metal,
> Metal brings about the hot taste,
> The hot taste brings about the lung,

---

29 See p. ex. the books by the authors Focks, P. Deadman, Nigel Wiseman and others. (See below).

30 As for characteristics, the trigram Qian and consequently the human character which is associated with Qian metal is bestowed with vitality, creativity, and leading qualities; he is a brilliant strategist but stubbornness and inflexibility are also part of his characteristics. Reactions may be violent though he is quite self-controlled. If the metal character cannot overcome mourning, he loses love of life and the contact to his environment. His skin is of alabaster color, his head is small, and his body slightly stocky.

31 For further information see also Frühauf. Frühauf gives an exhaustive explanation of the character *fei* 肺 on his homepage. See http://Classicalchinesemedicine.org.

32 *Zhi* 治 and *jie* 节 are translated as nouns here according to the parallel sentence which preceded the statement. Here it is question about the heart as the origin of *shenming* 神明 which may be interpreted as "spirit and intelligence". *Zhi* may moreover denote treatment, the correction or regulation of a disharmony in the organism; and *jie* also denotes a division of time and as a verb it may mean "to restrain".

33 *Suwen* (8); Yang Weijie, p. 76.

> The lung brings about the hairs,
> The hairs [metal] bring about kidney [water],
> The lung regulates the nose.
> In the heavenly influences it is dryness,
> On Earth it is metal,
> In the body it is the hairs,
> Among the inner organs it is the lung
> Among the colors it is white
> Among the music sounds it is shang
> Among the tones of voice it is drying
> Its counterflow brings about cough,
> In the orifices it is the nose,
> In the tastes it is hot
> Among the emotions it is mourning.
> Mourning impairs the lung,
> Joy overcomes mourning,
> The heat impairs the hairs,
> The Cold overcomes the heat,
> The hot impairs the hairs,
> The bitter taste overcomes the hot taste.[34]

Here we see the correspondences of the lung according to the system of the Five Phases and the relations between the lung and the kidney or the lung and the heart.

In the body there is a close relationship between the lung and the kidney. *Suwen* (61) states,

> "Why is the kidney responsible for water? (…) The kidney is highest Yin, the highest Yin is abundant Water. The lung is Taiyin, Shaoyin is the vessel of the winter. For this the root [of water] is in the kidneys, the end is in the lungs. They both store water."[35]

Both organs cooperate in the regulation of water metabolism. The kidney is responsible for *Qihua* (气化), the vaporizing of water. It sends vapor to the lung in order to moisten it, but for this work it needs the Qi of the lung; it has to absorb it (*na* Qi 纳气) because the lung is the "root of the Qi." Wang Tao (670–755) demonstrates this relationship in a metaphorical way. He states,

> The lung is the cover of the five viscera. When there is warm Qi below, it vaporizes upward and moistens the lung; when there is extreme cold below the Yang-Qi cannot rise upward, for this the lung dries up and becomes hot[…]

---

34 Yang Weijie, p. 52.
35 Yang Weijie, p. 449.

In a pot there is water and one heats it with fire. When one has covered the pot the hot vapor unfolds upward and the cover may be moistened. When the force of the fire lacks, water vapor does not rise upward and the cover cannot be moistened. The force of fire are strong loins and strong kidney Qi. Normally they have to take over the task of warming the Qi. The "vapor" is just the Qi of nutrition. When the Qi of nutrition is heated, then it nourishes the upper part and it is metabolized below. By this dryness and thirst can be avoided.[…][36]

The lung is a Qi-organ and together with the spleen it regulates the transport of Qi and fluids in the body. Both organs are also responsible for the immune system or – in terms of Chinese medicine – the *Zheng* Qi (straight Qi) and the *Wei* Qi (defense Qi) which flows between the skin and the muscles, and is the first blockage for pathogen factors. Nowhere in the classics is there a question about the waterways in relation to the lung; but in the Western literature we often find the statement, "The lung regulates the waterways". In his *Manual of Acupuncture*, Deadman even includes the therapeutic significance of the idea that the lung regulates the waterways. He states,

> […] treating oedema and obstructed urination when this is caused by impairment of the Lung's function of regulating the water passages and controlling disseminating and descending.[37]

He identifies the waterways in particular as ureter and urethra including the bladder and the lymph vessels. In the "Leitfaden Traditionelle Chinesische Medizin" by Focks and Hillenbrand, we also find the statement the lung "regulates the waterways"[38] and the authors' explanation is that the impure fluid particles of the body fluids are sent to the kidney by the lung and discharged via the bladder.

Even in Nigel Wiseman's translation *Fundamentals of Chinese Medicine* we find the statement "The lung ensures regular flow through the waterways".[39] As we may suggest that his translation was correct, this sentence must already be found in the original Chinese text which was a Taiwanese textbook.[40]

---

36 Wang Tao: *Waitai miyao*. Renmin weishengchubanshe: Beijing, 1987, p. 317.
37 Deadman, Peter: *Manual of Acupuncture*. University of California Press: Berkeley, 2006, p. 75.
38 Claudia Focks/Hillenbrand, Norman: *Leitfaden Traditionelle Chinesische Medizin*. Elsevier: München, 1997, p. 32.
39 Wiseman, Nigel: *Fundamentals of Chinese Medicine*. Southern Materials Center Inc.: Taibei, 1986, p. 71.
40 The original textbook is entitled *Zhongyixuejichu*.

3.1 Suwen (21) – Does the Lung Regulate the Waterways?

How could the idea of the lung regulating the waterways come into existence? The base for this theory can be found in the *Suwen* (21). We read:

飲入于胃，游溢精气上输于脾，脾气散精，上归于肺，通调水道，下输膀胱，水精四佈，五经併行。[...]⁴¹

Translation I:
The beverages enter the stomach, the floating abundant essence-Qi is transported upward to the spleen, the spleen Qi dissipates the essence, upward [it] returns to the lung, mixes up in the waterways and is transported downward to the bladder; [as long as] the fluid essence spreads in all directions the channels of the five viscera are in good accordance.
Unschuld:
Beverages enter the stomach.
Overflowing essence qi
Is transported to the spleen.
The spleen qi spreads the essence,
Which turns upward to the lung.
[The latter] frees and regulates the paths of the water,
It transports [the water] downward to the urinary bladder.⁴²

In this text it is a question about the distribution of the fluid essences from the stomach upward to the lung and downward to the bladder. The second part of the sentence is not quite clear. Is there a change of subject or not? Is it the lung which makes an "allover adjustment" *tong tiao* of the waterways and sends the essence down to the bladder?

Unschuld, referring to Wang Bing's comment,⁴³ introduces a change of subject for the second part of the sentence, making the lung the subject of this second part and interpreting the "lung regulates the paths of water". This interpretation seems plausible, of course, because of the lung's function of sending Qi downward to the periphery and to the kidney and its participation in the regulation of the water metabolism.

Seen from the point of view of the construction of the sentence, a change of subject (the subject I being the essence-Qi) in the second part of the sentence is not very probable for three reasons:

---

41 Yang Weijie, p. 189.
42 Unschuld, Paul: *Huang Di Nei Jing Su Wen*. University Press Group Ltd: Dhaka, 2011, pp. 375–376.
43 Ibid. p. 376.

1. In the first part of the sentence, the change of subject is indicated and the new subject – the spleen – is mentioned.
2. "*Tong*" 通 means "through" or, as a verb, "to pass through" or "to communicate". "*Tiao*" 调 may mean "to adjust, harmonize" but also "to mix up".
3. "To regulate" in the sense of the responsibility for something, we would expect the character *zhu* 主 instead of the two characters *tong tiao* 通调.

Nevertheless both interpretations are possible, but the introduction of the lung as a new subject produces a clarity which is not given in the original text.

In order to get more clarity here we may have a look at what the medical classics tell us about the waterways.

3.2 What Are the Waterways?

In the *Huangdi neijing* there is a question about the waterways in various chapters of the *Suwen* and the *Lingshu*. *Lingshu* (81) compares the waterways in the body to the waterways in nature such as rivers, channels, streams, etc. They may overflow or dry out when nature is out of balance. In the body we might find *shuidao* 水道 represented in the vessels transporting fluids like blood, Ying Qi and Wei Qi. In case of stagnation or obstruction in general these fluids do not flow and cause all kinds of swellings.[44] *Lingshu* (63) focuses on the tracts conducting the urine, i.e. ureter and urethra and even including the bladder. It states,

> When [the sour taste] resides in the stomach the inner of the stomach is harmonized and warm, the wrapper of the bladder being thin and weak shrinks when absorbing the sour taste. When there is an impairment and no passage the waterways do not flow, for this there is anuria.[45]

Where do the *shuidao* have their origin?

Lingshu (12) establishes a connection between the Huai river and the channel of the small intestine: "Hand-Taiyang [in nature] unites with the Huai waters, in the interior it pertains to the small intestine. The water ways start from here."[46]

But the main role is attributed to the Triple Burner. So *Suwen* (8) states, "The Triple Burner is the organ for drainage, the waterways start from here."[47]

And *Lingshu* (2) makes clear the role of the Triple Burner for the waterways and the regulation:

---

44 See *Lingshuyishi*, p. 620.
45 *Lingshuyishi*, p. 372.
46 *Lingshuyishi*, p. 133.
47 Yang Weijie, p. 78.

The kidney unites with the bladder, the bladder is the palace of the body fluids (*jinye*). The shaoyang channel [of the Triple Burner] pertains to the kidney, the kidney connects with the lung in the upper [burner], for this, it may direct the two organs [Triple Burner and the bladder]. The Triple Burner is the palace of the middle drains, the waterways start from here; it pertains to the bladder, it is a solely palace-organ, and it is part of the six palace-organs.[48]

The origin of the waterways is the Triple Burner, the organ which is responsible for the Triple Burner and the bladder is the kidney. The kidney is responsible for the regular flow of the waterways as *Suwen* (76) states,

> When [the pulse] is superficial but taut this means the kidney[Qi] is insufficient; if it is deep but like a stone it means that the kidney[Qi] is stagnating. When kidney[Qi] doesn't flow then the waterways don't flow; [if so the patient] gets afraid and short of breath and the Qi of his body scatters about.[49]

These statements make clear that the kidney is the main organ responsible for the waterways, i.e. the regular flow of all fluids in the body.

Water *shui* 水 may be interpreted as all the fluids which "moisten" the body. It may be water in the shape of urine, the body fluids *jinye*, the essence at least the fluid parts of it and the "heavenly water" *tiangui* as well as blood. As for the waterways, they pass through the skin, the muscles and the inner organs and they transport the fluids up and down in the body. In Western medicine we may see an anatomic correlation in the lymphatic vessels which are closely connected with the blood vessels, the blood vessels and the nerves, the peripherical nerves where the neurotransmitters flow from the periphery to the central nervous system or vice versa, and the spinal cord where the nerve fibers run up and down. The waterways also contain the ureter and urethra. The kidney's responsibility for the waterways may be seen in its responsibility for the water metabolism and in the fact that the kidney, in the sense of Chinese Medicine, is responsible for the neuroendocrine system.[50]

---

48 *Lingshuyishi*, p. 28.
49 Yang Weijie, p. 676.
50 For this theory see Riegel, Andrea: *Die Niereshen. Konzepte der klassischen chinesischen Medizin im Lichte der modernen Schulmedizin*. Bacopa: Schiedberg, 2010.

4 The Lung Regulates the Waterways: Consequences for the Therapy

Accepting the idea that the lung regulates the waterways or not may have far-reaching consequences for treatment.

Deadman and Focks state that edema or obstructed urination might be a result of a weak lung Qi. Though they do not make concrete proposals for acupuncture treatment, one can imagine the way:

One way could be to choose points of the lung channel like Taiyuan (Lu 9) as the *yuan*-point – which is also the earth point– of the lung channel or the *ben*-point of the lung channel, the metal point which is Jingqu (Lu 8).

The second way could be to apply the rule of mother and son. The lung is weak so one has to strengthen the metal's mother which is the earth, in the organ it is the spleen. Here one would choose the *yuan*-point of the spleen channel Taibai (Sp 3) which is also the earth point, or the metal point of the spleen channel which is Shangqiu (Sp 5).

Some therapists might also use points of the channel which is in the inner-outer relation with the lung, the large intestine. Here the *yuan*-point Hegu (LI 4) or the *luo*-point Pianli (LI 6) may seem useful. Of course one also may choose special points for drainage like the Shuifen (Ren 5) or Shuidao (St 28).

If one accepts the kidney and the Triple Burner as the regulators of the waterways, one would choose another way and prefer different points:

> points which do have edema in the scope of their indications like Yinlingquan (Sp 9) and Shuifen (Ren 5),
> points for drainage like Zusanli (St 36) or Shuidao (St 28) which has the "waterways" in its name.

Very important are points of the kidney channel or those which are effective for strengthening the kidney like Taixi (Ki 3), Guanyuan (Ren 4), Shenshu (Bl 23) or the Qi cleft point (*xi*-point) of the kidney channel which is Shuiquan (Ki 5). We also have to think of the *shu*-point of the Triple Burner which is Sanjiaoshu (Bl 22) or the *he*-point of the Triple Burner of the lower extremities which is Weiyang (Bl 39).[51] We get completely different acupuncture recipes depending on the theory which we accept. It would be the same for herbal treatment. In the first case, there is stress on the lung function; in the second case, herbs for strengthening the kidney will be the rulers in the recipe.

---

51 These are only special points the acupuncture recipe as a whole must be based on the disharmony pattern of the patient.

5 Conclusion

As was demonstrated, there are many misunderstandings of Chinese medical theories, not only in the Western world, due to mistakes in translations. The first expert who introduced misunderstandings of Chinese Medicine into the Western world was Soulié de Morant. Though Soulié de Morant's terminology is hotly debated, basically all of the terms he used have been adopted.

In the Western world, the difficulties of translating classical Chinese texts are often underestimated. Knowledge of classical Chinese grammar is indispensable for translation and one has to be aware of the fact that each classical text is full of allusions to works of classic philosophy in order to demonstrate the author's erudition. Medical texts are no exception. Here the Great Appendix is a main text of reference.

Experts with little knowledge of classical Chinese language who learnt Chinese medicine in Western organizations often just make their knowledge the standard for their translations. And another way for the dissemination of mistakes and misunderstandings is translations of old medical texts which are made from one Western language to another. The misunderstandings might even begin in Chinese Medicine's motherland for it might be the case that native speakers do not have sufficient command of the classical Chinese language.

There is no unalterable Chinese medicine. It is a living system which absorbs the predominant philosophies of each epoch. As there are no definite standards in the terminology of Chinese medical texts, one has to be even more careful in translation. This means a Latin translation of the Chinese medical terms does not help in the understanding of Chinese medicine because it is biunique and definite. And the teachings of doctrines which were adopted somewhere must necessarily be the wrong way in formation. To explore the "roots" and the characteristics of Chinese Medicine, one would have to carry out a retranslation without any prejudices of all the old original works. This requires close cooperation between experts in classical Chinese language, experts in Chinese medical practice and experts who are versed in Chinese cultural history.

References

Chan, Guying: *Zhuangzi jinzhujinshi*. Taiwan shangwuyinshu guan: Taibei, 1992, p. 341.

Chen, Guying: *Zhuang zijinzhu jinshi*. (Annotations and modern translation of the Zhuangzi). Taiwan shangwu yinshuguan goufen youxian gongsi: Taibei, 1975.

Deadman, Peter: *Manual of Acupuncture*. University of California Press: Berkeley, 2006.

Focks, Claudia/Hillenbrand, Norman: *Leitfaden Traditionelle Chinesische Medizin.* Elsevier: München, 1997.

Guangdi, Li: *Zhouyi zhezhong.* (The Analysis of the Book of Changes). Jiuzhou chubanshe: Beijing, 2003.

Jacquemin, Jeannine: "George Soulié de Morant, sa vie et son oeuvre d'écrivain et de Sinologue", *Revue française d'Acuponcture 42 Juin* 1985, pp. 9–31.

Jost, Franz: "Der Ursprung des Shen", *Zeitschrift für Akupunktur und Aurikulomedizin* (3), 2012, pp. 2–6.

Lehmann, Hanjo: "Am Anfang war ein Scharlatan". *Deutsches Ärzteblatt* 107(30) 2010, pp. A1454–A1457.

(*Huangdi neijing*) *Lingshu yishi* (The annotated and translated edition of the Holy Pivot of the Classic of Internal Medicine of the Yellow Emperor). Shanghai kexue jishu chubanshe: Shanghai, 1997.

Ren, Farong: *Daode jing shiyi* (Explanations of Dao De Jing). Santai chubanshe: Xian, 1988.

Riegel, Andrea-Mercedes: *Die Niere shen. Konzepte der klassischen chinesischen Medizin im Lichte der modernen Schulmedizin.* Bacopa: Schiedberg, 2010.

Schnorrenberger, Claus: *Lehrbuch der Akupunktur.* Area: Erftstadt, 2007.

Soulié de Morant, George: *Précis de la Vraie Acuponcture.* Mercure de France: Paris, 1934.

Unschuld, Paul: *Huang Di Nei Jing Ling Shu.* (The Ancient Classic on Needle Therapy) University of California Press: Oakland, 2016.

Unschuld, Paul/Tessenow, Herrmann: *Huang Di Nei Jing Su Wen.* (Annotated translation of Huang Di's Inner Classic Basic Questions). University Press Group Ltd.: West Sussex, 2011.

Wan, Quan: *Wan Mizhai yixue quanshu* (The Complete Works of Wan Mizhai). Zhongguo zhongyiyao chubanshe: Beijing, 1996 (orig. 1580).

Wang, Tao: *Waitai miyao* (The Medical Secrets of a Censor). Renmin weisheng chubanshe: Beijing, 1987 (orig. 752).

Wilder, George Durand/Ingram, James Henry: *Analysis of Chinese Characters.* Dover Publications Inc.: New York, 1974 (orig. 1922).

Wiseman, Nigel: *Fundamentals of Chinese Medicine.* Southern Materials Center Inc.: Taibei, 1986.

Yang, Weijie. *Huangdi neijing Suwen Shijie.* (Modern annotated translation of the Simple Questions of the Classic of Inner Medicine of the Yellow Emperor). Wenhua shuye gongsi: Taibei, 1990.

Zhongwen dacidian. (The Encyclopedic Dictionary of the Chinese Language). Zhongguo wenhua daxue chubanbu: Taibei, 1982.

Lixing Lao and Mingxiao Yang

Difficulties and Challenges Clinical Acupuncture Trials Are Facing

Abstract: This paper retrospectively analyzed the challenges presented in the choice of control, as well as patient and practitioner blinding. It also proposed several useful resolutions and recommendations to guide future clinical studies.

1 Introduction

In the domain of medical research, not all roads lead to Rome. Sometimes, there is only one optimal access to the goal. This is particularly true to the methods used in the attesting efficacy of medical intervention. Randomized controlled trial (RCT) has been considered the 'gold standard' of medicine for fulfilling such mission for many years[1]. It was introduced in clinical medicine when streptomycin was evaluated in the treatment of tuberculosis[2]. Now it is ranked together with systematic review and meta-analysis at the top of the hierarchy of evidence in the framework of evidence-based medicine (EBM)[3,4].

Clearly, its significance in acupuncture was not envisioned by early researchers and clinicians, so many early stage clinical studies in acupuncture were observational studies[5]. After EBM gained unprecedented welcome by mainstream medicine, researchers start to realize that most previous clinical studies of acupuncture were associated with methodological issues, including lack of randomization, inappropriate inclusion/exclusion criteria, lack of adequate treatment, no credible

---

1 Bothwell L E, Greene J A, Podolsky S H, et al. Assessing the Gold Standard—Lessons from the History of RCTs [J]. *New England Journal of Medicine*, 2016, 374(22): 2175–81.
2 Marshall G, Blacklock J, Cameron C, et al. Streptomycin Treatment of Pulmonary Tuberculosis: A Medical Research Council investigation [J]. *BMJ*, 1948, 2(4582): 769–82.
3 Concato J, Shah N, Horwitz R I. Randomized, Controlled Trials, Observational Studies, and the Hierarchy of Research Designs [J]. *New England Journal of Medicine*, 2000, 342(25): 1887–92.
4 Petticrew M, Roberts H. Evidence, Hierarchies, and Typologies: Horses for Courses [J]. *Journal of Epidemiology and Community Health*, 2003, 57(7): 527–9.
5 Linde K, Scholz M, Melchart D, et al. Should Systematic Reviews Include Non-Randomized and Uncontrolled Studies? The Case of Acupuncture for Chronic Headache [J]. *Journal of Clinical Epidemiology*, 2002, 55(1): 77–85.

controls, lack of patients blinding, and inappropriate endpoint[6]. Therefore, it is difficult to generate reliable evidence to support the use of acupuncture. The astringent situation was not changed until the 1997 NIH consensus conference of acupuncture, which stressed the importance of RCTs in acupuncture clinical research and granted many clinical trials to support its development[7]. Therefore, the following years saw a dramatic increase of published clinical trials since 1997 (Figure 1).

Fig. 1: Count of clinical acupuncture trials published since 1970.

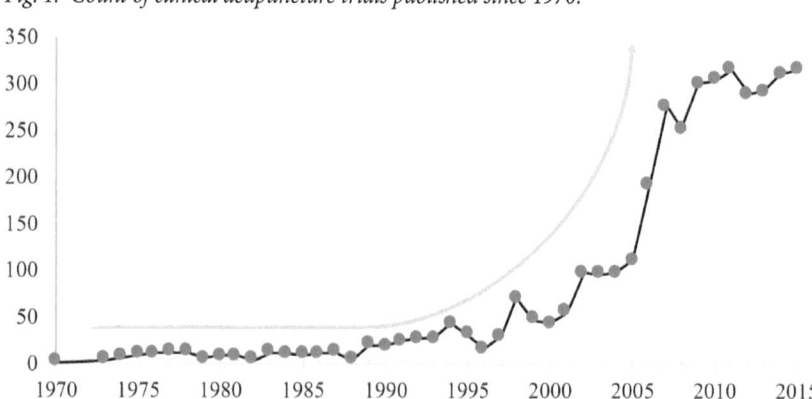

Note: *This figure showed that more clinical trials of acupuncture have been published since 1970, arriving at its peak in 2015. The primary data was obtained from PubMed. It used 'acupuncture' (MeSH) as the key word to search the PubMed database and the number of published clinical trials were obtained after adding a filter to get all clinical trials. The vertical axis indicates the number of publications; the transverse axis indicates the year.*

Although those trials clearly testified the effect of acupuncture, they also unanticipatedly brought many serious methodological considerations to the stakeholders of acupuncture. One of the significant issues is that, stakeholders constantly perceived inconsistency among results of different trials, leading to heated debates on

---

6   Ernst E, White A R. A Review of Problems in Clinical Acupuncture Research [J]. The *American Journal of Chinese Medicine*, 1997, 25(01): 3–11.
7   NIH Consensus Conference. Acupuncture [J]. *JAMA*, 1998, 280(17): 1518–24.

the effect of acupuncture[8,9]. It greatly hindered clinical decision-making process and consequently impeded its employment. Those issues also represent ubiquitous difficulties and challenges in current clinical acupuncture trials. Therefore, the suitability of using traditional RCTs in acupuncture research is questioned. Questions that has been commonly asked include: Is the classical RCT methods truly applicable to acupuncture therapy? Is it responsible to the inconsistency observed now? In order to address these questions, this part first made a direct comparison of the characteristics between Western Medicine (WM) and Chinese Medicine (CM) in which acupuncture is practiced based on its theory.

2 Is the Traditional RCT Applicable to Acupuncture?

Before the comparison, one must understand that those two medicines are built on the basis of two completely different logic systems (Table 1). WM targets at a specific disease, while CM aims to balance syndromes; Diagnosis in WM is often based on laboratory findings with specific diagnostic criteria while CM is based on four-diagnostic approaches such as observation, hearing and smelling, inquiring, and palpating to determine individualized condition; therefore, the WM emphasizes standardized treatment protocol while CM often offers individualized treatment based on individual patient condition.

Tab. 1: West meets the East–Western ruler and eastern distances

Western Medicine	Traditional Chinese Medicine
Disease Specificity	Differentiation (Syndrome)
Laboratory indications	Four diagnostic approach
Standard criteria	Individualized conditions
Standard treatment	Individualized treatment

Above comparison gives a direct impression that many discrepancies exist between the WM and CM logic systems. RCT was originally developed by WM to assess the effect of medications. It is a clinical research approach, which is devised

---

8   Roberts J R, Moore D. *Mapping the Evidence Base and Use of Acupuncture Within the NHS [M]*. University of Birmingham, Department of Public Health and Epidemiology, West Midlands Health Technology Assessment Collaboration, 2006.
9   Kim S-Y, Lee H, Chae Y, et al. A Systematic Review of Cost-Effectiveness Analyses Alongside Randomised Controlled Trials of Acupuncture [J]. *Acupuncture in Medicine*, 2012, 30(4): 273–85.

to compare an intervention (experimental arm) with a counterpart (control arm) in treating patients who have been randomized to different study groups, for assessing efficacy. Overall, drugs are designed with explicit bioactive chemical components. To assess efficacy, nonrelated factors in clinical practice can be ruled out by randomization in a RCT. Moreover, in order to peel off the psychological effect of a pharmacological agent, RCT under the umbrella of EBM is designed with an inactive and indistinguishable counterpart, known as a placebo control, such as sugar pills or starch pills. Moreover, a series of stringent procedures including allocation concealment, blinding, treatment and quality control, which are crucial to maintain the internal validity and external validity of the trial, are required to such studies.

However, acupuncture treatment is a procedure that is fundamentally different to modern drugs which are chemical compounds. Acupuncture as a monotherapy involves no pharmacological substances. It is a natural remedy that relies on motivating the innate healing ability of human body. According to traditional theories, *Qi* (vital energy) constituted by *Yin* and *Yang* is essential to life. The equilibrium between *Yin* and *Yang* is the premise to the healthy state of human body. When this equilibrium is interrupted, a disease would occur. Acupuncture designates its aim as to restore the balance of *Yin* and *Yang*, through puncturing acupuncture points/meridians in which *Qi* is circulating all over the body. As a consequence, in clinical practice it is necessary for a practitioner to carefully inquire, examine and diagnose a patient's condition, which includes many details of disease and patient's lifestyle. By using the information collected, a personalized traditional Chinese medicine (TCM) diagnosis can be made by acupuncturist, which is known as TCM syndrome differentiation. Based on the diagnosis, individualized treatment can be delivered accordingly to the patient.

Therefore, RCT may be applied in acupuncture trial to control several problems. For example, symptom improvement caused by environmental factors, temporal and spatial factors can be controlled through randomization. But one size doesn't fit all. Many problems inherited from the uniqueness of acupuncture is still hardly controlled by RCT (Table 2). Due to this, a great challenge in designing a variable control, blinding strategy and other aspects are faced with clinical acupuncture research. The challenges will be further discussed in next sections.

Tab. 2: Uniqueness of TCM and challenges posed to RCT and EBM

Unique aspect of TCM	Challenge to evaluation by conventional EBM
TCM diagnosis based on practitioner's subjective assessment of patient's state of disharmony, unlike technologically driven WM diagnosis	Eligibility requires consistent diagnosis, traditionally based on WM diagnostic criteria
Individualized treatment based on TCM syndrome; treatment may vary by patient or by visit	Traditional RCTs involve treatment standardized to WM diagnosis
CM involves complex array of treatments including (e.g., acupuncture, herbs, Tai Chi, etc...)	Traditional RCTs evaluate an isolated component (e.g. single drug), controlling for all non-specific effects

3 Major Challenges Presented to the Clinical Acupuncture

The control arm of a RCT is designed to eliminate the nonspecific components associated with an intervention. The paralleled arms should be identical in all aspects in order to control for any possible non-specific effects except for the treatment. A classical RCT is frequently equipped with a placebo control, which is a physically inert arm such as "a placebo control" in a drug trial, so that the true effect of the interventional arm won't get impaired during the comparison[10]. However, as mentioned in the above paper, a few well-design clinical trials stated that acupuncture is ineffective, even though numerous trials reported the effectiveness of acupuncture for a variety of diseases. By analyzing the studies with negative results, it is clear that experimental group always showed significant improvement after treatment as compared with baseline; however, such improvement was also observed in control group. This explains why in those trials the effect of verum acupuncture was not detected when compared with sham acupuncture. Because the controls used by those studies were not inert; they were with significant clinical effect, which represents a serious challenge facing clinical acupuncture trials. Therefore, many factors in acupuncture procedure needed to be controlled and different controls are used for different purposes. Currently, there are mainly four

---

10 White P, Lewith G, Hopwood V, et al. The Placebo Needle, is it a Valid and Convincing Placebo for use in Acupuncture Trials? A Randomised, Single-Blind, Cross-Over Pilot Trial [J]. *Pain*, 2003, 106(3): 401–9.

general types of control arms that are commonly used in RCTs of acupuncture[11]. Each form of control method has its own pros and cons (Table 3).

Tab. 3: Controls used in current RCTs of acupuncture

Type	Aim	Pros	Cons
Waitlist	To test if acupuncture is better than no treatment by controlling disease natural remission	Low resource input and easy to conduct	Unable to blind patients; Unable to address the efficacy of acupuncture
Non-insertion sham acupuncture	To test if acupuncture is more than a placebo	Can blind acupuncture-naïve patients; Effect associated with needle insertion can be minimized	Not physiologically inert; Not suitable for long-term use; Unable to address acupoint specificity
Insertion sham acupuncture	To test if acupuncture has specific effect by controlling the non-specific components	Patients can be fully blinded; Resembles real acupuncture	Not physiologically inert; Underestimates effect of acupuncture
Positive treatment/ usual care	To test if acupuncture in everyday practice is generally comparable to conventional treatment	All patients get immediate treatment; Able to determine the effectiveness and cost-effectiveness of acupuncture	Unable to blind patients; Unable to assess the efficacy of acupuncture

First of all, natural remission of disease is common to every disease. **Waitlist** is used to answer the question as 'Does acupuncture work?'. Patient in the waiting list commonly received no treatment at all during the study cycle. Therefore, in most cases, free acupuncture treatments were provided to patients at the completion of trial as a compensation for their participation of the study, so the waitlist group is also referred as delayed treatment group[12]. Moreover, for ethical considerations, it is commonly used for chronic diseases with no conventional treatment. Waitlist is not able to help address the efficacy or effectiveness of acupuncture, because it cannot blind patients or clinical researcher.

---

11 Vickers A J. Placebo Controls in Randomized Trials of Acupuncture [J]. *Evaluation & the Health Professions*, 2002, 25(4): 421–35.
12 Zhao L, Chen J, Li Y, et al. The Long-Term Effect of Acupuncture for Migraine Prophylaxis: A Randomized Clinical Trial [J]. *JAMA Internal Medicine*, 2017, 177(4): 508–15.

Psychological effects known as placebo and nocebo that are commonly associated with clinical trials need to be controlled in a RCT. Patients' beliefs and value systems, or researcher's preferences toward a specific arm could all lead to inappropriate justification of the intervention examined[13]. In most cases, if a patient was fully aware of the group allocation and he/she by any chance has been allocated to the preferable group, then they could easily report improved outcomes than those who has not been[14,15]. This is known as the 'placebo' effect. On the other hand, patient who has been assigned to a group they don't like may generate resentful emotions toward the treatment they received and hence often report worsened outcomes, which is the so-called 'nocebo' effect[16]. For clinicians, they may also have their own preference toward an intervention. Those who favor the experimental arm may choose to improve their clinical performance and thus lead to better outcomes.

To avoid such prejudices or bias, both patients and researchers are required to be strictly blinded to the allocation of patients[17]. Therefore, it is very important for a control arm to resemble the experimental arm no matter in shape, in flavor, or in other aspects, in order to realize double blinding (patient and clinical researchers). In such cases, patient can generate same amount of expectations when they were fully blinded and physicians perform similar treatment. However, considering the uniqueness of acupuncture, it is very challengeable to blind acupuncture practitioner as he or she is the one who performs the treatment procedure[18,19].

---

13 Witt C M, Liu J, Robinson N. Combining' Omics and Comparative Effectiveness Research: Evidence-Based Clinical Research Decision-Making for Chinese Medicine [J]. *Science*, 2015, 346(6216 Suppl): S10–S2.
14 Mahomed N N, Liang M H, Cook E F, et al. The Importance of Patient Expectations in Predicting Functional Outcomes After Total Joint Arthroplasty [J]. *Journal of Rheumatology*, 2002, 29(6): 1273–9.
15 Kalauokalani D, Cherkin D C, Sherman K J, et al. Lessons from a Trial of Acupuncture and Massage for Low Back Pain: Patient Expectations and Treatment Effects [J]. *Spine*, 2001, 26(13): 1418–24.
16 Torgerson D J, Sibbald B. Understanding Controlled Trials. What is a Patient Preference Trial? [J]. *BMJ*, 1998, 316(7128): 360.
17 Kaptchuk T J. The Double-Blind, Randomized, Placebo-Controlled Trial: Gold Standard or Golden Calf? [J]. *Journal of Clinical Epidemiology*, 2001, 54(6): 541–9.
18 Hammerschlag R. Methodological and Ethical Issues in Clinical Trials of Acupuncture [J]. *The Journal of Alternative and Complementary Medicine*, 1998, 4(2): 159–71.
19 White A, Filshie J, Cummings T. Clinical Trials of Acupuncture: Consensus Recommendations for Optimal Treatment, Sham Controls and Blinding [J]. *Complementary Therapies in Medicine*, 2001, 9(4): 237–45.

Ideally, patients should be blinded. But in what way can acupuncture be simulated to blind patient?

Non-insertion sham acupuncture is designed to mimic every procedure of acupuncture treatment except for the needle insertion. Clinical trials had applied nails, toothpicks, taped needles[20], and sham needle devices such as the Streitberger sham needle[21], the Park Sham Device[22], and the latest Takakura double-blind placebo needle[23], to prick the skin but without cutaneous penetrations. This type of control can be used to mask the placebo/nocebo effect. Therefore, it can be applied to answer the question 'Is acupuncture a placebo?'. However, it is not suitable for long-term use or patient with acupuncture experience. Because the study found that long-term use of such control may lead to incomplete blinding[24]. As to the double-blind placebo needles, there are also debates that the double-blinding is not satisfactory[25]. Another major drawback of this measure is that it cannot be used to address the specificity of acupuncture effect.

However, what are the nonspecific components that need to be controlled in an acupuncture trial? The Society of Acupuncture Research (SAR) proposed that the actions of acupuncture are generated by three major effect factors, including the needling components (specific), nonspecific components, and specific non-needling components[26] (Table 4). If the specificity of acupuncture effect is

---

20 Berman B M, Lao L, Langenberg P, et al. Effectiveness of Acupuncture as Adjunctive Therapy in Osteoarthritis of the Knee: A Randomized, Controlled Trial [J]. *Annals of Internal Medicine*, 2004, 141(12): 901–10.

21 Streitberger K, Kleinhenz J. Introducing a Placebo Needle into Acupuncture Research [J]. *The Lancet*, 1998, 352(9125): 364–5.

22 Park J, White A, Stevinson C, et al. Validating a New Non-Penetrating Sham Acupuncture Device: Two Randomised Controlled Trials [J]. *Acupuncture in Medicine*, 2002, 20(4): 168–74.

23 Takakura N, Yajima H. A Double-Blind Placebo Needle for Acupuncture Research [J]. *BMC Complementary and Alternative Medicine*, 2007, 7(1): 31.

24 White P, Lewith G, Hopwood V, et al. The Placebo Needle, is it a Valid and Convincing Placebo for use in Acupuncture Trials? A Randomised, Single-Blind, Cross-Over Pilot Trial [J]. *Pain*, 2003, 106(3): 401–9.

25 Vase L, Baram S, Takakura N, et al. Can Acupuncture Treatment be Double-Blinded? An Evaluation of Double-Blind Acupuncture Treatment of Postoperative Pain [J]. *PloS One*, 2015, 10(3): e0119612.

26 Langevin H M, Wayne P M, Macpherson H, et al. Paradoxes in Acupuncture Research: Strategies for Moving Forward [J]. *Evidence-Based Complementary and Alternative Medicine*, 2011, 2011(11).

Difficulties and Challenges Clinical Acupuncture Trials Are Facing   111

addressed, needling components must be retained in verum acupuncture; while, all the rest factors of acupuncture should be controlled by a sham control.

Tab. 4: *Components of the therapeutic effect of acupuncture*

Components	Corresponding procedures of acupuncture
Needling Components	Location, insertion depth, manipulation, needle texture, needle indices (length, diameter), needle number
Specific Non-Needling Components	*Psychological*: History, education, diagnosis *Physiological*: Palpation
Nonspecific Components	Patient beliefs and value system, expectation, credibility, time, reputation

Invasive sham acupuncture is commonly used in studies to address the question – 'is acupuncture a non-specific stimulation?' – because it was designed to resemble every nonspecific component and specific non-needling components of verum acupuncture[27,28]. However, this form of sham control has lately been disputed for incapable of being a valid control because it is not totally physiologically inactive[29]. It is argued that minimal acupuncture still triggers afferent nerves in the skin and consequently result in a 'limbic touch response' that is associated with salient functional connectivity changes in the brain. Therefore, this sham procedure that is meant to be inert may, in fact, still activate the C-fiber and consequently results in the alleviation of the affective components of pain[30]. Moreover, insertion sham acupuncture may also cause a non-specific diffuse noxious inhibitory control (DINC) effect, which also may alleviate pain and underestimate the clinical

---

27   Ma T, Yu S, Li Y, et al. Randomised Clinical Trial: An Assessment of Acupuncture on Specific Meridian or Specific Acupoint vs. Sham Acupuncture for Treating Functional Dyspepsia [J]. *Alimentary Pharmacology & Therapeutics*, 2012, 35(5): 552–61.
28   Zhao L, Chen J, Liu C-Z, et al. A Review of Acupoint Specificity Research in China: Status quo and Prospects [J]. *Evidence-Based Complementary and Alternative Medicine*, 2012, 2012: 1–16.
29   Lund I, Näslund J, Lundeberg T. Minimal Acupuncture is not a Valid Placebo Control in Randomised Controlled Trials of Acupuncture: A Physiologist's Perspective [J]. *Chinese Medicine*, 2009, 4(1): 1.
30   Lund I, Lundeberg T. Are Minimal, Superficial or Sham Acupuncture Procedures Acceptable as Inert Placebo Controls? [J]. *Acupuncture in Medicine*, 2006, 24(1): 13–5.

benefits of acupuncture[31,32]. An individual patient data meta-analysis-based study examined the influence of different controls on the effect size detected in clinical trials of acupuncture for chronic pain. It showed that in trials using penetrating acupuncture as sham control the effect size was smaller as compared with those using non-penetrating sham controls (difference in effect size: −0.45 (95% C.I. −0.78, −0.12; $p = 0.007$)[33]. Therefore, trials designed with an invasive sham control should have a large sample size if it aimed to reveal the specificity of acupuncture effect.

Those controls are designed to assess the efficacy of acupuncture which represents the genuine effect of acupuncture. But how 'large' on earth is the size of effect? In other words, how large is the 'real-world' effectiveness of acupuncture? For instance, most painkillers can be used to ease 70%–80% pain. Since acupuncture is also effective for pain management, is it superior to painkillers? In current trials, *Positive treatment/usual care* is applied in studies to address such question. Conventional medications and routine care are commonly used as positive controls by those trials. This type of RCTs are open-labeled because the differences between paralleled arms are too obvious to blind the patients or physician. Due to such reasons, this type of control group cannot be used to exclude the placebo effect of acupuncture. It can provide information about the general effectiveness of acupuncture, which is also of great significance to clinical decision making. For example, a pragmatic trial by AJ Vickers et al. compared acupuncture with usual care in daily use for treating chronic headache and found that acupuncture offers persistent and clinically relevant benefits for primary care patients. Based on the results of this study, the authors recommended acupuncture to the National Health Service (NHS) of UK[34].

4 Useful Resolutions and Recommendations

Based on the previous arguments, it is of great significance for future trials to be equipped with a valid control which is able to maximize the effect of acupuncture.

---

31 Zhang X, Ning Z, Chen H, et al. A Systematic Review of Acupuncture for Treating Osteoarthritis of the Knee: Results and Relationship with Control Design [J]. *Chinese Journal of Pain Medicine*, 2015, 10: 732–7.
32 Paterson C, Dieppe P. Characteristic and Incidental (Placebo) Effects in Complex Interventions such as Acupuncture [J]. *BMJ*, 2005, 330(7501): 1202–5.
33 Macpherson H, Vertosick E, Lewith G, et al. Influence of Control Group on Effect Size in Trials of Acupuncture for Chronic Pain: A Secondary Analysis of an Individual Patient Data Meta-Analysis [J]. *PLOS One*, 2014, 9(4): e93739.
34 Vickers A J, Rees R W, Zollman C E, et al. Acupuncture for Chronic Headache in Primary Care: Large, Pragmatic, Randomised Trial [J]. *BMJ*, 2004, 328(7442): 744.

Here, a 'step-by-step' approach is recommended for consideration when choosing a control for RCTs of acupuncture in future:

1. *Waitlist*: If a targeted disease was not commonly managed by acupuncture and the researchers hesitated about their interventional protocol, a pilot RCT using a waitlist control is recommended. Researchers may design and implement a large trial if the test results were positive. Statistically, a clinical outcome improvement over 50% is considered positive. Otherwise, the results will not be solid enough when challenged by a sham control. On the other hand, if acupuncture has been reported to be effective for the targeted disease, it is suggested that researchers should formulate an optimal treatment protocol through literature review and data mining.
2. *Non-insertion sham acupuncture*: With the preliminary results of waitlist-controlled trial, sample size estimation can be performed for a larger clinical trial with non-insertion sham acupuncture control. In this trial, many current sham acupuncture strategies as aforementioned can be employed, including toothpicks, taped needle, Streitberger needle, Park Sham Device (PSD), etc. Specifically, a taped needle is a noticeable non-insertion sham control which is initially reported in a study by Prof. Berman and Prof. Lao. This type of control can minimize the physiological response induced by acupuncture insertion; Moreover, it is a reliable dummy that mimics every procedure of acupuncture treatment except for needle insertion, and consequently capable of blinding patients. However, a small-scaled pilot study to validate the successfulness of this type of control would be recommended.
3. *Insertion sham acupuncture*: This type of control is recommended for non-painful diseases, or disease that is hard to implement blinding. Especially, for certain non-painful diseases, a significant statistical difference can also be exhibited by using insertion sham acupuncture. However, it is recommended with one condition for such disorders, that is positive preliminary results of a pilot study.
4. *Positive treatment/usual care*: If the trial focuses on the effectiveness instead of efficacy of acupuncture, then trial is recommended to be designed with a positive control/usual care, usually first-line medication or conventional therapy. This type of design is known as a pragmatic study, which generates clinical evidence close to 'real-world' practice. Therefore, pragmatic trials aim to better inform clinical decision-making, positive treatment/usual care can be used.

In addition, insulation of acupuncturist and allocation concealment to all other researchers should be strictly carried out in order to increase the blinding rate, as well as maximally secure the validity of RCTs. The insulation of acupuncturists can be achieved by standardizing their communications with the subjects/patients and also instructing independent researchers who do not know the treatment assignment to perform outcome assessment. Moreover, clinical training is recommended for physicians in order to quality control the standardized treatment procedure of acupuncture.

5 Conclusions

Preparing and conducting clinical acupuncture trials are always faced with serious challenges due to the uniqueness of acupuncture therapy. Rigorous scientific research methodology which preserves the essence of TCM practice should be employed. This paper further provides a useful 'step-by-step' approach to resolve the challenges for future clinical studies of acupuncture and maximize TCM effectiveness within the scope of rigorous Western scientific research.

References

Berman B M, Lao L, Langenberg P, et al. Effectiveness of Acupuncture as Adjunctive Therapy in Osteoarthritis of the Knee: A Randomized, Controlled Trial [J]. *Annals of Internal Medicine*, 2004, 141(12): 901–10.

Bothwell L E, Greene J A, Podolsky S H, et al. Assessing the Gold Standard—Lessons from the History of RCTs [J]. *New England Journal of Medicine*, 2016, 374(22): 2175–81.

Concato J, Shah N, Horwitz R I. Randomized, Controlled Trials, Observational Studies, and the Hierarchy of Research Designs [J]. *New England Journal of Medicine*, 2000, 342(25): 1887–92.

Ernst E, White A R. A Review of Problems in Clinical Acupuncture Research [J]. *The American Journal of Chinese Medicine*, 1997, 25(01): 3–11.

Hammerschlag R. Methodological and Ethical Issues in Clinical Trials of Acupuncture [J]. *The Journal of Alternative and Complementary Medicine*, 1998, 4(2): 159–71.

Kalauokalani D, Cherkin D C, Sherman K J, et al. Lessons from a Trial of Acupuncture and Massage for Low Back Pain: Patient Expectations and Treatment Effects [J]. *Spine*, 2001, 26(13): 1418–24.

Kaptchuk T J. The Double-Blind, Randomized, Placebo-Controlled Trial: Gold Standard or Golden Calf? [J]. *Journal of Clinical Epidemiology*, 2001, 54(6): 541–9.

Kim S-Y, Lee H, Chae Y, et al. A Systematic Review of Cost-Effectiveness Analyses Alongside Randomised Controlled Trials of Acupuncture [J]. *Acupuncture in Medicine*, 2012, 30(4): 273–85.

Langevin H M, Wayne P M, Macpherson H, et al. Paradoxes in Acupuncture Research: Strategies for Moving Forward [J]. *Evidence-Based Complementary and Alternative Medicine*, 2011, 2011: 1–11.

Linde K, Scholz M, Melchart D, et al. Should Systematic Reviews Include Non-Randomized and Uncontrolled Studies? The Case of Acupuncture for Chronic Headache [J]. *Journal of Clinical Epidemiology*, 2002, 55(1): 77–85.

Lund I, Lundeberg T. Are Minimal, Superficial or Sham Acupuncture Procedures Acceptable as Inert Placebo Controls? [J]. *Acupuncture in Medicine*, 2006, 24(1): 13–5.

Lund I, Näslund J, Lundeberg T. Minimal Acupuncture is not a Valid Placebo Control in Randomised Controlled Trials of Acupuncture: A Physiologist's Perspective [J]. *Chinese Medicine*, 2009, 4(1): 1.

Ma T, Yu S, Li Y, et al. Randomised Clinical Trial: An Assessment of Acupuncture on Specific Meridian or Specific Acupoint vs. Sham Acupuncture for Treating Functional Dyspepsia [J]. *Alimentary Pharmacology & Therapeutics*, 2012, 35(5): 552–61.

Macpherson H, Vertosick E, Lewith G, et al. Influence of Control Group on Effect Size in Trials of Acupuncture for Chronic Pain: A Secondary Analysis of an Individual Patient Data Meta-Analysis [J]. *PLOS One*, 2014, 9(4): e93739.

Mahomed N N, Liang M H, Cook E F, et al. The Importance of Patient Expectations in Predicting Functional Outcomes After Total Joint Arthroplasty [J]. *The Journal of Rheumatology*, 2002, 29(6): 1273–9.

Marshall G, Blacklock J, Cameron C, et al. Streptomycin Treatment of Pulmonary Tuberculosis: A Medical Research Council Investigation [J]. *BMJ*, 1948, 2(4582): 769–82.

NIH Consensus Conference. Acupuncture [J]. *JAMA*, 1998, 280(17): 1518–24.

Park J, White A, Stevinson C, et al. Validating a New Non-Penetrating Sham Acupuncture Device: Two Randomised Controlled Trials [J]. *Acupuncture in Medicine*, 2002, 20(4): 168–74.

Paterson C, Dieppe P. Characteristic and Incidental (Placebo) Effects in Complex Interventions Such as Acupuncture [J]. *BMJ*, 2005, 330(7501): 1202–5.

Petticrew M, Roberts H. Evidence, Hierarchies, and Typologies: Horses for Courses [J]. *Journal of Epidemiology and Community Health*, 2003, 57(7): 527–9.

Roberts J R, Moore D. *Mapping the Evidence Base and Use of Acupuncture Within the NHS [M]*. University of Birmingham, Department of Public Health and Epidemiology, West Midlands Health Technology Assessment Collaboration, Edgbaston, Birmingham, 2006.

Streitberger K, Kleinhenz J. Introducing a Placebo Needle into Acupuncture Research [J]. *The Lancet*, 1998, 352(9125): 364–5.

Torgerson D J, Sibbald B. Understanding Controlled Trials. What is a Patient Preference Trial? [J]. *BMJ*, 1998, 316(7128): 360.

Takakura N, Yajima H. A Double-Blind Placebo Needle for Acupuncture Research [J]. *BMC Complementary and Alternative Medicine*, 2007, 7(1): 31.

Vase L, Baram S, Takakura N, et al. Can Acupuncture Treatment be Double-Blinded? An Evaluation of Double-Blind Acupuncture Treatment of Postoperative Pain [J]. *PloS One*, 2015, 10(3): e0119612.

Vickers A J. Placebo Controls in Randomized Trials of Acupuncture [J]. *Evaluation & the Health Professions*, 2002, 25(4): 421–35.

Vickers A J, Rees R W, Zollman C E, et al. Acupuncture for Chronic Headache in Primary Care: Large, Pragmatic, Randomised Trial [J]. *BMJ*, 2004, 328(7442): 744.

White A, Filshie J, Cummings T. Clinical Trials of Acupuncture: Consensus Recommendations for Optimal Treatment, Sham Controls and Blinding [J]. *Complementary Therapies in Medicine*, 2001, 9(4): 237–45.

White P, Lewith G, Hopwood V, et al. The Placebo Needle, is it a Valid and Convincing Placebo for Use in Acupuncture Trials? A Randomised, Single-Blind, Cross-Over Pilot Trial [J]. *Pain*, 2003, 106(3): 401–9.

Witt C M, Liu J, Robinson N. Combining' Omics and Comparative Effectiveness Research: Evidence-based Clinical Research Decision-Making for Chinese Medicine [J]. *Science*, 2015, 346(6216 Suppl): S10–S2.

Zhang X, Ning Z, Chen H, et al. A Systematic Review of Acupuncture for Treating Osteoarthritis of the Knee: Results and Relationship with Control Design [J]. *Chinese Journal of Pain Medicine*, 2015, 10: 732–7.

Zhao L, Chen J, Li Y, et al. The Long-Term Effect of Acupuncture for Migraine Prophylaxis: A Randomized Clinical Trial [J]. *JAMA Internal Medicine*, 2017, 177(4): 508–15.

Zhao L, Chen J, Liu C-Z, et al. A Review of Acupoint Specificity Research in China: Status quo and Prospects [J]. *Evidence-Based Complementary and Alternative Medicine*, 2012, 2012: 1–16.

Fengli Lan

Women's Health: Fundamentals, Lifestyles and Acupuncture Approach

Abstract: The paper advances "the Axis of Brain – *Du* – Kidneys – *Tian Gui* – *Chong* & *Ren* – Uterus" as women's reproductive axis based on the interpretation of classical texts; elucidates vital significance of Yang Qi for women's health; investigates lifestyles which influence women's health; and discusses acupuncture treatment for women's diseases.

Women's health not only depends on their health in a gynecological sense, but more refers to their overall health condition which depends highly on their gynecological conditions. It is quite common that some diseases in women come and go or rise and fall in accordance with their menstrual cycles, e.g. premenstrual syndrome (PMS), migraine, acnes, or emerge during a specific period of women's life, e.g. postpartum depression, tinnitus, hypertension, cardiovascular diseases, sleep disorders, osteoporosis during or after the menopause. Thus, it is necessary to take women's health under consideration of women's specific physiology.

1 Fundamentals

1.1 *Huang Di Nei Jing Su Wen:* 7-Year Cycles and Beyond

"Discourse on the True [Qi Endowed by] Heaven in High Antiquity," the first chapter of *Huang Di Nei Jing Su Wen*, reads that

> In a female, at the age of seven, the Qi of the kidneys becomes abundant. The [first] teeth are replaced by [permanent ones] and the hair grows.
> At the age of two sevens (fourteen), the *Tian Gui* arrives, the Ren vessel is passable and the great Chong vessel abounds [with qi], the periods come regularly, and hence [she] may have children.
> At the age of three sevens (twenty one), the Qi of the kidneys has reached its normal level, and hence, the wisdom teeth emerge and [she] grows to her full size.
> At the age of four sevens (twenty eight), the sinews and bones are firm, the hair has grown to its full extent, and the body and the limbs are in a state of abundance and strength.
> At the age of five sevens (thirty five), the Yang-Ming vessels [begin to] weaken, the face begins to dry out, and the hair begins to fall off.
> At the age of six sevens (forty two), the three Yang vessels weaken [in the upper sections]. The face is all parched, the hair begins to turn white.
> At the age of seven sevens (forty nine), the *Ren* vessel is empty, the great *Chong* vessel is depleted, the *Tian Gui* is exhausted. The way of the earth is impassable. Hence, the physical appearance is spoilt and [she can] no [longer] have children.

女子七歲，腎氣盛，齒更髮長；二七，而天癸至，任脉通，太衝脉盛，月事以時下，故有子；三七，腎氣平均，故真牙生而長極；四七，筋骨堅，髮長極，身體盛壯；五七，陽明脉衰，面始焦，髮始墮；六七，三陽脉衰於上，面皆焦，髮始白；七七，任脉虛，太衝脉衰少，天癸竭，地道不通，故形壞而無子也。

The above passage describes a female's life based on 7-year cycles and the function of Kidney Qi, *Tian Gui*, Ren and Chong vessels on the uterus along with a female's development, maturation, reproduction, and aging process. *Tian Gui* exists on both female and male, becomes mature along with the abundance of the Qi in the kidneys, and functions to promote the development, maturation, and reproduction.

1.2 The Axis of Brain – *Du* – Kidneys – *Tian Gui* – *Chong* & *Re* – Uterus

"Three branching from one origin 一源三岐" indicates that the three vessels, Ren, Du, and Chong vessels all originate from the uterus in women, while from testes in men. The Ren and Du vessels also converge at perineum. Among them, Du vessel joins the interior of the spine, "ascending along the spinal column and homing to the kidneys," reaches the vertex, enters and homes to the brain and also meets the Kidney Meridian on Changqiang (GV1); while Chong vessel "joins the Shao Yin meridian of the foot.[1]" That "the brain is the sea of marrow," "the kidneys govern bone and engender marrow," and "all of the marrow homes to the brain" indicates that the Kidney Meridian has a direct physiological relationship with the brain. Besides, the kidneys govern birth, development, maturation, and reproduction, Ren vessel governs uterus and conception, and uterine collaterals connect to the kidneys. It is thus clear that the kidneys have an exceedingly close relationship with the uterus. Therefore, under the co-regulation of Ren, Du, and Chong vessels, there forms the menstrual physiological system, namely

Du   Ren
Brain → Kidneys → *Tian Gui* → Uterus → Menstruation,
Chong

which can be simplified and formulated as the Axis of Brain – Du – Kidneys – *Tian Gui* – Chong & Ren – Uterus.

---

1 Chapter 60 *Acupoints along Skeletal Indentations* of *Huang Di Nei Jing Su Wen*.

As Li Shizhen[2] said "the brain is the house of the original spirit," it is thus clear that the brain has a function of regulating and controlling tissues and organs of the whole body, including uterus, thus playing an important role in menstrual physiology.

In Western medicine, women's physiology is understood by the axis of Center – Hypothalamus – Hypophysis – Ovaries – Uterus, which can be associated with the Axis of Brain – Du – Kidneys – *Tian Gui* – Chong & Ren – Uterus in Chinese medicine. Thereby, the four phases of the menstrual cycle in both medical systems come to a common understanding: Endometrium-shedding – Follicular – Ovulation – Luteal phases in Western medicine and Menstrual – Postmenstrual – Intermenstrual – Premenstrual phases in Chinese medicine.

2 The Prime Importance of Yang Qi for Health Promotion

2.1 What Is Yang Qi?

In Chinese medicine, Yin refers to the physical body, and Yang refers to the energy of the body. If without energy transformed by Yang Qi, the body will be a dead body. The life is a process of Yang Qi declining. That's what "Comprehensive Discourse on Phenomena Corresponding to Yin and Yang," the Chapter 5 of *Huang Di Nei Jing Su Wen* states "Yang transforms into Qi, and Yin forms the physique 陽化气，陰成形."

Yang Qi, the opposite of Yin Qi, is the original power of the metabolism and all the physical activities, determines the growth, development, maturation, reproduction, and aging, and functions to warm the body and keep the viscera and all the other parts of the body working. If Yang Qi is deficient, the physiological activities will weaken and decline, and the body's ability of resisting cold lowers as well, and of course the being will be ill. If Yang Qi is depleted, the being will die.

Yang Qi comes from two sources, one is inherited from parents, and the other is transformed from the essence part of the food. All the activities, including the normal functioning of the body, work, sports, sex, emotional changes, adaptation to the temperature changes, trauma repair, etc. all consume Yang Qi.

---

2 Li Shizhen (李时珍, 1518–1593), one of the greatest naturalist, pharmacologists, and physicians in the world history, authored *Ben Cao Gang Mu* (本草纲目, "Compendium of Materia Medica"). *Ben Cao Gang Mu* and *Huang Di Nei Jing*, the two ancient classics from the field of Chinese medicine, were listed in the Memory of the World Programme by United Nations Educational, Scientific and Cultural Organization (UNESCO) in 2011.

Yang Qi is the root of life. Deficiency of Yang Qi manifests directly in a lower basic body temperature, a slower speed of flow of Qi and blood, reduced metabolism, accumulation and stagnation of pathological products like phlegm, fluids, blood stasis, stones, etc. and external pathogens like wind, cold, dampness, etc., finally resulting in occurrence of diseases. If Yang Qi is slightly deficient and the body still functions normally, people may feel cold in their extremities, gain weight, have lumbar pain, etc. If the deficiency of Yang Qi goes on, the flow of Qi and blood further stagnates, severe diseases like tumors, cirrhosis, may arise.

Moving is to cultivate Yang; Rest is to cultivate Yin. Wu Guozhong 武国忠 advances three ways to raise Yang Qi, i.e., mild exercises, being good (in wording, looking, and doing), and being happy.[3]

2.2 The Prime Importance of Yang Qi for Health Promotion

Yang Qi is of prime importance for the health of all the human beings. When a human being is ill, the body is just like a gloomy, cold, and damp weather, which needs the Yang qi, the sun of the being, to disperse it.

"Discourse on how the Generative Qi Communicates with Heaven," the chapter 3 of *Huang Di Nei Jing Su Wen* states that

> The Yang Qi [in the human being[4]] is just like the sun in the heaven. If [the sun in the heaven] loses its location, all things cannot exist; if the Yang Qi in the human being loses its location, the being cannot grow and will die early. The movements of the heaven require the normal shining of the sun; [accordingly] the Yang [qi] of the human being follows [the sun] and rises to protect the exterior [of the body].
>
> 陽氣者，若天與日，失其所，則折壽而不彰。故天運當以日光明，是故陽因而上衛外者也。

"Comprehensive Discourse on Phenomena Corresponding to Yin and Yang," the Chapter 5 of *Huang Di Nei Jing Su Wen* starts with

> Yin and Yang are the Way of heaven and earth, the fundamental principles [governing] the myriad beings, father and mother to all changes and transformations, the basis and beginning of generating life and killing, and the palace of spirit brilliance. To treat diseases, one must search for the basis.
>
> 陰陽者，天地之道也，萬物之綱紀，變化之父母，生殺之本始，神明之府也。治病必求於本。

---

3 Wu, Guozhong. *A Manual of Huang Di Nei Jing*. Shanghai: Jinxiu Wenzhang Press. 2009.

4 I use "being" instead of "body" to stress that the object in Chinese medicine is the "live being" which is composed of body and mind.

Zhang Jingyue 张景岳 (1563–1640) gave a note to "the basis and beginning of generating life and killing 生殺之本始:"
The way of generating life and killing is no more than Yin and Yang. The coming of Yang generates life, the going of Yang leads to death.

生殺之道，陰陽而已。陽来則物生，陽去則物死。

Dou Cai 窦材 (1127–1279), a famous physician of the Song Dynasty (960–1279), laid stress on the importance of supporting Yang for promoting health. The chapter of "Method of Living a Long Life" of his book entitled *Bian Que Xin Shu* 扁鹊心书 or *Bian Que's Precious Heart Book* records a famous story:

> Wang Chao 王超, an infantryman of the general Lui Wu 刘武 of the Shaoxing period (1131–1162) of the Southern Song Dynasty, was born in Taiyuan.[5] Later on he became a robber. He met an extraordinary person who taught him a method of how to live a long life. He then became very energetic with a rosy complexion and a well rounded out physique when he was ninety years old. In the year of XINMAO 辛卯 (1171), he deeply hurt many families in Yueyang[6] since he raped ten girls a day but still did not feel tired. Later on he was captured and [was sentenced to death]. A supervisor asked him before the execution, "You have an extraordinary method [of keeping healthy], don't you?" He answered, "Nothing special, just the power of fire. To apply 1,000 cones of moxibustion on Guanyuan (CV4) in every transition period from Summer to Autumn. Gradually I don't fear cold or summer heat anymore, nor feel hungry even without eating anything for some days. Up till today there is a mass under my umbilicus like the warmth of fire. Haven't you heard of making soil into brick, wood into charcoal, and brick and charcoal being not rotten for a thousand years, should all be contributed to the power of fire." After the execution, the supervisor asked the executioner to dissect the warmth spot of his lower abdomen, and got a mass which was not flesh nor bone, but congealed like a stone, i.e. the result from the moxibustion fire.

紹興間劉武軍中步卒王超者，本太原人，後入重湖為盜，曾遇異人，授以黃白住世之法，年至九十，精彩腴潤。辛卯年間，岳陽民家，多受其害，能日淫十女不衰。後被擒，臨刑，監官問曰：汝有異術，信乎？曰：無也，唯火力耳。每夏秋之交，即灼關元千炷，久久不畏寒暑，累日不饑。至今臍下一塊，如火之暖。豈不聞土成磚，木成炭，千年不朽，皆火之力也。死後，刑官令剖其腹之暖處，得一塊非肉非骨，凝然如石，即艾火之效耳。

In this story, applying moxibustion on Guanyuan (CV4) is recorded as a very secret, effective method to live a long and healthy life. Later on in the same chapter, he mentioned three methods to prolong lifespan: the first is moxibustion, the second is medicinal pills [made as a Taoist practice], and the third is Fuzi (Radix Aconiti Carmichaeli, 附子).

---

5 Taiyuan is now the capital city of Shanxi Province.
6 Yueyang is a big city of Hunan.

2.3 Inspirations of the School of Fire Spirit

Zheng Qinan 郑钦安 (1824–1911), a famous physician of Sichuan province of the late Qing Dynasty (1644–1911), developed a school named "School of Fire Spirit," also known as "School of Supporting Yang," which emphases the importance of Yang Qi and is good at using large dosages of hot herbs, especially Fuzi (Radix Aconiti Carmichaeli, 附子), Dried Ginger, Cinnamon, etc., to treat serious and stubborn diseases.

This school takes identification of Yin-Yang as the principle of pattern identification, which has been clinically proved to be reliable and practical. Many chronic diseases like prostatitis, diabetes, hypertension, tumors, and blood diseases (which are usually identified as pattern of damp-heat, excess heat, or deficient heat due to yin deficiency) are identified by this school as "Yang Deficiency and Yin Excess," and are treated by the method of "Supporting Yang" with reliable therapeutic effects. Tang Buqi 唐步祺 (1917–2004), another famous physician of this school, said that "My dozens of years of clinical experiences show that modified *Si Ni Tang* 四逆汤 or Frigid Extremities Decoction[7] achieves frequently satisfactory effects in treating all diseases due to Yang Deficiency, including nephritis, hepatitis, pulmonitis, myocarditis, gastritis, etc. If there is a solid evidence of Yang Deficiency in clinical manifestations, the inflammation can be ignored. This is Zheng's brilliant idea which I admire."

Besides, this school is also good at treating chronic pharyngitis, mouth ulcers, swollen and painful gums, tongue ulcers, red eyes, headache, fever due to internal damage, etc. which are traditionally known as conditions due to "fire flaming upward." Zheng named this kind of fire as "Yin Fire."

The "School of Fire Spirit" has been active in China until now since it was born in Sichuan province. Three books by Zheng Qin'an have been published and

---

[7] *Si Ni Tang* 四逆汤 or Frigid Extremities Decoction, a formula from *Shang Han Lun* 伤寒论 or *The Treatise on Cold Damage* by Zhang Zhongjing 张仲景 (150–219) of the Eastern Han Dynasty. Please be aware the differences between *Si Ni Tang* 四逆汤 or Frigid Extremities Decoction and *Si Ni San* 四逆散 or Frigid Extremities Powder. Both formulas are from *Shang Han Lun*. They are both for frigid extremities but due to different causes so share the same name but have different compositions and in different preparation forms. *Si Ni Tang* is listed as the first formula in the "Section 3 Formulas that Rescue Devastated Yang (Bensky and Barolet, 1990: 226–228)," while *Si Ni San* is listed as the first formula in the "Section 2 Formulas that Regulate and Harmonize Liver and Spleen" of the book "*Chinese Herbal Medicine: Formulas and Strategies*" (Bensky and Barolet, 1990: 145–146) published by Eastland Press compiled and translated by Bensky and Barolet in 1990.

reprinted many times in many editions from 1869 to 1996. Dozens of works from physicians of this school have got published and spread since 1869.

Here I would like to mention another legendary physician of this school, Zhu Weiju 祝味菊 (1884–1951), also known as Zhu Fuzi 祝附子 for he was very good at using large dosages of Fuzi (Radix Aconiti Carmichaeli, 附子) to relieve very serious diseases. As a young man in Sichuan province, he was exposed to a variety of medical schools, and he was heavily influenced by the "School of Fire Spirit." He first learned Chinese medicine with his father, later graduated from Sichuan Military Medicine Academy after studying Western medicine there for two years, and then traveling to Japan with his Japanese teacher for one year to learn about the medical system in Japan. He first practiced medicine in Sichuan province, later on moved to and settled down in Shanghai since 1917. He was regarded as a representative of both integrative medicine and the "School of Spirit" since he advocated "supporting Yang" and was very good at using large dosages of Fuzi (Radix Aconiti Carmichaeli, 附子) to relieve many serious diseases. There is an interesting story about him:

Zhu's boldness, his skill in using the warming and hot herbs and formulas from *Shang Han Lun* or *The Treatise on Cold Damage*, his notoriety for defying the Jiangnan predilection for gentle, cooling therapies, earned him much acclaim. His reputation – and the issues that motivated his reformist comrades – are captured in a memorable encounter with the famous pediatrician, Xu Xiaopu 徐小圃 (1887–1959). A Warm Illness advocate, i.e. warm illness should be relieved by cool herbs, Xu Xiaopu believed that the "pure yang 純陽" of the child must not be disturbed by the use of warming herbs. Zhu and Xu's competing medical philosophies were put to the test when Xu's son, Xu Boyuan 徐伯遠, became gravely ill (perhaps with typhoid fever) at the age of nineteen. Despite meticulous medical attention from the father, Boyuan grew sicker each day, until he was in critical condition. As the son's condition deteriorated, friends and family urged Xu Xiaopu to invite Zhu Weiju for a consultation. Xu was reluctant. Believing his son was dying of a warm illness and knowing Zhu Weiju's proclivity for Cold Damage formulas, he feared that Zhu's treatment would be the final blow. But with his son's life seemingly beyond hope, he finally agreed. True to his nickname, Aconite Zhu's first prescription contained a large dose of the very hot and toxic herb, Aconiti Radix lateralis praeparata 附子. Zhu Weiju stayed by Xu Boyuan's side throughout a difficult night. By the next day, Boyuan had stabilized; a week later his fever was gone; one month later he had made a full recovery (https://www.ncbi.nlm.nih.gov/pmc/articles/PMC4765078). In the aftermath of this case, Xu Xiaopu was so awed with Zhu Weiju's clinical abilities and disappointed with his own failures that he effectively "converted" to the Cold Damage school. Both of his sons became disciples of Zhu Weiju, and he went on to become one of the most respected pediatricians in Shanghai, skillfully marshaling the very Cold Damage formulas he had once feared, helping countless children with yang warming herbs that he had once believed anathema to pediatric medicine.[8]

Yin and Yang as the guiding principle of pattern identification is surely correct. I also agree with that Yang Qi is much more important than Yin in respect to maintaining, cultivating, and promoting health in Chinese medicine. But please keep in mind: Yin and Yang depend on each other and exist on each other; Yin-Yang Balance and Harmony has always been the goal of treatments of Chinese medicine. As some famous quotations reads that,

> *Huang Di Nei Jing Su Wen · Comprehensive Discourse on Phenomena Corresponding to Yin and Yang*:
> When Yin predominates, Yang will be diseases; When Yang predominates, Yin will be diseased.
>
> 陰勝則陽病，陽勝則陰病。
>
> Yin is in the interior and is the material foundation of Yang; Yang is on the exterior and is the manifestation of Yin. *Huang Di Nei Jing Su Wen*
>
> 陰在內，陽之守也；陽在外，陰之使也。
>
> Wang Bing's 王冰 (710?–805) annotation of *Huang Di Nei Jing Su Wen· Comprehensive Discourse on Regulating the Spirit [in Accordance with] the Qi of the Four [Seasons]*:
> Yang Qi roots in Yin; Yin Qi roots in Yang. Without Yang there would be no production of Yin; Without Yin there would be no transformation of Yang.
>
> 陽气根於陰，陰气根於陽。無陽則陰無以生，無陰則陽無以化。
>
> *Jingyue's Complete Works* 景岳全书 by Zhang Jingyue:
> Who is good at supplementing Yang must seek Yang in Yin, and Yang will be endlessly generated and transformed with the aid of Yin; Who is good at supplementing Yin must seek Yin in Yang, and Yin will never exhaust its source with the ascending of Yang.
>
> 善補陽者，必于陰中求陽，則陽得陰助而生化無窮；善補陰者，必于陽中求陰，則陰得陽升而泉源不竭。

---

8   Karchmer, Eric I. Ancient Formulas to Strengthen the Nation: Healing the Modern Chinese Body with *The Treatise on Cold Damage*. Asia Medicine. 2013, 8(2): 394–422.

2.4 Comments

Many schools developed in the history of Chinese medicine, e.g., the Four Great Schools of Jin (1115–1234) & Yuan (1271–1368) Dynasties, i.e., School of Nourishing Yin, School of Invigorating Earth (Spleen and Stomach), School of Attacking Pathogens, and School of Cooling, which all have their underlying rationality and developed under different conditions.

The School of Fire Spirit developed initially in Sichuan, where damp is prominent and spicy foods are popular. I have been living in Shanghai for almost 20 years, and notice that Shanghai is also a place where damp is prominent. The dampness being prominent in the weather may play a part in the success of this school in Sichuan and Shanghai. Remember practice Chinese medicine and institute treatment in accordance with the climatic and seasonal conditions, geographical locations and the individual conditions.

Generally speaking, practice based on modern textbooks is more reliable than that based on ancient texts and specific schools. A safe and lawful practice is the most important. Think over and over carefully, do a detailed research, and prepare a consent form for your patient before you are going to distinguish yourself – try something new from ancient texts or specific schools.

As for dosages of herbs, especially of toxic herbs or herbs with prominent features, observe the suggested dosages from the modern textbooks. For example, if you are going to try to use a larger dosage of Fuzi (Radix Aconiti Carmichaeli, 附子) by following the School of Fire Spirit, first study carefully how famous physicians of this school used it, including the combination of herbs, the preparation methods, for which conditions, etc., then increase the dosage gradually, and observe the patient's response and adjust your prescription and treatment plans, etc.

If you are going to try to apply moxibustion on Guanyuan (CV4) for a patient to promote his/her health, do it in accordance with the local laws and regulations first, e.g., scarred moxibustion may be prohibited in some places, then do it carefully and increase the dosage step-by-step, and please don't apply moxibustion on Guanyuan (CV4) continuously 1,000 moxa cones in one transition period from Summer to Fall by following the ancient text, *Bian Que Xin Shu* 扁鹊心书! Or try what you are going to do on the patient first on yourself!

Practice based on modern textbooks could be very successful in the reality. Chen Haixin 陈海新 (01/1970–02/2007) graduated from Shanghai University of Traditional Chinese Medicine in July 1993 after 5 years of undergraduate study with a Bachelor's degree in medicine, which is sometimes paralleled to an MD in the USA. She practiced at a Community Health Center near her home because of physical disability due to serious congenital diseases. If without disabilities, she may practice at one of the best hospitals in Shanghai. In her 14 years of practice of the primary level, she had seen over 20 million times of patients, average 50–60 patients a day with the highest record at 118 patients a day. Many patients came very early in the morning from very far away to line up to see her because she was famous for relieving many problems with herbal remedies.[9,10,11] You may see one patient in one hour or even two hours, and you will doubt the quality of her medical service. But remember she practiced in Shanghai – a city with over 24 million permanent residents (2015)!

To sum up this part, Yang Qi is of the prime importance in respect to maintaining, cultivating, and promoting health in Chinese medicine for all the beings. Seek Yang in Yin when caring and supporting Yang Qi. And always keep in mind: Yin and Yang depend on each other and exist on each other; Yin-Yang Balance and Harmony has always been the goal of the treatments of Chinese medicine.

3 Lifestyles which Influence Women's Health

3.1 Specific Vital Significance of Yang Qi for Women

In Chinese medicine, females are attributed to Yin, and so theoretically caring and supporting Yang Qi is extremely important for women. The normal menstruation, ovulation, sex, delivery, postpartum recovery, and lactation, etc. all depends on the abundance of Yang Qi. The women's physiological system all depends on the nourishment from the blood. Blood needs Yang Qi to warm and flow smoothly. Women take blood as their root of life. The flow of Qi and blood in the vessels is just like the flow of water in the rivers. If it is too cold, the river will be icebound. As *Huang Di Nei Jing* states, "Blood moves when it gets warm, and stagnates when it gets cold." Pain results from blockage of the flow of Qi and blood; if the flow of Qi and blood is smooth, there would be no pain.

---

9   Official website of State Administration of Traditional Chinese Medicine, P. R. China: http://www.satcm.gov.cn/e/action/ShowInfo.php?classid=140&id=1145; Date of last access: May 1, 2018.

10 Official website of Shanghai University of Traditional Chinese Medicine: http://www.xn--fhq2cw7qj9gf4c062b4e6a.net/shutcm/xuanchuanbu/jswm/chxjs/15896.shtml. Date of last access: May 1, 2018.

11 Publicity Department of Shanghai Municipality, et al. *Chen Haixin: Angel on Wheelchair*. Shanghai University of TCM Press, 2007.

Women's diseases are always attributed to cold, including deficient cold due to Yang deficiency and excess cold due to cold invasion in different ways. External cold pathogen or deficient cold due to deficiency of Yang Qi may lead to stagnation of Qi and Blood. This may result in many problems for women, especially during the menstrual period when the stagnation and stasis are hard to expel. That is why warming herbs like dried ginger and Folium Artemissiae Argyi (Ai Ye, 艾叶) are so common in formulas of Gynecology of Chinese Medicine – the uterus needs to be warmed even when there is pathogenic heat! You may go to check the gynecological formulas from *Jin Gui Yao Lue* 金匮要略 or *Essential Prescriptions from the Golden Cabinet* by Zhang Zhongjing.

3.2 Lifestyles Which Consume Yang Qi Impair Women's Health

Lifestyles which consume women's Yang Qi all impair their health. In the clinical practice, diseases like cancer, infertility, obesity, endocrine disorders, and kidney problems, etc. may all result from deficiency of Yang Qi.

3.2.1 Clothing: Exposing Key Points to Cold

In ancient China, a woman, especially a virgin, rarely went out. As *Shi Gu* 释诂 or *Explaining the Old [Words]*, the first chapter of *Er Ya* 尔雅 or *Approaching to the Standard*, explains "安 An", an associative compound being composed of "Mian 冖, a deep room" and "Nǚ 女, a virgin," reflecting the image of "a maiden staying in a deep room," indicating that the original meaning of the sinogram is "free from any danger", "calm", "safe", and "peaceful", etc.

The ancient Chinese women's clothing in the last thousands of years is mostly like a long-sleeve maxi dress or a long-sleeve top with a maxi skirt of different styles, which covers very well the women's body. While today is very different in different ways.

First of all, almost all females need to go out for different reasons, e.g. for school, work, date, shopping, and exercises, etc., no matter in freezing cold winter or terribly hot summer.

Second, cold pathogen is much more popular than before because of the widespread use of air conditioners. Before the time of air conditioners, cold pathogen emerged only under natural conditions. For example, people had no time to wear enough warm clothes when the weather suddenly became extremely cold or the very cold weather lasted for a very long period of time, and then this extreme cold weather may become cold pathogen to attach people of weak constitutions. Over thousands of years human beings have developed the ability of adaptation to cold in the winter, and heat in the summer, etc.

But with the arrival of the time of air conditioners, it is very common for people to alternate between shivering with cold in the air-conditioned spaces including offices, shopping malls, buses, metros, homes and sweating with outside summer heat. This is very typical in the summer of many places, for example Shanghai. People sweat a lot in the natural summer heat, but sweating immediately stop upon entrance of a cold air-conditioned space. The sweats which are going to excrete are finally kept inside. This is a condition named "Interior Heat and Exterior Cold" and "Disharmony between Ying and Wei" in Chinese medicine. The cold pathogen impairs women more than men because they expose more key points than men.

Exposing ankles: Women like to wear capri-pants or skirts to expose their ankles and lower legs. But this may lead to the cold pathogen invading Sanyinjiao (SP6), damaging Yang Qi. As we know, Sanyinjiao (SP6) is located at 3 cun above the inner ankle, and is the crossing point of the three-foot yin meridians, i.e. Spleen, Liver, and Kidney meridians. Spleen controls blood, Liver stores blood, and Kidneys store essence. The three-foot yin meridians are all injured by this lifestyle! While Sanyinjiao (SP6) is the most important for women's health: According to my study on 33 ancient books and 1,196 journal papers since 1950 on acupuncture treatment for women's diseases, Sanyinjiao (SP6) has gradually come to the first point for women's diseases since Tang, Song and Jin Yuan Dynasties; and modern literature shows that Sanyinjiao (SP6) is the most frequently used as the chief point, followed sequently by Zusanli (ST36), Ciliao (BL32) and Shenshu (BL23), mostly as supplementary points.[12]

Exposing the waist and umbilicus: This is regarded as a kind of fashionable and sexy look for women. Designers also like to offer more and more styles of low waist pants for women. But as we know, Mingmen (GV4), the point named the Life Gate, is just located below the spinous process of the second lumbar vertebra. The kidneys are the foundation of the prenatal existence, while the life gate stores the true fire. The Qi of the kidneys and the fire of the life gate warm the Yang Qi of the whole being. If the being is abundant in Yang Qi, the being will be surely a well being, happy and healthy, and can resist the invasion of the pathogens.

The umbilicus itself is also a very important point, Shenque (CV8) or Spirit Palace, a point which is very susceptible to cold. It can only be applied moxibustion

---

12 Lan, Fengli. "Acupuncture Treatment for Women's Diseases: History and Rational Interpretations". In: Lan, F.L./Wallner, F.G./Wobovnik, C. (eds.): *Shen, Psychotherapy, and Acupuncture: Theory, Methodology and Structure of Chinese Medicine*. Peter Lang: Frankfurt a. M. 2011, pp. 233–296.

not a needle. The meridians of Spleen, Stomach, Kidneys, Liver and Ren all pass through the abdomen, and can be invaded by cold and thus are somehow blocked.

If cold invades the lumbar and abdomen, the Yang Qi of the kidneys, Liver, Spleen, Ren and Du meridians will be impaired. If Yang Qi is deficient, the blood flow will be stagnant, dysmenorrhea may develop, and the patient may feel cold, pain, or numbness in her lower extremities.

Exposing neck and shoulders: This is very popular for women, too. As we know there are three points named after wind in this area:

> Fengfu (GV16) or Wind Palace: 1 cun directly above the midpoint of the posterior hairline, directly below the external occipital protuberance, in the depression between m. trapezius of both sides;
> Fengchi (GB20) or Wind Pool: In the depression between the upper portion of m. sternocleidomastoideus and m. trapezius, on the same level with Fengfu (GV16) or Wind Palace; and
> Fengmen (BL12) or Wind Door: 1.5 cun lateral to the Du meridian, at the level of the lower border of the spinous process of the second thoracic vertebra.

These three points are not only key points for various diseases caused by wind, but also are most vulnerable to wind pathogen. As Chapter 29 "Discourse on the Taiyin and Yangming [Meridians]" of *Huang Di Nei Jing Su Wen* states that

> Hence, if one was harmed by wind, the upper [parts of the body] receive it first. If one was harmed by dampness, the lower [parts of the body] receive it first.
>
> 故傷於風者，上先受之；傷於濕者，下先受之。

Therefore, please keep your shoulder and neck warm with a shawl or a scarf; and avoid exposing your shoulder and neck directly to the cold air current from the air conditioner or the nature no matter during the day or night. Otherwise, you may easily get a cold, cervical spondylosis, or even stroke.

3.2.2 Diets: Too Much Cold Drinks and Foods

Many women believe more vegetables and fruits in the diet can supplement various vitamins, help keep a young look and reduce weight. Ice cream is also very popular, even in the winter. In the USA, many people eat raw vegetables or salad. Anyway the temperature of these foods is much lower than that of the human stomach. Having too much cold foods and drinks, especially during period may injure Yang Qi of the Spleen and Kidneys. Dysmenorrhea, oligomenorrhea, or even amenorrhea due to too much cold food or drinks during period is not uncommon in the clinical practice. Many women's diseases, for example, menstrual disorders, infertility, postpartum regulation, etc. can be relieved or alleviated by supplementing Yang and warming the uterus in Chinese medicine.

Traditional Chinese diets are generally healthy. A balanced diet, which may include tea, stir-fried vegetables, Tofu, meat, and grains, is traditionally served as warm or hot, which do not need the stomach to warm them first to the body temperature, then to digest them. To digest ice-cold foods and drinks consume much more Yang Qi, which impairs people's health.

As for modern diets, modern China is no big difference from the West. People like tasty and rich foods. Many people just eat what they like, especially when they can afford.

Some specific formulas which are warm in nature are somehow popular and used like a kind of dietary therapy for women in China. For example, a dish or hot pot based on Mutton Stew with Danggui (Angelika) and Fresh Ginger 当归生姜羊肉汤 from *Jin Gui Yao Lue* 金匮要略 or *Essential Prescriptions from the Golden Cabinet* by Zhang Zhongjing 张仲景 (150–219) for dysmenorrhea and postpartum abdominal pain of cold pattern, etc; fresh ginger and brown sugar tea, a folk recipe, for dysmenorrhea and common cold; brown sugar and Shan Zha (haw) tea, a folk recipe, for promoting the discharge of lochia after the childbirth; Fermented Glutinous Rice Dumpling with Eggs Soup 酒酿鸡蛋圆子羹 for promoting the discharge of lochia and lactation after the childbirth; and Generation and Transformation Decoction 生化汤, from *Gynecology & Obstetrics by Fu Qingzhu* 傅青主女科 (1826), is so commonly prescribed for postpartum women for promoting the discharge of lochia and cold pain in the lower abdomen, etc.

Here I want to mention a research on a statement from *Ling Shu* 灵枢 or *Miraculous Pivot* that "Physical cold and cold drinks harm the lungs 形寒饮冷则伤肺:"

Fifty-six healthy Wistar male rats were randomly grouped into 4 groups with 14 rats in each group: control group, group of physical cold, group of cold drinks, and group of physical cold and cold drinks. The rats were treated accordingly for 7 days, during which their general conditions, skin, hair, appetite, quality of stool, and behavior were carefully observed. After 7 days, samples from their lungs were tested, including observation of the pathological changes of the lung tissues, the serum C-reactive protein (CRP) detected by radioimmunoassay, changes of Interleukin 8 (IL-8) in lung tissue homogenate, the expression of β-defensin in lung tissue detected by enzyme immunoassay, and the expression of transforming growth factor-beta 1 (TGF-β1)-mRNA in lung tissue and bronchial epithelium detected by in situ hybridization CRP. The results proved the close correlations between "physical cold" and/or "cold drinks" and the injuries of the lungs.[13]

Do the people who alternate between the air-conditioned cold air current and the heat in hot summer and have cold food and drinks resemble the rats in the above-mentioned research? But people take this as a kind of lifestyle not just for 7 days.

3.2.3 Work, Rest and Exercise: Overexertion

Mental or Physical overwork has always been regarded as an origin of disease. Nowadays, it is so common that some women sit all day long before the laptop or computer in the office, which is a lifestyle lack of sunshine and activity (Yang); some work out too much in the gym or do too much exercise in order to lose weight or keep a good body shape, or stay up too late in the night, either of which consumes too much Yang Qi. This lifestyle over a long period of time may result in many problems, including cervical spondylosis, lumbar pain, insomnia, chronic fatigue syndrome, cancer, etc.

As *Further Discourse on Meridians* 经脉别论, the 21st chapter of *Huang Di Nei Jing Su Wen* 黄帝内经素问, reads that

> Hence, whenever in spring, autumn, winter, and summer, [i.e.,] during the four seasons with their [rise and fall of] yin and yang [qi], a new disease emerges because of overuse, [then] this is the rule.[14]

故春秋冬夏四時陰陽，生病起於過用，此爲常也。

"*Wide Promulgation of the Five Qi*," the 23rd chapter of *Huang Di Nei Jing Su Wen* 黄帝内经素问 reads that

> The harms caused by the five kinds of overexertion:
> Seeing for a long time harms the blood.
> Lying down for a long time harms the qi.
> Sitting for a long time harms the flesh.
> Standing for a long time harms the bones.
> Walking for a long time harms the sinews.

13　Zhang, Yang. *Simulation Study and Substantive Analysis about Physical Cold and Cold Drinks Harming the Lungs*. Master Thesis, Shandong University of Traditional Chinese Medicine. 2009.

14　This translation is based on the translation from Prof. Paul U. Unschuld. For 过用, I choose "overuse" instead of "overexertion."

These are the so-called "harms caused by the five kinds of overexertion".

五勞所傷：久視傷血，久臥傷氣，久坐傷肉，久立傷骨，久行傷筋。是謂五勞所傷。

As for when to go to rest, the general guideline of Chinese medicine is to go to rest when darkness has fallen. As "*Comprehensive Discourse on Regulating the Spirit [in Accordance with] the Qi of the Four [Seasons]*," the 2nd chapter of *Huang Di Nei Jing Su Wen* 黄帝内经素问 reads that

> In the three months of Spring, … go to rest when darkness has fallen and rise early, ….
> In the three months of Summer, … go to rest when darkness has fallen and rise early.
> In the three months of Autumn, … go to rest early and rise early, get up together with chicken.
> In the three months of Winter, … go to rest early and rise late until the sun to shine.
>
> 春三月，……，夜臥早起，……。
> 夏三月，……，夜臥早起，……。
> 秋三月，……，早臥早起，與雞俱興，……。
> 冬三月，……，早臥晚起，必待日光，……。

Nowadays it seems impossible to go to rest when darkness has fallen. But try to go to sleep before 11:00 PM since the time from 11:00 PM to 1:00 AM is the transition period from Yin to Yang, when Yin is in its highest extreme and Yang is in its lowest extreme. This is the best time for sleep. Staying up beyond 1:00 AM will surely consume Yang Qi.

A reasonable amount of exercise is surely good and beneficial to the health. As Hua Tuo 華佗 (?–203), who created the Five-Animal Mimic Exercise 五禽戲, stressed that

> Moving and shaking help digest food, circulate blood in the vessels, and so disease does not rise. This is just like a moving door hinge, which is never stick.
>
> 動搖則穀氣消，血脈流通，病不得生。譬如戶樞，終不朽也。

Moving can raise Yang Qi. Strenuous exercise will consume Yang Qi. Do some mild exercises like jogging, walking, Yoga, Qigong, Taiji, and some other forms of traditional exercises until the body slight sweats.

3.2.4 Emotional Strains: Origin for Various Diseases for Women

Seven affects, i.e. joy, anger, worry, pensiveness, sadness, fear, and fright, as internal causes of diseases, are well discussed in all the textbooks on fundamental theories of Chinese medicine. Women take blood as their prenatal foundation, while Qi is the motive force of blood. Emotional strains disorder Qi, as the Chapter 39 "Discourse on Pain" of *Huang Di Nei Jing Su Wen* reads that

> [Huang] Di: "Good! I know that the hundred diseases are generated by the qi.
> When one is angry, then the qi rises.
> When one is joyous, then the qi relaxes.
> When one is sad, then the qi dissipates.
> When one is in fear, then the qi moves down.
> In case of cold the qi collects; in case of heat, the qi flows out.
> When one is frightened, then the qi is in disorder.
> When one is exhausted, then the qi is wasted.
> When one is pensive, then the qi lumps together."[15]
>
> 帝曰：善。余知百病生於气也。怒則气上，喜則气緩，悲則气消，恐則气下，寒則气收，炅則气泄，驚則气亂，勞則气耗，思則气結。

When Qi is in disorder, blood will be surely affected. Disorder of Qi and blood results in the occurrence various diseases in women. Tan Yunxian 谈允贤 (1461–1556), a famous female physician and gynecologist of the Ming Dynasty (1368–1644), recorded some cases with emotional strains as the origin of women's diseases in her book entitled *Nu Yi Za Yan* 女醫雜言 or *Female Physician's Miscellaneous Words:*

> A married woman, 43 years old. Her husband took a concubine because of no child [with her], and lived outside with the concubine. This woman was ill due to being sad and angry, and erysipelas erupted seriously on the two thighs.
>
> 一婦人，四十三歲，其夫因無子，取一妾，帶領出外。婦憂忿成疾，兩腿火丹大發。
>
> A married woman, 32 years old. She delivered four babies before, but she didn't get pregnant in the last ten years, and so she had been so depressed. I asked her for the underlying reason. This was because her husband went to sleep with prostitutes frequently. On one occasion, she made a terrible scene to give vent to her anger during her period, which consumed a lot of Qi and blood and finally resulted in stranguria.
>
> 一婦人，三十二歲，生四胎，後十年不生，因無子，甚是憂悶。某詢其故，乃因夫不時宿娼，偶因經事至，大鬧乘時，多耗氣血，遂成白淋。
>
> A married woman, 32 years old. Her husband was a middleman. Her husband, who was formerly a businessman, cheated her on financial affairs. She was a hot-tempered person, so she made a terrible scene to give vent to her anger. She vomited two bowels of blood right away, and later had coughing for three years. The medications she took didn't work.
>
> 一婦人，年三十二歲，其夫為牙行，夫故商人，以財為欺，婦性素躁，因與大鬧，當即吐血二碗，後兼咳嗽，三年不止，服藥無效。

---

15 This translation is from Paul U. Unschuld.

According to Tan Yunxian's records, sadness, anger, depression caused erysipelas, infertility, stranguria, vomiting of blood, coughing, etc. Nowadays emotional strains for women may come from work, family, and relationship with men, etc. Desire may also become an origin of women's diseases, especially when desires are too many and strong and can't be satisfied. A 2008 study by the University of Michigan indicated that, while humans experience desire and fear as psychological opposites, they share the same brain circuit.[16]

Stress may also trigger many problems such as hypertension and migraine. Stress management is a big topic.

Emotional strains, too many and strong unsatisfied desires, and stress all consume Yang Qi, and can be origins of women's diseases.

The "Discourse on the True [Qi endowed by] Heaven in High Antiquity," the first chapter of *Huang Di Nei Jing Su Wen* suggests people of nowadays to follow the way of the people of high antiquity to live a healthy and long life, which can be summarized as follows:

> Model [behaviors] on yin and yang and comply with the arts and the calculations; 法於陰陽，和於術數;
> Moderate in eating and drinking; 食飲有節;
> Regular in working and resting; 起居有常;
> Avoid any kind of overstrain; 不妄作勞;
> Avoid invasion of external pathogens at specific times; 虛邪賊風，避之有時;
> Quiet peacefulness, free from avarice and desires, and the true qi follows [these states]. When essence and spirit are guarded internally, where could a disease come from?
> 恬惔虛无，真氣從之，精神內守，病安從來？

4 Women's Health: Acupuncture Approach

Women's diseases are composed of two parts: gynecological and obstetrical diseases, and "women's miscellaneous diseases" as stated in ancient Chinese texts. Acupuncture has been used to treat women's diseases for thousands of years in China.

---

16 "Changing stress levels can make brain flip from desire to dread." March 19, 2008. http://ns.umich.edu/new/releases/6419-changing-stress-levels-can-make-brain-flip-from-desire-to-dread. Date of last access: May 1, 2018.

4.1 The General Principle of Acupuncture Treatment

The general principle of acupuncture treatment is stated in the Chapter 10 "Meridians" of *Ling Shu* 灵枢 or *Miraculous Pivot* that

> If excess, reinforce; if deficiency, reduce; if heat, use quick technique; if cold, retain [the needles]; if sinking, apply moxibustion; if neither excess nor deficiency, select points in accordance with meridians.
>
> 盛則瀉之，虛則補之，熱則疾之，寒則留之，陷下則灸之，不盛不虛，以經取之。

The chapter 73 "Qualifications of Acupuncturists" of *Ling Shu* 灵枢 or *Miraculous Pivot* that Deficiency of Yin and Yang should be treated by mixubustion.

> 陰陽皆虛，火自當之。

As women's Yang Qi needs to be cared and supported particularly and many of women's diseases are caused by deficiency of Yang Qi, so moxibustion and reinforcing need to be used more in the modern healthcare setting. As stated in most of the textbooks, moxibustion has the functions of warming meridians and expelling cold, inducing smooth flow of Qi and blood, strengthening Yang from collapse, and preventing disease and keeping healthy.

In *Bian Ques's Precious Heart Book* (Bian Que Xin Shu, 扁鹊心书, 1146) by Dou Cai, all prescriptions were single-point prescriptions with moxibustion as the treating method, and acupoints on the controlling vessel were much more frequently used.

One famous example is to apply moxibustion on Zhiyin (BL67) to correct fetus malposition. Thousands of clinical reports showed that restitution rate of breech presentation in cases performing moxibustion or laser radiation on Zhiyin (BL67) (usually before 32 weeks or even after 32 weeks but before 34 weeks of gestation) was significantly higher than the spontaneous restitution rate. The difference has a statistical significance.

Actually, moxibustion can be used more extensively for women's health: apply moxibustion on Shenque (CV8) for diarrhea or dysentery for women during pregnancy; on Shenmen (HT7) for insomnia; on Zusanli (ST36), Guanyuan (CV4), Dazhui (GV14) or Zhongwan (CV12) for tumor patients; and on Sanyinjiao (SP6) for dysmenorrhea, etc.

4.2 The Principles of Formulating Point Prescriptions

4.2.1 The General Principle: Balancing

The general principles of combination of points are all applicable for acupuncture treatment for women's diseases, which are known as balancing between Inside and Outside 内外相应, between Left and Right 左右相对, between Exterior and Interior 表里相合, between Upper and Lower Parts of the body 上下相通, between Distal and Local Points 远近相引, between Front and Back 俞募相配, and between Yin and Yang 阴阳相和. Briefly speaking, balancing helps to reestablish balance and harmony.

4.2.2 Disease Diagnosis, Pattern Identification, Symptom Consideration: Foundation of Acupuncture Treatment

In ancient literature, a point or a group of points are recorded in the format that "**point is indicated for ** disease or ** symptom." The modern education advocates selecting points based on pattern identification. Pattern identification is somehow a new invention proposed by Ren Yingqiu 任应秋 in 1955.[17,18] Research on *Bian Zheng Lun Zhi* 辨证论治 shows that disease diagnosis, symptom consideration, and meridian or visceral pattern identification should be comprehensively considered as the foundation for individualized treatment in Chinese medicine.[19] Take climacteric syndrome for instance: It is a syndrome caused by gradual debilitation of kidney Qi, deficiency of Thoroughfare and Controlling Vessels, and gradual exhaustion of Tiangui; as for visceral pattern identification, it is attributed to non-interaction between the heart and kidneys together with depression and stagnation of liver Qi. Therefore, the therapeutic principle is formulated as tonifying and nourishing the kidney and the heart, pacifying the liver and regulating Qi, dredging and regulating Controlling and Thoroughfare Vessels, with a basic effective prescription of Shenmen (HT7), Shenshu (BL23), Taichong (LR3), Guanyuan (CV4) and Sanyinjiao (SP6), which can be modified according to patient's chief sufferings.

---

17 Ren, Yingqiu: Great Homeland Medical Achievements. *Journal of Traditional Chinese Medicine* (2), 1955, p. 1; 1955(4): 19.
18 Ren, Yingqiu: The System of Pattern Identification and Treatment in Chinese Medicine. *Journal of Traditional Chinese Medicine* (4), 1955, p. 19.
19 Lan, Fengli: *Metaphor: The Weaver of Chinese Medicine*. Verlag Traugott Bautz GmbH. 2015, pp. 242–259.

4.2.3 Effects of Acupoints Resembling that of Medicinals: Monarch, Minister, Assistant, and Guide

Li Xintian 李心田 wrote a book entitled *The Merging of Acupuncture and Herbal Medicine* (Zhen Yao Hui Tong, 针药汇通),[20] in which he advocated that effects of acupoints resemble that of medicinals, and that effects of herbal remedies could be achieved merely by acupuncture. This viewpoint opens a way to understand and formulate acupoint prescriptions. Each acupoint has its own comparatively independent actions. That "effects of acupoints resemble that of medicinals" has its rationality. For example, Sanyinjiao (SP6) has the effect of moving Qi, activating and nourishing blood, just like angelica (Dang Gui, 当归); Zusanli (ST36) dredging and activating meridians and collaterals, tonifying and supplementing Qi and blood, like ginseng (Ren Shen, 人参) and astragalus (Huang Qi, 黄芪); Guanyuan (CV4) warming the kidney and invigorating yang, dredging and regulating controlling vessel and thoroughfare vessel, like antler (Lu Rong, 鹿茸), eucommia (Du Zhong, 杜仲), cistanche (Cong Rong, 苁蓉) and morinda (Ba Ji Tian, 巴戟天); Zhongji (CV3) draining water, regulating menstruation and checking abnormal vaginal discharge, like poria (Fu Ling, 茯苓), achyranthes (Niu Xi, 牛膝) and lycopus (Ze Lan, 泽兰); and so and so forth. Thereby you may work out the point prescription according to the same principle of composing herbal prescriptions: Monarch, Minister, Assistant, and Guide.

4.2.4 Formulating Acupoint Prescription According to Four Phases of a Menstrual Cycle

As elucidated in part 1, the four phases of the menstrual cycle are a common understanding in both Western medicine and Chinese medicine: Endometrium-shedding – Follicular – Ovulation – Luteal phases in Western medicine and Menstrual – Postmenstrual – Inter-menstrual – Premenstrual phases in Chinese medicine.

Based on Chinese understanding of the four phases, acupoint prescription can be formulated according to the pattern identified in each phase for different patients.

Take acupuncture treatment for anovulatory menstrual disorders as an example. Anovulatory menstrual disorders involve ovulation failure, luteal phase

---

20 The draft of the book was completed in 1945, supplemented later by his son, Li Shizhen 李世珍, and renamed *Practical Elaboration of Commonly Used Acupoints* (Chang Yong Shu Xue Lin Chuang Fa Hui, 常用腧穴临床发挥), which was published in 1985 by People's Medical Publishing House in Beijing

defect (LPD), polycystic ovarian syndrome, fallopian tube obstruction, ovarian hypofunction, hyperprolactinemia, and endometriosis, etc. Currently, the time for acupuncture is generally chosen from the 12th to the 15th day of a menstrual cycle, namely the ovulation or inter-menstrual phase to promote ovulation. Giving treatment in each phase of the menstrual cycle accordingly will surely improve both the patient's constitution and therapeutic effects. For example, Tonifying kidney – Coursing liver – Warming Yang – Activating Blood, Tonifying kidney – Supplementing Qi – Tonifying kidney – Activating blood, Tonifying kidney – Resolving Phlegm – Tonifying kidney – Activating blood for Menstrual – Postmenstrual – Inter-menstrual – Premenstrual phases respectively, then compose different point prescriptions accordingly.

4.2.5 Formulating Acupoint Prescription According to Dermatomes

It is clear from the above analysis that no matter choosing acupoints along the meridian according to the theory that "a meridian can treat diseases of where it goes by", or using specific points according to functional characteristics of five transport, crossing, Back-Shu and Front-Mu points, or even selecting acupoints according to disease diagnosis, pattern identification, and symptom consideration and "the effects of acupoints resemble that of medicinals", indications of an acupoint are almost all closely related to its segmental innervations, i.e., dermatomes.

Studies on the relationship between acupoint actions and dermatomes started since the end of 1950s and the beginning of 1960s. As morphological researches progressed, very few people studied the substantive essence of meridians and acupoints in respect to dermatomes after 1980s. In the recent years, this approach seems to be revived.

It is believed in this approach that the range of indications of an acupoint is mainly decided by its corresponding dermatomes. Hereafter is a table (Table 1) of commonly used acupoints for women's diseases and their dermatomes.

Women's Health: Fundamentals, Lifestyles and Acupuncture Approach 139

Tab. 1: *Indications of commonly-used points for women's diseases and dermatomes*

Acupoint	Location	Dermatomes	Innervation	Indications of Acupoint
Sanyinjiao (SP6)	Lower Limb	L_{2-4}, $L_4 \sim S_3$	saphenous nerve, tibial nerve	Disorders of genitourinary system and intestinal tract, lumbocrural disorders
Guanyuan (CV4)	Lower Abdomen	T_{12}	anterior cutaneous ramus of intercostal nerve	Disorders of kidneys, uterus, ovary and large intestine
Zhongji (CV3)	Lower Abdomen	T_{12}	iliohypogastric nerve	Disorders of genitourinary system and rectum
Qihai (CV6)	Lower Abdomen	T_{11}	anterior cutaneous ramus of intercostal nerve	Disorders of small intestine, large intestine, kidneys, testis and ovary
Ciliao (BL32)	Lumbosacral Region	S_2	posterior ramus of sacral nerve	Disorders of pelvic organs
Taichong (LR3)	Lower Limb	$L_4 \sim S_2$, $L_5 \sim S_3$	deep peroneal nerve, tibial nerve	Lower limb paralysis, disorders of genitourinary system
Shenshu (BL23)	Lumbosacral Region	L_2	posterior ramus of lumbar nerve	Disorders of kidneys and pelvic organs
Rugen (ST18)	Chest	$C_5 \sim T_1$, T_5	anterior thoracic nerve, intercostal nerve	cough with dyspnea, palpitation, breast diseases, pain in chest and hypochondrium
Xuehai (SP10)	Lower Limb	L_{2-4}	Obturator nerve, Muscular ramus of femoral nerve, saphenous nerve	Disorders of genitourinary system, articular dyskinesia of the knee
Zhiyin (BL67)	Lower Limb	$L_4 \sim S_2$	superficial peroneal nerve, sural nerve	Lumbocrural Pain, diseases of genitourinary system
Qugu (CV2)	Lower Abdomen	$T_{12} \sim L_4$	Iliohypogastric nerve	Disorders of genitourinary system
Guilai (ST29)	Lower Abdomen	$T_{12} \sim L_4$	Iliohypogastric nerve	Disorders of large intestine and genitourinary system

Acupoint	Location	Dermatomes	Innervation	Indications of Acupoint
Pishu (BL20)	Lumbodorsal Region	T_{11}	posterior ramus of thoracic nerve	Disorders of small intestine, colon, kidneys, testis and ovary
Mingmen (GV4)	Lumbosacral Region	L_2	posterior ramus of lumbar nerve	Disorders of genitourinary system, rectum, pain long spinal column
Yinbai (SP1)	Lower Limb	L_5~S_2, $L_{2~4}$	dorsal digital nerves of superficial peroneal nerve, saphenous nerve of femoral nerve	Disorders of genitourinary system and large intestine
Daimai (GB26)	hypochondrium	T_{11}	intercostal nerve	Disorders of upper urinary system (kidneys & ureter), testis, ovary, small intestine and colon
Yaoshu (GV2)	Lumbosacral Region	L_2	posterior ramus of sacral nerve	Disorders of pelvic organs

Now take chronic pelvic inflammation as an example to illustrate how to select acupoints according to this theory.

The 1st Group – Acupoints in the Lumbar Neural Section: Weishu (BL21), Sanjiaoshu (BL22), Shenshu (BL23), Qihaishu (BL24), Dachangshu (BL25), Zhishi (BL52);

The 2nd Group – Acupoints in the Abdominal Neural Section: Zhongji (CV3), Qugu (CV2), Shuidao (ST28), Fushe (SP13), Guilai ((ST29), Dahe (KI12);

The 3rd Group – Acupoints in the Sacral Neural Section: Baliao (BL31 through BL 34), Pangguangshu (BL28), Zhonglvshu (BL29), Baihuanshu (BL30);

The 4th Group – Acupoints on the Lower Limbs of the Above Neural Sections: Sanyinjiao (SP6), Diji (SP8), Yinlingquan (SP9), Gongsun (SP4), Taixi (KI3), Ququan (LR8).

Then we make a prescription by combining acupoints of the 1st group with those of the 3rd group, combining those of the 2nd group with those of the 4th group. Four to six points are selected each time with moderate or strong stimulating methods.

Explanations: Women's internal genitals and their peripheral tissues are mainly distributed by the nerves from L1-3 and S2-4 neural sections, therefore acupoints in the corresponding controlling areas should be selected to treat women's diseases.

The acupoints of the 1st and 2nd groups are distributed in the controlling regions of L1-3, while those of the 3rd and 4th groups in the controlling regions of S2-4.

Comments: This theory should not be taken as the leading theory in selecting acupoints for treating diseases. Connecting function of acupoints with dermatomes can illustrate at a certain level the functional relationship between needling points and the regulated parts, and can only be used as an auxiliary guide to acupoint selection.

It is advisable to comprehensively consider the above-mentioned theories when you select points. Generally speaking, apply small prescriptions for simple conditions, big prescriptions for complex conditions.

4.3 Frequently Used Acupoints for Women's Diseases

4.3.1 Frequently Used Acupoints for Women's Diseases in Qing Dynasty

The Source of Acupuncture and Moxibustion (Zhen Jiu Feng Yuan, 针灸逢源), *The Classic f Miraculous Moxibustion* (Shen Jiu Jing Lun, 神灸经论), and *A Collection of Acupuncture and Moxibustion at Mian Xue Tang* (Mian Xue Tang Zhen Jiu Ji Cheng, 勉学堂针灸集成), three works of acupuncture in the Qing Dynasty, may stand for the achievements of acupuncture treatment for women's diseases in the ancient China before 20th century. A general survey of the three works shows that menstrual disorders and postpartum diseases were common diseases treated by acupuncture; use of moxibustion was stressed for women; and 131 acupoints of 14 meridians were used for treating women's diseases with Sanyinjiao (SP6), Zhongji (CV3), Guanyuan (CV4), Qihai (CV6), Hegu (LI4), Zhaohai (KI6), Yinjiao (GV7), Zusanli (ST36), Shimen (CV5), Qichong (ST30), Shenshu (BL23), Zhiyin (BL67) as frequently used points.

4.3.2 Frequently Used Acupoints for Women's Diseases in Modern China

A comprehensive analysis of 1,196 journal papers on acupuncture treatment for women's diseases published in China since 1950 shows that:[21]

① Most Commonly used acupoints were meridian points on Controlling Vessel, Spleen, Bladder, or Stomach Meridian;
② Sanyinjiao (SP6) was most frequently used as the chief point, followed by Zusanli (ST36), Ciliao (BL32) and Shenshu (BL23), mostly as supplementary

---

21 Lan, Fengli. 2011, pp. 233–296.

points, reflecting the importance of caring and protecting Stomach Qi and Back-Shu Points in the treatment of women's diseases.
③ Most of the meridian points selected for women's diseases are specific points, among which five transport points (e.g. Jing-Well point and He-Sea point), Back-Shu and Front-Mu points [e.g. Zhongji (CV3), Guanyuan (CV4), Shenshu (BL23) and Pishu (BL20)] and crossing points (e.g. crossing points of extraordinary vessels and Three-Foot Yin meridians as well as eight confluent points) are commonly used;
④ Most points selected for women's diseases are located on the lower limbs, lower abdomen and lumbosacral portion, mainly points on meridians;
⑤ Single-point prescriptions mainly take distal points.

Here are some examples of common understanding of point selection for women's diseases: Zhiyin (BL67) for correcting malposition of the fetus, Yinbai (SP1) for spotting (metrostaxis) and flooding (metrorrhagia), Zusanli (ST36), Shaoze (SI1) and Danzhong (CV17) for promoting lactation, Hegu (LI4) and Sanyinjiao (SP6) for relieving pain during delivery, etc.

Sanyinjiao (SP6) is the most frequently used point for women's diseases, namely for abnormal vaginal discharge of damp-heat type, malposition of the fetus, postpartum retention of urine: with Hegu (LI4) for treating amenorrhea, inducing abortions, and relieving pain during delivery; with Zhongji (CV3) for treating amenorrhea, postpartum retention of urine, postpartum pain due to contraction of the uterus, infertility; with Guanyuan (CV4) for inducing abortions and promoting delivery; with Qihai (CV6), Guanyuan (CV4) and Yinbai (SP1) for dysmenorrhea and infertility; etc.

4.3.3 Master Tong's Extra Points for Women's Diseases

Master Tong's extra points are a kind of multi-layered holographic acupuncture. It is different from the most popular style of classical acupuncture but shares the same source – *Nei Jing* or *Inner Classic* and follows the same theoretical foundation – the meridian theory. For example, for pains, it is advisable in Master Tong's acupuncture system to needle the contra-lateral or the opposite side or the healthy side, to use the upper for the lower, and vice versa, which follows principles advised in the *Nei Jing* or *Inner Classic*. The chapter *On Miu Ci* or *On Misleading Piecing* 缪刺论 of *Huang Di Nei Jing Su Wen* discusses the method of piecing the healthy side to treat diseases of the other side: "Disease in the right, select points on the left [to treat it]; Disease in the left, select points on the right [to treat it]." The chapter *Beginning and Ending* 终始 of *Ling Shu Jing* also advises that

"Disease in the upper, select points on the lower [part of the body treat it];"
"Disease in the lower, select points on the upper [part of the body to treat it];"
"Disease in the head, select points on the foot [to treat it];"
"Disease in the lumbar, select points on the popliteal fossa [to treat it]."

病在上者，下取之；病在下者，高取之；病在頭者，取之足；病在腰者，取之膕。

Most of the Master Tong's points are located on the four extremities, safe, convenient and very effective in relieving pains and treating various types of diseases.

The founding father of Master Tong's extra points is Jingchang Tong 董景昌 (1916–1975). He was originally from Shandong province, and then moved to Taiwan with Kuomintang in around 1949. His style of acupuncture which was inherited from his family was flourishing in Taiwan first, and then was transmitted to America and back to mainland China, and is now extensively used in the practice worldwide. Based on my personal experiences, frequently used Master Tong's extra points for women's diseases may include Fuke (Gynecology, 11.24), Huanchao (Returning to Nest, 11.06), Three Emperors (77.17, 77.19, 77.21), Ling Gu (Spiritual Bone, 22.05), etc.[22]

Combining Master Tong's extra points with the classical Chinese acupuncture may exert a better therapeutic effect. Evidence of the efficacy of Master Tong's extra points based on clinical trials needs to be provided to support its extensive use in the practice.

4.4 Mechanism of Acupuncture Treatment for Women's Diseases

The mechanism of acupuncture treatment for women's diseases is the same as that for other diseases: positive double-direction regulating effect. Modern studies demonstrate that the mechanism of acupuncture treatment for women's diseases lies in the following three aspects:

① Activating the axis of center-hypothalamus-pituitary-ovary, thus exerting double-direction regulating effect on women's reproductive system, which is the most important mechanism;
② Activating the body's immunity system, thus influencing the nervous-reproductive and endocrine-immunological controlling system, thus taking therapeutic effects;
③ Promoting release of opioid peptides, thus relieving menstrual pain.

---

22 Lee, Miriam: *Master Tong's Acupuncture: An Ancient Alternative Style in Modern Clinical Practice*. Blue Poppy Press: Boulder. 1992 1st ed.; 2005 8th printing.

To sum up, effects of acupuncture treatment for women's diseases is mainly achieved through regulating the nervous-endocrine-immunological system, partly through the nervous-humor system.[23]

As for update progress in the field of acupuncture treatment for women's diseases, you may refer to the official website of WHO on evidence- based acupuncture at: http://www.evidencebasedacupuncture.org/who-official-position/.

5 Conclusion

Women in classical China live in a very different "life world" from the "life world" in which European women live. As for women's health from Chinese perspective, lifestyle matters. Acupuncture is good at treating women's diseases including annovulatory menstrual disorders, infertility, dysmenorrhea, fetus malposition, menopausal syndrome, lactation promotion or delactation, chronic pelvic inflammation, menstrual migraine, endometriosis, etc. The effectiveness and efficacy of acupuncture treatment for women's diseases evidence that acupuncture, as a part of Chinese medicine which is rooted in classical Chinese culture and philosophy, is working and thus real and true in the polymedical systematic world.

References

Bensky, Dan and Barolet, Randall. *Chinese Herbal Medicine: Formulas and Strategies*. Washington: Eastland Press. 1990.

Dou, Cai. *Bianque's Precious Heart Book* (Bian Que Xin Shu, 扁鹊心书). 1146. Reprinted with annotations by China Medical Science Press in Beijing in 2011.

Lan, Fengli. "Acupuncture Treatment for Women's Diseases: History and Rational Interpretations". In: Lan, F.L./Wallner, F.G./Wobovnik, C. (eds.): *Shen, Psychotherapy, and Acupuncture: Theory, Methodology and Structure of Chinese Medicine*. Peter Lang: Frankfurt a. M. 2011.

Karchmer, Eric I. Ancient Formulas to Strengthen the Nation: Healing the Modern Chinese Body with *The Treatise on Cold Damage*. Asia Medicine. 2013, 8(2): 394–422.

Lan, Fengli. *Metaphor: The Weaver of Chinese Medicine*. Nordhausen: Verlag Traugott Bautz GmbH, 2015.

Lee, Miriam. *Master Tong's Acupuncture: An Ancient Alternative Style in Modern Clinical Practice*. Boulder: Blue Poppy Press, 1992 1st ed.; 2005 8th printing.

---

23 Lan, Fengli. 2011, pp. 233–296.

Li, Shizhen. *Practical Elaboration of Commonly Used Acupoints* (Chang Yong Shu Xue Lin Chuang Fa Hui, 常用腧穴临床发挥). Beijing: People's Medical Publishing House, 1985.

Publicity Department of Shanghai Municipality, et al. *Chen Haixin: Angel on Wheelchair.* Shanghai University of TCM Press, 2007.

Ren, Yingqiu. Great Homeland Medical Achievemnts. *Journal of Traditional Chinese Medicine.* 1955 (2):1.

Ren, Yingqiu. The System of Pattern Identification and Treatment in Chinese Medicine. *Journal of Traditional Chinese Medicine.* 1955 (4):19.

Tan, Yuxian. *Female Physician's Miscellaneous Words* (Nu Yi Za Yan, 女医杂言). 1510. Reprinted with annotations by China Press of Traditional Chinese Medicine in Beijing in 2016.

Unschuld, Paul U. *Huang Di Nei Jing Su Wen: An Annotated Translation of Huang Di's Inner Classic.* California: University of California Press, 2011.

Wu, Guozhong. *A Manual of Huang Di Nei Jing.* Shanghai: Jinxiu Wenzhang Press. 2009.

Zhang, Yang. *Simulation Study and Substantive Analysis about Physical Cold and Cold Drinks Harming the Lungs.* Master Thesis, Shandong University of Traditional Chinese Medicine. 2009.

Andrea-Mercedes Riegel
Acupuncture Treatment for Lifestyle Related Diseases

Abstract: In mainland China and Taiwan one everywhere sees western hospitals which all have at least one department for Chinese medicine the consultations offered being not the traditional indications but modern diseases related to an inadequate lifestyle. In this field of lifestyle-related diseases acupuncture has proven to be an effective method of treatment in combination with a change of lifestyle.

1 Introduction

Over the course of Chinese history, acupuncture and herbal treatments were used to treat all kinds of diseases and health problems from pain symptoms to epidemic diseases. But when the Western medicine entered China, the old native medical system gradually fell into oblivion and was ridiculed for not being scientific. During the Cultural Revolution Mao Zedong, needing a cheap medical supply for the people, revived the Chinese medical system and called it "a treasure of Chinese culture worth being unearthed". Owing to his encouragement, a new Chinese medical system developed that was less complicated than the old one and without any kind of "superstition". New textbooks based on Marxist dialectics and poor in theories were written. During the 1970s, acupuncture became an article for export to Western countries whereas in China it was not highly appreciated. Nowadays acupuncture treatment is popular again and is used for all kinds of diseases and symptoms except infectious diseases and – of course – diseases which require surgical operation or strong medication. Even in modern hospitals for Western medicine, in the midst of numerous small departments, one generally finds a department for acupuncture or Traditional Chinese Medicine. The scope of indications for acupuncture treatment is rather astonishing. For example, consultations are offered for obesity, giving up smoking, sterility/infertility and diabetes.

In the Western world, acupuncture is currently only recognized by health insurance companies for pain treatment (headache, back pain and knee pain). The argument for these restricted indications is the lack of scientific studies proving the efficiency of acupuncture, but experience has taught us that – single or adjuvant – acupuncture treatment for lifestyle-related diseases such as allergies, high blood pressure or diabetes and obesity shows good results.[1]

2 The Pathogen Factors and Lifestyle

In Chinese medicine, all kinds of diseases and disorders of the organism are correlated with an impaired flow of Qi. The flow of Qi might be impaired by pathogen factors. In Chinese medicine we are aware of different factors which – if strong or long-lasting enough – may attack our health. As they are harmful to our "straight Qi" (*zheng* Qi 正氣) they are called the "oblique influences" *xie* Qi 邪气 and since Chen Yan (1131–1198), they have been divided into three categories: the exogenous factors (*wai yin* 外因) which are mostly climatic factors; the endogenous factors (*nei yin* 內因), which subsume the emotional disorders; and the factors which are neither exogenous nor endogenous (*bu nei wai yin* 不內外因). These are not pathogen factors themselves and they do not influence health in a direct way but they bring about pathogen factors in the interior of the body and they are mostly related to an inadequate lifestyle.

Within the category of exogenous factors, specifically climatic factors, the most important one is wind, and wind may transport the other factors: heat, cold, dampness, wetness and dryness. These may penetrate the body via the skin pores and the body's defense system Qi – *Wei* Qi.

Emotional or mental disorders such as mourning (lung), stress (liver), sorrow (spleen) and fear (kidney) on a long-term basis may harm the viscera in which they are stored and, according to the five phases theory, the balance between the viscera will be disturbed. The pathogen factors which emotional disorders bring about are mostly: heat in the interior; wind; and phlegm because of an impaired flow of Qi.[2]

The most important factors in modern life are heterogeneous factors which are related to malnutrition, overwork, inactivity and biorhythmic disturbances. But symptoms and diseases such as diabetes (type II), allergies, major mental depression, maniac depression, nervousness, fear or hysteria may be the result of heterogeneous and of endogenous factors.

---

1   See p.ex. the publications by Eich et al. 2000 and 2003, Hollifield, Michael 2007, Maric-Oehler, Walburg 2000 and Schnyer, Rosa 2007 which are listed in the reference works.
2   Though the factors wind, dampness and heat may be subsumed under the exogenous and the endogenous factors, one has to make a clear distinction between them for treatment. See also the statement of Zhang, Jiebin: *Jingyue quanshu*. Shanghai kexue jishu chubanshe: Shanghai, 1996, pp. 22–23.

Acupuncture Treatment for Lifestyle Related Diseases 149

2.1 The Ideal Lifestyle for Health

The *Suwen* (1) and (2) ask a question about fertility and the way of prolonging the fertile period of man. Normally the span of reproduction lasts from 2 × 7 to 7 × 7 (14–49) years in women and 2 × 8 to 8 × 8 (16–64) years in man. But it should be possible for a man to delay the exhaustion of the *tiangui*, the substance which bestows man with fertility, and the decay of the body and spirit for decades by means of an adequate lifestyle. So the *Suwen* (1) states,

> Now, those [who follow] the **Way**,
> they can drive away old age and they preserve their physical appearance.
> Although their body has lived a long life,
> They are [still] able to produce children.[3]
> Man is healthy enough when he goes "along with the Way".
> What does this mean?

In the initial part of the first chapter and in the very next chapter (2) of the *Suwen*, we find the description of the Daoist Way to longevity which is a lifestyle marked by asceticism, peace and harmony *he* 和 with Heaven and Earth, the four seasons, the patterns of the eight winds, in the emotions and between Yin and Yang. Harmony with Heaven and Earth includes adapting to the climate where one lives and the actual climatic conditions. And in a specific climatic zone, there are soil conditions. One therefore has to adapt agriculture to these conditions in order to have a rich harvest and the nutrition which fits to the people living there. The four seasons also require adaption in nutrition and clothing and for work. Spring is the time of seeding the fall is the time of the harvest and in winter the harvest is stored in the house. The activity of man also adapts to the seasons: in spring, one gets up early and goes to bed late at night and it is the same for the three summer months. In the three months of the fall, one gets up early in the morning and goes to bed early with the hens whereas in the three months of winter one goes to bed early and gets up late in the morning. One concentrates on one's duties during the corresponding seasons and respects the times of activity and rest. Irregularities in lifestyle do have their impact on human health: the corresponding organs are impaired, liver (spring), the heart (summer), the lung (fall) and the kidney (winter) and the health impact of non-compliant behavior will also be felt in the next season.

The adaption to Yin and Yang includes the adaption of activity and rest to the seasons, to the time of the day and to the actual climatic conditions. The "harmony

---

3   Unschuld, Paul/Tessenow, Herrmann: *Huang Di Nei Jing Su Wen*. University of California Press: Berkeley, 2011, pp. 36–42.

in the emotions" means that all the emotions have to be present in man, and man has to show emotional reactions in an adequate manner. It does not mean an absolute lack of emotions, an "empty heart" in the Buddhist sense, but that all emotions are in balance, in the sense of the Confucian *Zhong Yong*. This is understandable because the emotions are stored in the viscera and overflowing emotions or lack of emotion in one organ first impairs the organ function and then the balance between the inner organs, according to the five phases model. This is the ideal situation which helps man to stay healthy.

But *Suwen* (2) also states that only "the wise man can follow [this way] and therefore his body is free of extraordinary diseases, the [mechanism] of the ten-thousand things doesn't get lost and his Qi for life doesn't become exhausted."[4]

2.2 The Role Nutrition Plays in Health

Nutrition may be one of the most important factors for health. The most important criterion for nutrition is first of all harmony; harmony between Yin and Yang.

Firstly, nutrition must take the season into consideration and adapt to all the inner organs. The foods are divided into categories, called the *xing* 性 of the food. This corresponds to the division of herbal drugs. There are Yin-Yang criteria like the temperature behavior and the taste, which provoke different actions in the organism. The temperature behavior describes the action which the food develops in the organism: cooling, cold, warming or hot. During summer time, the food should be cooling by tendency, and during the cold winter months it should be warm in order to get a balance between Yin and Yang. The extreme hot (Yang) and cold (Yin) should be avoided or balanced by the addition of foods or spices which tend to harmonize the meal.

Other categories of foods are the taste and its action, the action on the inner organs and their channels. A meal always has to be harmonious concerning temperature and taste.

Each organ has its requirements and not only concerning the taste. For example, the spleen loves dryness, the stomach likes dampness and the kidney needs water. Though the kidney is at the base of all the inner organs, the spleen is the center of the body and is the most important organ for the nourishment of body and soul. In the Ming Dynasty (1368–1644) it was even described by Sun Yikui as the *Taiji*, the Great Eternal One, of man. This is because the spleen is responsible for the selection of the essence of nourishment and the essence is the base for the

---

4   *Suwen* (2); Yang, Weijie: *Huangdi neijing Suwen shijie*. Yuejun wenhua shuye gongsi: Taibei, 1990, p. 17.

blood, the marrow including the brain and the bones. And it also has to distribute it, to send fluid and solid particles to the lung so that they may become blood or Qi; whereas the stomach has to send the waste particles downward to the kidney and intestines. The spleen Qi flows upward; the stomach Qi flows downward. It becomes clear that stomach and spleen need good food rich in nutrients to fulfill their tasks. The taste of foods should be rather neutral. The earth organs need the *gan* 甘 taste, which is not necessarily "sweet" but only a little "sweetish" flavor. But the sweetish taste tends to last and float in the middle burner so that the addition of harmonizing tastes, spicy and sour taste becomes necessary. And man must avoid too much water for the spleen loves dryness. In order not to disturb the Qi of the spleen, which is the base for health, some rules must be respected:

- regular meals and no snacks between the main meals
- no raw fruits or vegetables because their metabolism needs too much energy
- no icy meals because they are too cold for the kidney which has to warm the spleen
- no foods which might be apt to produce phlegm like fresh milk or raw bananas

It becomes obvious that nutrition is an important factor for health and may sustain any treatment whereas the wrong nutrition may disturb every success of treatment.

3 Acupuncture for Diabetes

Suwen (1) and (2) traced the way to a long-lasting and healthy life, free from extraordinary diseases. But it was also clear that only the sages could follow this way of life in perfect harmony; and the practitioners had made the experience that an excessive lifestyle – a situation which they encountered in the upper classes – could harm the inner organs and cause diseases. One saw that malnutrition with sweet and fatty foods and alcohol could harm the spleen Qi and produce heat in the interior; but not only malnutrition was recognized as being dangerous for health but also the consumption of "hot" substances destined for the prolongation of life like cinnabar or mercury, mental stress and body exhaustion may be caused by sexual over-activity.

Suwen (47) introduces the impairment of the spleen function caused by malnutrition:

When someone suffers from a sweet taste in the mouth, what do we call it? Where does it come from?> Qibo answered: <This is a surplus of the five tastes, its name is *pibi* [obstruction of the spleen]. The five tastes come into the mouth and they are first stored in the stomach. The spleen makes their essence and Qi

start to flow, but when [the fluids] accumulate in the spleen [because of spleen Qi deficiency] the mouth taste becomes sweet. This happens when eating fatty and opulent dishes, when man often consumes rich sweet foods and a lot of fat. Fat causes heat in the interior, the sweet taste causes fullness in the middle burner; for this the Qi of the concerned person accumulates in the upper burner and results in *xiaoke*, exhaustion – thirst.>[5]

What this little text section introduces may be understood as the diabetic syndrome as a result of malnutrition. Malnutrition impairs the spleen Qi and makes the spleen unable to fulfill its metabolic task of *yunhua* ("transport and change"). The main symptom is thirst caused by heat and the result is an exhaustion of the inner organs and the body fluids.

Lingshu (46) introduces emotional disorders as pathogen factors causing heat in the interior which may result in the diabetic syndrome:

When the viscera are weak the result not being seldom is *xiaobi*. The yellow Emperor asked: <Where do we know from that the viscera are weak?> Shaoyu answered: <Weakness has to along with extreme hardness, with extreme hardness and a lot of anger; and when the organs are weak they are vulnerable.> The Yellow Emperor answered: <How do we diagnose weakness caused by hardness? Shaoyu answered: <Such a person has thin skin, but the eyes are rigid and piercing, the long eyebrows rise, the heart is hard this hardness causes a lot of anger, anger makes the Qi flow upward against its direction and it accumulates in the thorax, Qi and blood stay contrary to their direction, they expand in the skin, they fill the muscles, the blood vessels don't flow any more, by this heat develops when heat has developed the muscles and the skin exhaust and by this *xiaobi* develops.[…]

This text also explains the pathomechanism of weakness and atrophy of muscles in the diabetic syndrome: an adverse flow of Qi and blood and the undernourishment of muscles and skin.

What was mostly observed in patients suffering from *xiaobi* 消痹 was polyphagia, polyuria, thirst, and a loss of weight; and so the unity of these symptoms was called *san duo yi shao* 三多一少 (three times much one time little). The *Huangdi neijing* mentions several synonyms for the diabetic syndrome like *xiaobi* (exhaustion and obstruction), *pibi* (obstruction of the spleen), *pixiao* 脾消 (exhaustion of the spleen), *gexiao* 隔消 (exhaustion of the diaphragm) and *xiaozhong* 消中 (exhaustion of the middle burner).

During later times, several theories about the pathomechanisms for heat symptoms such as thirst, polyuria and polyphagia developed. During the Tang dynasty

---

5   *Suwen* (47); Yang Weijie, p. 356.

(618–905), Wang Tao (670–755) introduced a threefold division of the diabetic syndrome *xiaoke* 消渴 *xiaozhong* 消中 and *shenxiao* 肾消; and he postulated that in the end, the *xiaoke* syndrome was mostly caused by weakness of the kidney. By the time of the Tang dynasty, the attendant symptoms of the diabetic syndrome were already known. Sun Simiao p. ex. described fatigue, headache, pain in the lower extremities, exhaustion, dyspnea, amenorrhea and abscesses.[6]

During the Yuan dynasty on the base of Wang Tao's three types of *xiaoke*, the division in the three types of the three burners came up which should prevail until the Qing dynasty; and even in some modern textbooks we find this division.

The three types of *xiaoke* are:

Shang xiaoke (Exhaustion-thirst of the upper burner)
Main symptoms: dry throat, thirst, frequent urination with large amounts of urine
Zhong xiaoke (Exhaustion-thirst of the middle burner)
Main symptoms: ravenous appetite, dry stool, dry mouth, weight loss
Xia xiaoke (Exhaustion-thirst of the lower burner)
Main symptoms: frequent urination with fatty urine, dry mouth and lips, thirst, feverish feeling, weak knees and lumbalgia

Nevertheless one recognized that, for clinical practice, these three types were not useful because most patients showed mixed symptoms of all three types and one recognized that these types could even be seen as different states of the same disease.

Since the discovery of the pancreas and its function, the point of view of diabetes in Chinese medicine changed. Nowadays in the field of diabetes, the two medical systems are normally combined and in Chinese medicine one differentiates between three types, based on the duration of the disease and the function of the islet cells.

I Yin deficiency with heat
The latent or initial state of diabetes, normal function of the islet cells and insulin resistance; duration of the diabetic situation is 1 to 5 years.
II Yin and Qi deficiency
The manifest diabetes, reduced function of the islet cells; duration of the diabetic situation is 10 about years.

---

6 See also Riegel, Andrea-Mercedes: *Diabetes und TCM: Traditionelle chinesische Medizin als adjuvante Therapie bei Diabetes mellitus*. Pflaum: München, 2004a, ch. 2. For further information on the history of diabetes in Chinese medicine, see ibid.

III Yin and Yang deficiency
The late state of diabetes, exhaustion of the islet cells; duration of the diabetic situation is over 10 years.[7]

In the first two stages, regulation of metabolism is still possible. After that, only the complications may be treated successfully. Important principles for the diabetes treatment are:

- activation of the blood circulation from the very beginning
- care for the kidney from the very beginning
- treatment either of the metabolism or of the complications

3.1 How Can Acupuncture Help in the Treatment of Diabetes?

In 1974 the point *yishu* 胰输, the *shu*-point of the pancreas, was discovered. It is located on the bladder channel on the level of TH 8.[8] This point may be useful in the case of weak function of the islet cells. Besides this point there are other useful points:

- points resolving phlegm: (these are points which are used in cases of insulin resistance and for the regulation of the metabolism).
  Zhangmen (Liv 13), Zhongwan (Ren 12), Fenglong (St 40) (together with Zusanli St 36)
- points for the activation of the blood circulation
  Zusanli (St 36), Sanyinjiao (Sp 6), the Four Gates Hegu (LI 4) and Taichong (Liv3)
- points for strengthening the Qi
  Zusanli (St 36), Qihai (Ren 6), Qihaishu (Bl 24)
- points for the stabilization of the spleen and the kidney
  Taixi (Ki 3), Shenshu (Bl 23), Zusanli (St 36), Sanyinjiao (Sp 6), Fenglong (St 40), Guanyuan (Ren 4)
- points for the causes
  - stress: Qimen (Liv 14) left side, Taichong (Liv13) left side, Neiguan (Pc 6), Zusanli (St 36)
  - obesity (malnutrition): Zhangmen (Liv 13), Zhongwan (Ren 12), Zusanli (St 36), Liangqiu (St 34)

---

7 Several subtypes are defined but these are rather artificial and the subtype should be defined for every patient individually. In case of the first state, there are normally no corresponding symptoms because the diabetic situation is compensated. The best way is just to adhere to the main principle valid for the corresponding state of diabetes.

8 This point was already mentioned in the *Qianjin yaofang* by Sun Simiao.

The acupuncture treatment for diabetes has been recognized in China since the 1990s owing to the positive results of studies which were carried out in the 80s. As for the treatment of complications such as polyneuropathy or diarrhea, the studies also showed significant ameliorations. The number of sessions was 30 on average.[9] For effective therapy, an adequate dietary regimen is indispensable.

4 Acupuncture for Major Mental Depression

In the modern western world and not only here, mental disorders such as anxiety disorders or major mental depression do occur rather often and they may even be the main reason for absenteeism from work and employees seeking medical advice. The reason is often high physical strain and psychological stress and the fear of not being able to meet all the demands of daily life. Another factor which may be interdependent with mental stress is hormonal disturbances: hormonal disturbances may be the result of mental stress or the reason for mental disturbances. Even malnutrition or food allergies may be responsible for mental disturbances.

In Western medicine, major mental depression and anxiety disorders are strictly defined by the International Classification of Diseases (ICD)-10 (F 30–F 39 for mental depression, F 40–42 for anxiety disorders).

For mental depression we have typical symptoms such as:

- depressive mood
- loss of interest
- fatigue and exhaustion

The additional symptoms are:

- loss of affection
- lack of self-estimation
- lethargy
- sorrow and grief
- lack of concentration, restlessness, anxiety
- pain and sleeplessness

4.1 Emotional Disorders Seen from the Point of View of Chinese Medicine

How does Chinese medicine interpret emotional disorders? The basic substances of the human organism are Qi (Yang) and blood (Yin), whose free flow is essential

---

9   Ibid.

for the body and mental health. Health means free flow of Qi and blood, harmony of Yin and Yang and perfect harmony in the interaction of the inner organs according to the five phases theory. The function of the inner organs and the harmony between them is largely dependent on the emotional balance because emotions are stored in the inner organs and each exaggeration or deficiency in emotions may cause imbalances between the inner organs.[10]

Mental disturbances may cause stagnations in the flow of Qi and blood but the opposite way is also possible: emotional disorders may be the result of Qi stagnation and Qi stagnation may be caused by all kinds of metabolic disorders. "Metabolic disorders" may refer to metabolic processes in the inner organs and in the brain (neurotransmitters). The metabolism in the brain may be influenced by the metabolism in the inner organs. This is the reason why the treatment of mental disorders by the regulation of the metabolism in the inner organs is possible. And this is also understandable from the point of view of Western medicine.

Most kinds of mental depression are associated with the liver, the heart, the spleen and the kidney. As the liver is responsible for the free flow of energy (Qi) this organ may be affected by anger, and stress (*nu* 怒) may cause stagnation of Qi, i.e. – in terms of Western medicine – it might result in metabolic problems even in the metabolism of the neurotransmitters which might impair psychological health. The heart is the organ which stores the *shen*, the consciousness. A weak heart impairs the consciousness, causes lethargy, anxiety and palpitations. The spleen is responsible for the selection of essence which is needed in the brain and partly for the production of Qi and blood. The kidney – in the sense of Chinese medicine – represents the endocrine pivots[11] and the deficiency of its Yin or Yang aspects may be interpreted in different ways.[12]

4.2 Patterns of Disharmony for Mental Depression

The major mental depression pertains to the scope of the Chinese "depression syndrome", *yusheng* 郁症. In the *Great Encyclopedia of Chinese Medicine*, we find a summary of the *yuzheng*:

Yuzheng are diseases which are caused by oppressed emotions and suppressed Qi mechanism. One makes a difference between syndromes of fullness and deficiency. In the syndromes of fullness we find the three categories "suppressed

---

10 See above.
11 For this theory, see Riegel, Andrea-Mercedes: *Die Niere shen. Klassische Konzepte der chinesischen Medizin im Lichte der modernen Schulmedizin.* Bacopa: Schiedberg, 2010.
12 See below.

liver-Qi", "suppressed Qi causes fire", and "suppression of phlegm-Qi".[…] In the syndromes of deficiency there are two types: "Impairment of the shen by long-term suppression of Qi" and "uprising fire caused by Yin-Deficiency".[13]

The *yuzheng* are nevertheless ancient syndromes known in Chinese medicine since the Yuan Dynasty. It was Zhu Zhenheng (1282–1358), one of the famous Four great medical doctors of the Yuan dynasty (1280–1368), who described six different kinds of depression syndromes: the depression syndrome of Qi, blood, dampness, phlegm, heat, and food. All of them are associated with emotional disorders and they influence one another.[14] During the Ming dynasty (1368–1644), the famous physician Zhang Jiebin (1563–1640) added three "emotional depression syndromes": sorrow, mourning and the stress syndrome; and the monograph *Yixue rumen* (Introduction to Chinese medicine) describes the main symptoms of and interdependence between the nine depression syndromes.[15]

We can divide the patterns for mental depression into patterns of fullness (stagnation of Qi) and deficiency (lack of Qi, Yin or Yang).

The most common patterns of fullness are associated with the liver and are based on liver-Qi stagnation. They may be independent from one another or be interpreted as different stages of severity:

Patterns of fullness for mental depression:

	Body symptoms	Mental symptoms	Pulse/tongue
Liver-Qi stagnation	Menstrual disorders, flatulence	Irritability, depression, "burn-out" frustration, resignation, PMS	Livid, slippery border of tongue; chordal pulse
Liver-Qi transforms to heat	Palpitation, thirst, chest pain, headache, bitter taste, constipation	Violent temper, sleeplessness	Chordal rapid pulse
Liver wind	Headache, dizziness, tinnitus, constipation	Viciousness, inability to make decisions	
Liver heat produces phlegm	Headache, dizziness, cough with phlegm, chest pain	Irritability, sleeplessness, vexation restlessness	Dark tongue, red border of tongue, yellow slippery fur; chordal slippery pulse

---

13 *Zhongyi mingci shuyu xuanshi*. Renmin weisheng chubanshe: Beijing, 1989, p. 365.
14 See Riegel, Andrea-Mercedes: "Xianwei jiroutong zonghezheng shu yu yuzheng", Lecture in Beijing, September 5, 2011.
15 Ibid.

	Body symptoms	Mental symptoms	Pulse/tongue
Liver heat attacks the heart	Headache, high blood pressure, red eyes and red face, heat sensation in the head, palpitations	Confusion, irritability, sleeplessness, restlessness, compulsive ideas	Red tongue yellow fur, hard slippery and rapid pulse
Phlegm heat in the heart	Vexation, chest pain,	Confusion, nervousness, restlessness, irritability, sleeplessness, maniac depressive psychosis, laughing without motivation	Red tongue, yellowish slippery fur and rapid tense pulse

Seen from the point of view of modern psychology, we may interpret the patterns as the development of severe depressive episodes on the basis of light depressive episodes. In the event that *shen* cannot be stored by the heart, we may be dealing with mania, maniac depression or hysteria.

The most common patterns of deficiency:

	Body symptoms	Mental symptoms	Pulse/Tongue
Spleen Qi deficiency produces phlegm	Loss of appetite, fatigue, exhaustion, loss of energy, loose stools with phlegm	Progressive confusion, compulsive ideas	Pale tongue with white slippery fur, slippery pulse
Heart-Qi deficiency	Exhaustion, loss of energy, palpitation, dizziness	Mental instability, nervousness, jumpiness	Pale thin tongue, white slippery fur, weak small pulse

The most common Yin or Yang deficiency patterns:

	Body symptoms	Mental symptoms	Pulse/Tongue
Kidney Yin deficiency	Loss of hair, dizziness, osteoporosis, night sweats, lumbago, tinnitus	Depression, anxiety, restlessness, sleeplessness, phobic fear,	Red tongue without or little fur, deep rapid and small pulse
Kidney Yin deficiency with uprising fire	Profuse night sweats, dizziness, palpitations, yellow urine, dry throat,	Anxiety, restlessness, hypersensitivity, insomnia, poor concentration	Red tongue with little yellow fur, thin and rapid pulse

	Body symptoms	Mental symptoms	Pulse/Tongue
Kidney Yang deficiency	Lack of interest, exhaustion, cold sensation, cold limbs, lumbago, edema, nocturnal urge to void bladder, loose stools	Depression, lethargy, poor will, anxiety	White edematous tongue with white fur, slow and deep pulse
Heart blood/Yin deficiency	Dizziness, palpitation, low energy, dreams, paleness, exhaustion	Nervousness, sleeplessness, lack of concentration, confusion, anxiety	Thin and pale tongue, light white fur, thin pulse

Whereas the patterns of deficiency in the Qi aspect mostly concern the Qi organs (spleen and heart), Yin and Yang deficiency in particular concerns the kidney. Here we may find depressive episodes due to old age, chronic disease or to hormonal disturbances. This is because the kidney in Chinese medicine is responsible for the development of the human organism and the whole neuro-endocrine system.[16] We may find depression here due to the climacteric disorders, to dysfunction of the thyroid gland, disturbances in the hypothalamus – pituitary gland – thyroid gland (HPT) pivot or due to a chronic activation of the stress pivots. We may also think of trauma during childhood. Yin deficiency in general (kidney – Yin, liver – Yin and heart – Yin) also concerns an overload of the sympathetic nervous system.

4.3 Acupuncture Treatment for Major Mental Depression

Mental depression and anxiety disorders are mostly treated with acupuncture in combination with Chinese herbs.

In China the effect of the stimulation of acupoints on mental health and behavior must have been known since the times of the compilation of Huangfu Mi's (215–282) *Zhenjiu jiayi jing* (Classic of Acupuncture in Categories), one of the oldest classics on acupuncture, because here we find hints in a lot of acupoints' names on their mental effect; most of them have the word "*shen*" (spirit) in their name.

Additionally we have points and extra points such as Yingtang (Ex 1), Pc 6 (Neiguan), Pc 7 (Daling), St36 (Zusanli), Lv3 (Taichong) and Tianshu (St 25).

Indeed during the previous 20 years, many randomized studies have been carried out to prove the value of acupuncture in psychotherapy. Many of them used standard recipes combining points which are described in medical literature

---

16 This is one of the main theories of Riegel, Andrea-Mercedes 2010.

as effective on the autonomic nervous system and the limbic system such as He 7, Pc 6, Ex 6, Gb 20, Bl 62) [4,5,7] or Ex 1(Yingtang) combined with Du 20.[17] The results were mostly positive, that is, acupuncture treatment or acupuncture combined with Chinese herbs or antidepressants showed a better effect than conventional treatment.[18]

In Chinese pharmacology, many herbs are highly effective in cases of mental depression and anxiety disorders.

The most important herbs for mental depression:

Name	Effects	Symptoms
Longanae arillus Longyanrou 龙眼肉	Regulates blood Strengthens heart and spleen	Anxiety, palpitations, insomnia, vertigo, exhaustion
Polygalae Radix Yuanzhi 远志	Smoothes liver-Yang, nourishes the kidneys	Palpitations, insomnia, restlessness, lack of consciousness
Platycladi Semen Baiziren 柏子仁	Strengthens liver-Yin and heart-Yin	Palpitations, insomnia, restlessness, transpiration
Poria cocos Fuling 茯苓	Strengthens the kidneys, heart and spleen, calms the spirit	Nervousness, palpitation, vertigo
Jujubae Fructus Dazao 大枣	Nourishes the spleen, calms the spirit	Nervousness, mania, irritability, depressive mood, exhaustion
Ziziphi spinosae Semen Suanzaoren 酸枣仁	Replenishes heart-Yin	Insomnia, anxiety, palpitation
Curcumae longae Tuber Yujin 郁金	Delivers liver-Qi, activates the Qi-circulation	Mental depression
Cyperi rotundus Rhizoma Xiangfu 香附	Activates and regulates Qi	Fullness of the chest, depression, irritability, insomnia
Paeoniae albae Radix Baishaoyao 白芍药	Smoothes the liver, activates Qi	Mental depression, irritability, pain, vertigo

---

17 See Andreescu, Carmen, et al.: "Acupuncture for the Treatment of Major Depressive Disorder: a Randomized Controlled Trial": *Journal of Clinical Psychiatry* 72 (8), 2011, pp. 1129–1135.
18 See He, Qingyong, et al.: "A Controlled Study on Treatment of Mental Depression by Acupuncture plus TCM Medication". *Journal of Traditional Chinese Medicine* 27 (3), 2007, pp. 166–169.

Name	Effects	Symptoms
Citri reticulatae Pericarpium Chenpi 陈皮	Resolves phlegm, activates Qi	Depression, nervousness, fullness of chest
Acori Rhizoma Shichangpu 石菖蒲	Regulates Qi, delivers liver-Qi	Depression, phobia, mental disturbances in general
Albiziae Cortex Hehuanpi 合欢皮	Calms shen, activates Qi	Nervousness, irritation, anxiety, insomnia
Tritici Fructus Xiaomai 小麦	Replenishes heart-blood	Nervousness, insomnia, palpitation

The main principles for treatment are:
Selection of

- body points which are known for their mental effects
- scalp points
- body points with no mental effect but fitting for the corresponding disharmony pattern

The selection of herbs is made according to the disharmony pattern and herbs with effects on mental disturbances are added to the recipe.

5 Acupuncture for Female Sterility

Acupuncture is very effective in treating female sterility. It is a fact that, during the previous twenty years, female sterility has become an increasing problem and a main reason for this may be the lifestyle changes that have occurred over the previous thirty years, particularly stress and mental pressure.

As early as the Song-Jin-Yuan-Dynasty (960–1367), practitioners recognized that anger, jealousy and emotional disorders in general could impair fertility in women.[19] This is still true for women in modern times. Which factors are responsible for the female fertility?

Chinese medicine says the woman is dominated by blood. One sees this in the menstrual blood which flows once in a month. Regularity, quality, consistence, odor and color of the so-called Yin blood are the factors which give information on the female organism and determine the female fertility. So the first principle

---

19 This basic knowledge became a main topic of the new literary genre in Ming time's medicine, the *Guangsi* 广嗣 literature which deals with the question of how to increase progeny.

for treatment an unfulfilled desire for children was and still is the regulation of the menstruation (*tiao jing* 调经).

5.1 What Are the Preconditions for a Regular Menstruation?

Menstruation depends on the organs which are responsible for the production of blood, the kidney and the spleen; the liver stores the blood and is responsible for the regular flow of blood. Chongmai and Renmai are the two vessels which are the "sea of blood" (Chongmai) and the "sea of all channels" (Renmai), respectively. They have their origin in the *baozhong* 胞中 which, in the female organism, might be interpreted as the uterus. It is the liver which opens this sea of blood every 28 days.

To make this Yin blood fertile it needs the *tiangui* 天癸, the "heavenly water". *Tiangui* is part of the essence of preheaven and it "arrives" (*zhi* 至) in the female organism at the age of fourteen and in the male organism at the age of sixteen.[20] The arrival of the *tiangui* in the female body becomes visible in the first menstruation; at the age of 49 it is exhausted. *Tiangui* loses its influence on the production of the Yin blood, the surplus in Chongmai and Renmai is absent and so menstruation stops.

Sterility may first be caused by a deficiency of blood and deficiency of blood may be caused by:

- a weak function of the organs responsible for the blood production (spleen and kidney)
- weak function of the liver
- exhaustion or blockage of Chongmai and Renmai
- lack of *tiangui*

Other blood disorders or menstrual disorders which, according to Chinese medicine, may result in sterility are: cold blood in the uterus, blood heat, and stagnation of blood caused by Qi stagnation.

Factors which may impair the function of the inner organs are those which impair the flow of Qi and blood, for example – as mentioned above – malnutrition, obesity, emotional disorders such as anxiety disorders, mental depression, stress and anger.

---

20 See *Suwen* (1).

The main patterns for female sterility which may be lifestyle-related are:

- blood deficiency caused by weakness of the kidney or the spleen or lack of heart blood
- cold in the uterus caused by deficiency of kidney Yang
- blood heat mostly caused by liver fire
- Qi stagnation mostly caused by liver-Qi stagnation or Qi deficiency

Main points for all types of female sterility are:
  Guilai (St 29), Guanyuan (Ren 4), Qihai (Ren 6), Sanyinjiao (Sp 6), Zusanli (St 36), Taichong (Liv 3).

5.2 Main Patterns for Female Sterility

5.2.1 Blood Deficiency

Main symptoms: little menstruation, pale blood color, prolonged cycle, paleness, "emptiness" in the vagina, fatigue, vertigo
Pulse-tongue diagnosis: pale thin tongue, fine rapid pulse
Causes: malnutrition, malabsorption, weakness of the kidney and/or the spleen
Interpretation: anemia, insufficiency of the corpus luteum
Acupuncture: Guilai (St 29), Guanyuan (Ren 4), Geshu (Bl 17) – Pishu (Bl 20) (the four blossom points), Zusanli (St 36) and Sanyinjiao (Sp 6), Xuehai (Sp 10)

5.2.2 Cold in the Uterus

Main symptoms: prolonged rhythm, dysmenorrhea heat application improves the pain, the color of menstrual blood is violet; cold extremities
Pulse-tongue diagnosis: white tongue, deep and stingy pulse
Causes: absorption of cold by frequent bathing in cold water, extreme light clothing, malnutrition with cold food
Interpretation: lack of Yang may be interpreted as a lack of progesterone which brings about arise in body temperature. The violet blood color also indicates a lack of progesterone (insufficiency of the corpus luteum)
Acupuncture: Guilai (St 29), Guanyuan plus moxa (Ren 4), Shenshu (Bl 23), Taixi (Ki 3), Zusanli (St 36), Sanyinjiao (Sp 6)

5.2.3 Blood Heat

Main symptoms: great amount of blood during menstruation, burning pain, powerful red color of the blood of thick consistency, short rhythm; nervousness, thirst

Pulse-tongue diagnosis: dark red tongue with yellow coat, rapid and stingy pulse
Causes: liver fire by emotional disorders (stress and anger)
Acupuncture: Guilai (St 29), Dadou (Sp 1), Rangu (Ki 2), Xuehai (Sp 10), Zusanli (St 36), Sanyinjiao (Sp 6)

5.2.4 Liver-Qi Stagnation

Main symptoms: irregular cycle, dark lumpy menstrual blood, dysmenorrhea and the passing of lumps relieves pain; depressive mood, internal unrest, irritability, fullness of chest and abdomen.
Pulse-tongue diagnosis: livid tongue, smooth tongue frenulum, overfilled sublingual veins, stingy pulse
Cause: stress, depression
Acupuncture: Danzhong (Ren 17), Qimen (Liv 14), Taichong (Liv 3), Neiguan (Pc 6), Zusanli (St 36), Sanyinjiao (Sp 6)

5.2.5 Kidney Deficiency

Main symptoms: small amount of menstrual blood, thin consistency; pain in the lower abdomen and the knees, lack of concentration, weakness in the loins and knees, light tinnitus
Pulse-tongue diagnosis: pale tongue with white coat, deep weak pulse
Cause: mainly body and emotional exhaustion, long time use of the contraceptive pill, malnutrition
Acupuncture: Guanyuan (Ren 4), Shenshu (Bl 23), Pishu (Bl 20), Guilai (St 29), Taixi (Ki 3), Zusanli (St 36), Sanyinjiao (Sp 6)

It takes about three cycles of acupuncture with treatment twice a week; the days of menstruation are free. Moreover it is useful to add herbal treatment and adequate nourishment to the acupuncture treatment. After three cycles of treatment the quality of menstrual blood and the general situation of the woman should have significantly improved.

6 Acupuncture for High Blood Pressure

High blood pressure is the most common symptom in modern life. It is mostly the consequence of stress and overburden in work. Further risk factors are malnutrition, nicotine and alcohol. Other causes may be seen in hormonal disturbances (hyperthyreosis) or in renal dysfunction or stenosis of the renal artery. This stenosis might be caused by plaques ("phlegm"); and high blood viscosity – caused, for example, by high cholesterol – is another factor which may be subsumed under the concept of phlegm. From the point of view of Chinese medicine, we see the involvement of the liver and the kidney and as a main factor we also see "phlegm".

The main disharmony patterns for – lifestyle-related – high blood pressure may be:

- uprising Liver-Yang
- liver wind causing heat in the heart and phlegm
- heat phlegm annoying the heart
- weak kidney water doesn't extinguish heart fire

The main points for high blood pressure may be divided into different categories:
Points soothing the liver:
> Fengchi (Gb 29)
> Yanglingquan (Gb 34)
> Xingjian (Liv 2)
> Taichong (Liv 3)
> Ganshu (Bl 18)
> Neiguan (Pc 6)

Points resolving phlegm:
> Zhong wan (Ren 12)
> Juque (Ren 14)
> Fenglong (St 40)
> Jiexi (St 41)

Points reinforcing the kidney:
> Shenshu (Bl 23)
> Taixi (Ki 3)
> Zhaohai (Ki 6)
> Sanyinjiao (Sp 6)

Points activating the flow of Qi:
> Zusanli (St 36)
> Danzhong (Ren 17)

6.1 The Different Main Patterns for High Blood Pressure

6.1.1 Uprising Liver Yang

Main symptoms: high blood pressure (systolic and diastolic), choleric behavior, palpitation, irritability, red face, headache (migraine), thirst
Pulse-tongue diagnosis: red tongue with yellow coat, stringy pulse
Causes/interpretation: stress, anger

Acupuncture: Fengchi (Gb 20), Yanglingquan (Gb 34), Xingjian (Liv 2), Sanyinjiao (Sp 6), Neiguan (Pc 6), Shenmen (He 7)

6.1.2 Liver Wind Causing Heat in the Heart and Phlegm

Main symptoms: high blood pressure (systolic and diastolic), dizziness, vertigo, headache, fullness in the chest, difficulty in breathing
Pulse-tongue diagnosis: stiff and vibrating tongue, slippery tongue
Causes: plaques, emotional disorders, stress and anger and/or high blood fat
Interpretation: precursors of a heart attack; blockage of the coronary vessels
Acupuncture: Fengchi (Gb 20), Yanglingquan (Gb 34), Sanyinjiao (Sp 6), Juque Ren (14), Neiguan (Pc 6), Jiexi (St 41), Zusanli (St 36)

6.1.3 Heat Phlegm Annoying the Heart

Main symptoms: high blood pressure (systolic and diastolic), difficulty in breathing, fullness in the chest, unrest, palpitations, extra systoles
Pulse-tongue diagnosis: red tongue, red tip of tongue, slippery yellowish coat, slippery rapid pulse
Causes/Interpretation: high blood fat, vegetative disorders
Acupuncture: Danzhong (Ren 17), Juque (Ren 14), Shenmen (He 7), Fenglong (St 40), Zusanli (St 36), Sanyinjiao (St 6), Neiguan (Pc 6)

6.1.4 Weak Kidney Water Doesn't Extinguish Heart Fire

Main symptoms: high blood pressure (systolic), nervousness, palpitation, exhaustion, heat sensation, night sweat, sleeplessness
Pulse-tongue diagnosis: red tongue red tip of tongue, little whitish coat
Causes/Interpretation: Exhaustion, vegetative dystonia
Acupuncture: Guanyuan (Ren 4), Taixi (Ki 3), Shenmen (He 7), Zusanli (St 36), Danzhong (Ren 17), Zhaohai (Ki 6)

Successful treatment requires at least 15 sessions and changes in lifestyle.

7 Conclusion

In China it appears that the scope of indications for classical acupuncture treatment has either changed or been widened to include lifestyle-related diseases. The treatment of lifestyle-related diseases has become very popular in China, either as a single treatment or alongside Western medication. The main indications are: diabetes and its complications; sterility/infertility; high blood pressure;

psychosomatic pain; and major mental depression in less severe cases. Studies have proved acupuncture's efficiency but nevertheless a change of lifestyle such as eating habits or the reduction of stress is compulsory.

References

Andreescu, Carmen, et al.: "Acupuncture for the Treatment of Major Depressive Disorder: A Randomized Controlled Trial". *Journal of Clinical Psychiatry* 72 (8), 2011, pp. 1129–1135.

Eich, H., et al.: "Akupunktur bei leichten bis mittelschweren depressiven Episoden und Angststörungen; Ergebnisse einer experimentellen Untersuchung". *Fortschritte der Neurologie Psychiatrie* (68) 2000, pp. 137–144.

Eich, H, et al..: "Beeinflusst Akupunktur die autonom kardiale Regulation bei Patienten mit leichten depressiven Episoden oder Angststörungen? Eine randomisierte, placebokontrollierte Verlaufsstudie" *Fortschritte der Neurologie. Psychiatrie* 71, 2003, pp. 141–149.

Fu, Wen-bin, et al.: "Depressive Neurosis Treated by Acupuncture for Regulating the Liver – A Report of 176 Cases". *Journal of Traditional Chinese Medicine* 29 (2), 2009, pp. 83–86.

He, Qingyong, et al.: "A Controlled Study on Treatment of Mental Depression by Acupuncture plus TCM Medication". *Journal of Traditional Chinese Medicine* 27 (3), 2007, pp. 166–169.

Hollifield, Michael, et al.: "Acupuncture for Posttraumatic Stress Disorder – A Randomized Controlled Pilot Trial". *The Journal of Nervous and Mental Diseases* 195 (6), 2007, pp. 504–513.

Li, Ting: *Yixue Rumen.* (Introduction to Medicine). Zhongguo zhong yiyao chubanshe: Beijing, 1995 (orig. 1575).

(*Huangdi neijing*) *Lingshu yishi.* (The Translated and Annotated Edition of the Heavenly Pivot of the Classic of Internal Medicine of the Yellow Emperor). Shanghai kexue jishu chubanshe: Shanghai, 1997.

Maric-Oehler, Walburg: "Akupunktur bei depressiver Verstimmung". *Zeitschrift für Komplementärmedizin* 4, 2010, pp. 42–4.

Qi Hao: *Zhongyi mingci shuyu xuanshi* (Explanations of Selected Terms of Chinese Medicine). Renmin weisheng chubanshe: Beijing, 1989.

Riegel, Andrea-Mercedes: *Das Streben nach dem Sohn. Fruchtbarkeit und Empfängnis in den medizinischen Texten Chinas von der Hanzeit bis zur Mingzeit.* Utz: München, 1999.

Riegel, Andrea-Mercedes: *Diabetes und TCM: Traditionelle chinesische Medizin als adjuvante Therapie bei Diabetes mellitus.* Pflaum: München, 2004a.

Riegel, Andrea-Mercedes: "Kidney and Psyche". Wallner, Friedrich/Lan, Fengli (eds.) *Shen, Pschotherapy and Acupuncture. Theory, Methodology and Structure of Chinese Medicine.* Peter Lang: Frankfurt, 2004b.

Riegel, Andrea-Mercedes: *Die Niere shen: Klassische Konzepte der chinesischen Medizin im Lichte der modernen Schulmedizin.* Bacopa: Schiedberg, 2010.

Riegel, Andrea-Mercedes: "Xianwei jiroutong zonghezheng shu yu yusheng" (Fibromyalgia: An Example for Yuzheng), Lecture in Beijing, September 5, 2011.

Riegel, Andrea-Mercedes: "Yuzheng, ein vergessenes Syndrom der chinesischen Medizingeschichte". *Report Naturheilkunde* 15 (6), 2011, pp. 47–54.

Schnyer, Rosa N./Allen, John: *Akupunktur bei Depressionen.* Urban & Fischer: München, 2007.

Unschuld, Paul/Tessenow, Herrmann: *Huang Di Nei Jing Su Wen.* University of California Press: Berkeley, 2011.

Xu Guoqian: *Zhenjiu jiayi jing jiaozhu* (Revised edition of the Classic of Acupuncture) et al. Renmin weisheng chubanshe: Beijing, 1996.

Yang, Weijie: *Huangdi neijing Suwen shijie* (Modern Translation and Explanations of the Classic of Internal Medicine of the Yellow Emperor). Yuejun wenhua shuye gongsi: Taibei, 1990.

Zhang, Jiebin: *Jingyue Quanshu* (The Collected Works by Zhang Jingyue). Shanghai kexue jishu chubanshe: Shanghai, 1996.

Zhang, Zhang-Jin: "The Effectiveness and Safety of Acupuncture Therapy in Depressive Disorders: Systematic Review and Meta Analysis". *Journal of Affective Disorders* 124 (1–2), 2010, pp. 9–21.

Zou Hua/Riegel, Andrea-Mercedes: *Akupunktur bei Blutungsstörungen und Zyklusanomalien.* Haug: Heidelberg, 2001.

Kwon Jong Yoo

Acupuncture and Placebo Effect

Abstract: This research compares different theories of placebo effects of acupuncture, traditional Chinese medicine (TCM), in experiments reported from countries in Europe, Australia, China, and Korea and to discuss whether acupuncture is an effective medicine or not.

1 Study Design

Target: This research compares different theories of placebo effects of acupuncture, Chinese traditional medicine, in experiments reported from countries in Europe, Australia, China, and Korea and to discuss whether acupuncture is an effective medicine or not. Some opinions insist that acupuncture is just a placebo and cannot be counted as an effective treatment. Others argued that in some cases there is little difference between real acupuncture (RA) and sham acupuncture (SA), while in other cases there have been a clear difference between the two.

Approach: First it is to compare different opinions of acupuncture. In this study, at least three different opinions are studied, each of which is backed up by designed experiments or empirical data. The most extreme opinion established in the United Kingdom is that acupuncture is not effective at all, because it cannot guarantee any physical and physiological effect even after long-term acupuncture. But the other opinion in Australia, China, and Korea, accept acupuncture as an effective medicine, even though each of them has different results from placebos in their experiments.

Argument:

1) Is acupuncture a placebo or not?
2) What is/are the real factor(s) of acupuncture efficacy, if the acupuncture has actual efficacy in treatment of illness, disease, disorder, sickness, etc.?
3) Is the meridian system acceptable to non-Asian people?

2 Research Motive and Direction of Discussion

Acupuncture is plainly one of the very influential and popular medicines in the East Asian countries. Many people still seek acupuncture clinics to treat their sufferings from various kinds of illness, disease, pain, etc. In Korea, most acupuncture clinics treat patients not only for acupuncture but also for moxibustion and traditional medication. But after Western medicine established itself as the most effective medicine in East Asian societies, acupuncture and other treatments, for example moxibustion, medication, acupressure, etc., became less popular than Western medicine. Even though many people use acupuncturists as a remedy for their suffering, most recognize the limitations of acupuncture in treating incurable diseases, i.e., kinds of cancer, cardiac disease, etc. On the other hand, diseases for which the acupuncture is effective include paraesthesia that comes from nervous function acceleration, muscle pain, tonic pain, desensitization that comes from visceral function acceleration and functional disorder of nerve, myoparalysis, visceral hypofunction, etc.

In addition, most Koreans share a common belief that the 'gi/qi' (氣/气) exists and flows inside a body to keep a balance in the whole body, and even the body-mind system. This belief is supported by the meridian system that has been developed and accepted by traditional Korean medicine (TKM) that shares most ideas with traditional Chinese medicine (TCM). This meridian system is in fact not only backs up the acupuncture, moxibustion, and medication theory but also acupressure, meridian massage, and even the Daoist regimen, etc. According to this belief in the meridian system, East Asian medicine and ancillary therapies have their own traditions of medical therapies that are very different from Western traditions.

Recently, in the 1970s, acupuncture and moxibustion have again drawn the West's attention after a journalist, James Reston, in the *New York Times* described his experience of acupuncture for postoperative pain. Because of this, they have become more popular aided by active researchers on TCM as well as operations at TCM in clinics. Acupuncture and even the whole TCM have developed a very different methodology from Western medicine and based on a very different etiology. One of the most typical ideas of etiology in TCM and TKM is the meridian system in which the gi/qi is flowing everywhere in a body. However, the flow of gi/qi is not easily accepted by the Westerners, including many medical doctors, because the flow of gi/qi seems impossible to prove. Therefore, the use of them still incurs suspicion in European and American medical expert groups as well as in patients. Some specialists suggest that acupuncture is a theatrical placebo for which the idea of meridians is purely imaginary.[1] This idea shows that the acupuncture may be quackery or pseudoscience. Although some scholars refuted

---

1 Colquhoun, D./Novella, SP.: "The Acupuncture is Theatrical Placebo". *Anesthsia & Analgesics*, Vol. 116, No. 6: 1360–1363, the International Anesthesia Research Society, June 2013.

such a negative idea about acupuncture,[2] arguments on the efficacy and justification of the theoretical basis of the efficacy in the European culture of medicine continue.

Such conflicts between support and non-support of acupuncture efficacy are serious also in contemporary Korean society, because most doctors of Western medicine in Korea do not believe in acupuncture efficacy and even true the value of TKM/TCM. What is worse, they are blocking patients from seeing acupuncturists for treatment and citing extremely negative cases of failure in acupuncture treatment. The conflicts are supposedly based on the same reasons as in Western societies.

For removing possible misunderstanding or a lack of appreciation, it is necessary to implement not only experiments that verify real effects of acupuncture but philosophical studies that make Western people understand the TCM theory of the meridian system. Of course, many of them have become widespread in the East and West. While many of these experiments should supply medical evidence for justification of the meridian system, the philosophical studies of the meridian system, such as the type of the arguments, is linked to the conception on human body and health. In fact, no amount of the experiments would place them into compliance without convincing them of the conception of gi/qi or the meridian system.

For this reason, acupuncture and the placebo effect should be linked to make it clear the origin of the Western people's misunderstanding or lack of the effect of the acupuncture and simultaneously how to advance people's understanding of the acupuncture and meridian system.

3 Arguments on the Placebo Effect in Acupuncture

Opinions of the placebo effect in acupuncture could be divided into three categories: Firstly that acupuncture is a placebo that has no real effect in curing, secondly it is effective regardless of real and sham or negative results against deqi sensation, and finally it is effective only in RA and very positive for the deqi sensation. But one has to realize that every experiment is only a partial approach to the whole meridian system and that some of them used functional magnetic resonance imaging (fMRI), positron emission tomography (PET), SPECT, electroencephalogram (EEG), etc., in order to check physiological change and real

---

2   Wang, S-M./Harris, RE./Lin, Y-C./Gan, T-J.: "Acupuncture in 21st Century Anesthesia: Is There a Needle in the Haystack?". *Anesthesia & Analgesics*, Vol. 116, No. 6: 1356–1359, June 2013.

medical effect. But some of them, whether or not using such approved measuring devices, emphasized 'deqi' (得氣/得气) effect as the direct evidence of the acupuncture effectiveness. Let me describe experiments in the three categories by paying attention to their methods, results, opinions, and conclusions.

3.1 The First Category: Acupuncture is Totally Placebo with no Real Effect

An article, "The Acupuncture is Theatrical Placebo",[3] published in 2013 by David Colquhoun and Steven P. Novella made an extremely negative opinion as the title showed. The authors insist that:

[The outcome of this research, we propose, is that the benefits of acupuncture are likely nonexistent, or at best are too small and too transient to be of any clinical significance. It seems that acupuncture is little or no more than a theatrical placebo.] (Colquhoun, David/Novella, Steven P.: "The Acupuncture is Theatrical Placebo". *Anesth Analg*, Volume 116, Number 6, the *International Anesthesia Research Society*, June 2013, P. 1360.)

Their opinion is supported with roughly two kinds of strong evidence. Whereas the first kind embraces historical evidence that acupuncture efficacy was denied by Chinese leaders themselves, the second is a meta-analysis of experiments on acupuncture operations to some special body problems under controlled conditions.

According to the authors, the acupuncture has been present in China for thousands of years, it has not been always popular. The decisive evidences in Chinese history that denied the acupuncture efficacy are the cases of Emperor Dao Guang in Qing Dynasty and Mao Zedong in modern China. The Emperor issued an imperial edict stating that acupuncture and moxibustion should be banned forever from the Imperial Medical Academy. And in the case of Mao Zedong, they stated that Mao Zedong and the Communist Party he led ridiculed TCM including acupuncture as superstitious. In addition Mao personally preferred Western medicine, even though he as Chairman of the party revived TCM as part of the Great Proletarian Cultural Revolution. He is reported to have siad, "[Even though I believe we should promote Chinese medicine, I personally do not believe in it. I do not take Chinese medicine.]" (Colquhoun, David/Novella, Steven P., "The Acupuncture is Theatrical Placebo", 2013, P1360.)

The authors do not recognize that acupuncture has enough evidence to check the effectiveness by fMRI or endorphin release studies, and would not acknowledge most individual studies could be proper evidence because 'inconsistency'

---

3   Colquhoun, D./Novella, S.P., ibid.

is a prominent characteristic of acupuncture research. And the heterogeneity of results from every individual research, according to them, poses a problem for meta-analysis. Though such heterogeneity and inconsistency, they considered only meta-analysis for development of their negative idea.

Only one thing that is unanimously accepted is that the benefits of acupuncture are for analgesia, but they are too small to be helpful to patients according to the authors. Rather, the authors insisted that the apparent improvement after acupuncture is merely a placebo effect invoking statistical evidence as follows:

[Large multicenter clinical trials conducted in Germany and the United States consistently revealed that verum (or true) acupuncture and sham acupuncture treatments are no different in decreasing pain levels across multiple chronic pain disorders: migraine, tension headache, low back pain, and osteoarthritis of the knee.] (Colquhoun, David/Novella, Steven P., "The Acupuncture is Theatrical Placebo". P. 1361.)

The main reason why apparent improvement after acupuncture is merely a placebo effect lies in the statistical fact that RA and SA treatments are no different in decreasing pain levels. Even though some meta-analyses have found that there may be a small difference between sham and RA and a somewhat bigger difference between the acupuncture group and the no-acupuncture group, they ignored the difference as a 'minimal' or 'little change' that is corresponded to only a 10-point improvement on a 100-point pain scale. Thus, it is not big enough for the patient to notice much effect.[4] They cited a few more experimental results that similarly supported their opinion besides those above.

According to the authors, acupuncture should, ideally, be tested separately for effectiveness for each individual condition for which it has been proposed (like so many other forms of alternative medicine, that is a very large number). Good quality trials, however, according to them, have not been done for all of them, but results suggest strongly that it is unlikely that acupuncture works for rheumatoid arthritis, stopping smoking, irritable bowel syndrome, or for losing weight. There is also no good reason to think it works for addictions, asthma, chronic pain, depression, insomnia, neck pain, shoulder pain or frozen shoulder, osteoarthritis of the knee, sciatica, stroke or tinnitus, and many other conditions. They highly regard official judgment of authority. Even though in 2009 the United Kingdom's National Institute for Clinical Excellence did recommend acupuncture for back pain, another organization, the Oxford Centre for Evidence-Based Medicine, came up with its updated verdict as follows: "[**Clinical bottom line.** Acupuncture

---

4   Ibid., p. 1361.

is no better than a toothpick for treating back pain.]" (Colquhoun, David/Novella, Steven P.: "The Acupuncture is Theatrical Placebo". P. 1361.)

In conclusion, they insist it is clear from meta-analyses that results of acupuncture trials are variable and inconsistent, even for single conditions, and after thousands of trials of acupuncture and hundreds of systematic reviews, arguments continue unabated. They thought that any more trials are not useful, because it has proved impossible to find consistent evidence after more than 3000 trials. According to them, the best-controlled studies show a clear pattern, with acupuncture the outcome does not depend on needle location or even needle insertion. They emphasized that since these variables are those that define acupuncture, the only sensible conclusion is that acupuncture does not work.

They don't believe that the efficacy of acupuncture for the following reasons:

"[Everything else is the expected noise of clinical trials, and this noise seems particularly high with acupuncture research. The brief conclusion is that for acupuncture there is no signal, only noise.]" (Colquhoun, David/Novella, Steven P., "The Acupuncture is Theatrical Placebo", P. 1362.)

3.2 The Second Category: Acupuncture Is Effective Regardless of Deqi Sensation

An article, "Different Responses to Acupuncture in Electroencephalogram according to Stress Level: A Randomized, Placebo-Controlled, Cross-Over Trial",[5] has a different conclusion from the above. It reports the result of an experiment designed to examine how acupuncture treatment at Shenmen (HT7) affects brain activity and the automatic nervous system (ANS) by using EEGs and heart rate variability (HRV). The results in the report show a very positive function and effect of acupuncture by measuring changes in brain activities, ANS, and HRV with acupuncture at the point of HT7. And methodologically this research has a feature that it applied a stress level to establish an unbalanced condition, instead of a pain model, which had been used in previous acupuncture studies.[6] A main hypothesis of the study is that stimulations of HT7, which is used on the psychological and nerve problems would have an effect on the stress levels of the participants.[7] Why the research team chose the HT7 as their acupuncture point

---

5   Kim, S-Y./Kim, S-W./Park, H-J.: "Different Responses to Acupuncture in Electroencephalogram according to Stress Level: A Randomized, Placebo-Controlled, Cross-Over Trial". *Korean Journal of Acupuncture*, Vol. 31, No. 3: 136–145, 2014.
6   Ibid., p. 142.
7   Ibid.

lies in that the HT7 has been used for neurological or psychiatric disorder, clinically.[8] According to their references, acupuncture treatment at the HT7 activates parasympathetic nerve works on stress levels with decreasing tachycardia induced by stress, decreases the rising heart rate, improves insomnia, and is effective for depression-induced maternal separation in animal studies and for anxiety-like behavior following nicotine withdrawal.

Methods used in the experiment are as follow. Eighteen healthy volunteers participated in two separate experiments. In each experiment, either RA or non-penetrating SA was applied at HT7 in random sequences to each person. The EEG and HRV measurements were conducted simultaneously before and during the acupuncture stimulation for five minutes, respectively. Resulting EEG and HRV parameters were compared between RA and SA groups. To assess differences according to the stress levels for participants, subgroup analysis was performed based on the results of the stress response index questionnaire.

The results are as follow: In the results, acupuncture stimulation at HT7 increased α-frequency in EEG. In the HRV analysis, heart rate was decreased significantly but HF band (high-frequency component; 0.15–0.40 Hz) and root mean square of the successive differences (RMS-SD) were increased in the RA group, compared to those of the SA group. In the subgroup analysis by stress level, participants in the RA group with high stress exhibited an increase in the α-band in their EEG while the low-stress participants showed a decrease or small increase in the band. For the SA group, the α-band reported relatively moderate changes in all channels.[9]

This research concludes that acupuncture induces changes in brain activation and the ANS, and acupuncture was related to the activation of the parasympathetic nervous system, but the brain activities of the participants were different depending on the stress level.[10]

As introduced above, the research team confirms the efficacy of acupuncture depending on the brain activation, and activation of parasympathetic nervous system. But the team paid attention to the variation depending on the stress level. What the team importantly observed shows little difference between RA patients group and SA group and rather more difference relying on individual patient's condition, i.e., stress level. According to the team, the individual patient's

---

8   Ibid.
9   Ibid.
10 Ibid., p. 136.

variations might be due to the unbalanced Yin-Yang in the individuals, which can be rebalanced by readjusting the participant's qi.[11]

One of the important ideas that the study disclosed is that there was no correlation between deqi sensation and the EEG or HRV results. The reason why they had no meaningful consequence of the deqi sensation on the acupuncture point HT7 is attributed to the fact that there was some needle stimulation in the SA groups (although the needle was blunt) or may be due to the weak stimulation of acupuncture in the RA group.[12] However, the reason why they did not get meaningful data of deqi from their experiments is related to distinct characteristics of the HT7 point. The article shows some references about such characteristics and among them some persuasive as follow: "[The HT7 acupuncture point's anatomical position is known for the likelihood of inducing less deqi sensation compared with other points such as LI4 and ST36 which widely used in deqi studies.]" (Kim, Song-Yi/Kim, Sang-Woo/Park, Hi-Joon: "Different Responses to Acupuncture in Electroencephalogram according to Stress Level: A Randomized, Placebo-Controlled, Cross-Over Trial". Korean Journal of Acupuncture, Vol. 31, No. 3, 2014. P. 143.) A study which compared the deqi sensation using HT7 and S16 showed that both have deqi sensation, that the brain responses were different for each. Therefore, the research team said, direction of further studies could be to compare and further elucidate deqi sensation for the different acupoints instead of grouping them together.

The findings of the study showed that acupuncture affects one's autonomic nervous system functions and brain activity in specific ways, and that participants' EEG and HRV result are different in the RA and SA groups depending on their stress level. But the study failed to show the precise relationship or reason for EEG changes in the autonomic nervous function.[13]

The study concluded that acupuncture is a means to control balance of the human body, and therefore, treatment of symptoms depends greatly on the individual patient's physiology and condition.[14]

---

11 Ibid., p. 142.
12 Ibid., p. 143.
13 Ibid.
14 Ibid.

3.3 The Third Category: It Is Effective Only in RA and Positive for the Deqi Sensation

Being different from the study in the second category, another research article, "Characterization of Deqi Sensation and Acupuncture Effect",[15] is important because it shows the interrelationship of neuro-imaging on the deqi sensation and acupuncture effect and discusses the physiological mechanism of deqi. Also it emphasizes the relation between deqi and clinical efficacy.

This article focuses on a discussion of deqi, a composite of unique sensations that arises when acupuncture needles stimulate certain acupoints on the body. According to this article, the application of acupuncture through stimulating certain acupoints is to activate the qi and blood of meridians and collaterals and to regulate the function of internal organs so as to prevent and treat diseases in TCM theory. Deqi in the article is literally defined as 'the arrival of vital energy' that acupuncture stimulation elicits and is regarded as a prerequisite for clinical effects, also an important judgment of the exuberance and decline of meridian qi and the prognosis of diseases.[16]

According to the article, in recent years, evocation of deqi has been paid increasing attention in clinical trials of acupuncture, but the physiological mechanisms that produce deqi effect are still not well understood. To elucidate more about the deqi, for example, a description of deqi from both the patients' and the acupuncturists' perspective and examination of the relationship between deqi and therapeutic effect, clinical characterization of the deqi, qualitative and quantitative measurement of deqi, and physiological mechanisms of deqi effect are focused in this study.

Though the literal definition mentioned above, deqi is commonly translated as "needle sensation," sometimes as "arrival of qi" or "needling response", and current view holds that there is no significant difference between them. However, these three meanings are often differently understood as follow. Needling sensation mainly means subjective feelings and perceived responses of patients and acupuncturists; arrival of qi means a healing process, which activates the antipathogenic qi to expel the pathogens; needling response suggests the final aim of acupuncture.[17] Generally deqi is a description of the subjective sensations felt

---

15 Yang, X-Y./Shi, G-X./Li, Q-Q./Zhang, Z-H./Xu, Q./Liu, C-Z.: "Characterization of Deqi Sensation and Acupuncture Effect". *Evidence-Based Complementary and Alternative Medicine*, Vol. 2013, Hindawi Publishing Corporation, 2013.
16 Ibid., p. 1.
17 Ibid.

by the patients during acupuncture treatment, but some others argue that deqi comprises not only the patients' sensations but also the acupuncturists' senses.[18] Furthermore, there are few people suggesting that denials include propagated sensation along meridians and the externally visible signs due to acupuncture treatment.[19] As such, deqi can be understood in diversity, but the most important and main idea is the subjective sign of the patient during acupuncture treatment that can be felt or observed by the acupuncturist.

Therefore in this article, characterization of deqi is separated into three situations; felt by the patients, felt by the acupuncturists, and physical signs due to acupuncture treatment. In fact it is said that the patients' sensations and the acupuncturists' senses are closely linked.[20]

[When the acupuncturists feel tense or tight, the patients usually experience soreness, numbness, fullness, or heaviness at the same time. Under the circumstances that the qi has not arrived, the patients have no special sensation or response and acupuncturists feel slow, slipping, or empty. It has been vividly described in classical prose named "biao you fu" (标幽赋).] (Yang, Xing-Yue/Shi, Guang-Xia/Li, Qian-Qian/Zhang, Zhen-Hua/Xu, Qian/Liu, Cun-Zhi: "Characterization of Deqi Sensation and Acupuncture Effect". *Evidence-Based Complementary and Alternative Medicine*, Volume 2013, Hindawi Publishing Corporation, 2013. P. 2.)[21]

Following the quoted sentences above, it introduces a generally recognized idea as follows:

[Acupuncture through stimulating certain acupoints may contract intraspindle muscle and then produce myoelectricity. Secondary impulse reaching to central brain produces the patients' needling sensation, and the contraction of local muscle fibers through needle body to needle handle causes the deqi sensation of acupuncturists' hands.] (Yang/Shi et al., "Characterization of Deqi Sensation" 2013, P. 2.)[22]

These sentences might be used, by the authors, to maintain that the deqi can be shared by both of the patients and the acupuncturists.

The most attractive approach in the study is neuroimaging studies on deqi sensation and acupuncture effect in chapter 4. Several tests about relationships between deqi sensation and acupuncture effect using fMRI or PET are reviewed.

---

18 Ibid.
19 Ibid.
20 Ibid., p. 2.
21 Ibid.
22 Ibid.

The fMRI and the PET are among the revolutionary tools to monitor the dynamic response of the whole brain to acupuncture with specific regional localization, and fMRI and PET studies on acupuncture at commonly used acupoints, according to the article, have demonstrated the limbic system and paralimbic, hypothalamus, and subcortical gray structures as the important components in mediating the acupuncture effects and deqi.[23]

Nonetheless it is still in the process to accumulate data of the relationships and thus it is too early to certainly and totally explain the relationships. Some very persuasive research is reviewed to show important advance in gathering the data. Hereby, some researches reviewed in the article are quoted.

[Over the past decade, Hui et al. have built a database of fMRI scans of the brain response to acupuncture at multiple acupoints, LI4 (*hegu*), ST36 (*zusanli*), and LV3 (*taichong*) in healthy adults. Their studies showed that acupuncture deqi evoked deactivation of a limbic-paralimbic-neocortical network, which encompassed the limbic system as well as activation of somatosensory brain regions. Importantly, Hui et al. consistently observed distinct patterns of limbic network hemodynamic response in the brain, mainly deactivation in deqi and activation in sharp pain.] (Yang/Shi, et al., "Characterization of Deqi Sensation", 2013. P. 4.)[24]

[Hsieh et al. showed via PET that elicitation of deqi resulted in a significant increase of blood flow in the hypothalamus and insula with an extension to the midbrain when compared with minimal or no stimulation after needle insertion at LI4.] (Yang/Shi, et al., "Characterization of Deqi Sensation", 2013. P. 4.)[25]

[Lai et al. revealed a significant difference in activated brain areas and brain metabolic changes when deqi was achieved by proper needle manipulation in SJ5 (*waiguan*) using PET in healthy volunteers.] (Yang/Shi, et al., "Characterization of Deqi Sensation", 2013. P. 4.)[26]

In chapter 5, the physiological mechanism of deqi is discussed with some related research results that show physiological mechanism correspondent with the central brain. And research that compared SA to laser acupuncture reported that after acupuncture placebo (sham) acupuncture showed a universal increase of transcutaneous CO_2 emission, while deqi acupuncture showed a significant increase of transcutaneous CO_2 emission specifically at acupoints located on the same meridian.[27]

---

23 Ibid., p. 4.
24 Ibid.
25 Ibid.
26 Ibid.
27 Ibid., pp. 4–5.

However, the relation between deqi and clinical efficacy is not easy to be prove, because of some contradicting research results as follow.

[Enblom et al. found that verum acupuncture, eliciting deqi, was no more effective than SA in reducing emesis in cancer patients receiving radiotherapy. White et al. indicated that the presence and intensity of deqi, using the subscale of the Park questionnaire, had no significant influence on the pain relief for the treatment of osteoarthritis of the hip and knee.] (Yang/Shi, et al., "Characterization of Deqi Sensation", 2013. P. 5.)[28]

Depending on the contradicting research results, the authors took a cautious attitude to make their decision and only said that traditional Chinese acupuncture intentionally elicits deqi sensations in patients and regards them as signs of treatment efficacy, but this is not true for all forms of acupuncture. The conclusion is that deqi is of great importance to clinical effects and mechanisms of acupuncture treatment, which also needs a lot of effort to deeply understand although some progress has been made.

The task ahead for the development of acupuncture is to clarify the mechanism of deqi and to explain the subjectivity of deqi more scientifically and objectively.

4 Argument on the Placebo Effect of Acupuncture

Through comparison of each different opinion on the acupuncture efficacy, we contacted the concept of placebo many times. The concept of placebo is defined in the Wikipedia as follow.

[A placebo is a substance or treatment with no active therapeutic effect. It may be given to a person in order to deceive the recipient into thinking that it is an active treatment. In drug testing and medical research, a placebo can be made to resemble an active medication or therapy so that it functions as a control; this is to prevent the recipient(s) and/or others from knowing (with their consent) whether a treatment is active or inactive, as expectations about efficacy can influence results. This phenomenon, in which the recipient perceives an improvement in condition due to personal expectations, rather than the treatment itself, is known as the **placebo effect** or **placebo response**.]

In acupuncture, the placebo concepts reviewed above in the articles are respectively used with different meanings. According to the article in the first category, whole acupuncture has no real effect and thus acupuncture itself is a placebo. In this sense, the concept of a placebo has been used to predicate no efficacy

---

28 Ibid., p. 5.

in acupuncture. This prediction has made its basis on a judgment of inconsistency and heterogeneity. Of course, there exist many research results that tried to prove efficacy of acupuncture each of which was performed at each different acupuncture point(s) and measured kinds of changes in blood flow, brain activity, autonomic nerve response, sympathetic nerve and parasympathetic nerve, etc., with some devices as fMRI, EEG, PET, etc. Nevertheless, all the results from such research cannot establish a consistent and homogeneous judgment on whether acupuncture is effective or not. Consequently, meta-analyses of such inconsistent and heterogeneous results make the statement, "acupuncture is a theatrical placebo", inevitable.

Instead, the other research in the second and third categories and another research have tried to substantiate efficacy of acupuncture by implying methods for medical measurements on a living body. Most of the researchers believe the reality of qi and meridian system in every body, but they have no actual and direct way to show the reality of qi and meridian system. Therefore, they used indirect methods such as fMRI, EEG, PET, etc., to explain and show the reality of qi and meridian system and to prove the efficacy of acupuncture.

In this research SA was extensively used to many controlled patient groups for verifying the limit of placebo acupuncture. SA is defined as an intervention, which mimics the sensation of acupuncture stimulation; however, it is thought to lack the analgesic and antiemetic effects of acupuncture.[29] The SA used in the researches has no penetrating stimulation on acupoints, but only stimulation on the skin at each acupoint. Some results of RA compared to SA were considered as proof of the efficacy of acupuncture, while some other results showed that there is no difference between each of them[30]: Some of them took verification of acupuncture effect regardless of the real or the sham as in the study discussed in the second category. On the other hand, there was a study to introduce both of them have no effect in a case of acupuncture to the radiotherapy-induced nausea.[31]

---

29 Wang, S-M./Harris, RE. et al., "Acupuncture in 21st Century Anesthesia", 2013, p. 1356.
30 Ee, C./Xue, C./Chondros, P./Myers, SP./French, SD./Teede, H./Pirotta, M.: "Acupuncture for Menopausal Hot Flashes: A Randomized Trial". *Annals of Internal Medicine*, Vol. 164, No. 3: 146–154, American College of Physicians–American Society of Internal Medicine, 2016 Feb 02. This study has a conclusion that Chinese medicine acupuncture was not superior to noninsertive sham acupuncture for women with moderately severe menopausal hot flashes.
31 Enblom, A./Johnsson, A./Hammar, M./Oneloev, E./Steineck, G./Boerjeson, S.: "Acupuncture compared with placebo acupuncture in radiotherapy-induced nausea—a randomized controlled study". *Annals of Ontology*, Vol. 23: 1353–1361, 2012.

In fact, many diverse research results to test and verify the efficacy of acupuncture are not consistent and homogeneous. This fact might induce a meta-analysis that acupuncture is a theatric placebo as David Colquhoun and Steven P. Novella titled their article. Until now this opinion cannot be easily challenged because no amount of trials to verify acupuncture efficacy will examine consistency and homogeneity. Even though many studies show the lack of effectiveness of acupuncture in many special diseases, it seems reasonable to have serious doubts on the acupuncture efficacy as a complete medicine. Even though many researches found some meaningful effect of acupuncture checking by medical measuring devices, it doesn't seem easy to convince Westerners of acupuncture efficacy that is based on flow of qi.

Nevertheless, many other studies have been making persistent efforts to prove the efficacy of acupuncture using empirical data that were produced by many medical measuring devices and questionnaires. Some studies could not get meaningful value from their experiments that used both RA and SA. On the other hand many others contributed to accumulation of meaningful empirical data that can prove the efficacy.

In fact, the opinion of David Colquhoun and Steven P. Novella looks more reasonable than the opposite opinion that still trusts in the efficacy of acupuncture. However, a total ignorance on acupuncture efficacy depending on decision by David Colquhoun and Steven P. Novella seems unwise. In spite of some ineffective cases of acupuncture, many acupuncture treatments, for example, pain treatment, neuropathic pain treatment, migraine treatment, sprain treatment, stress-reduction treatment, etc., are still acknowledged as being very effective.

In those positive cases for acupuncture efficacy, what is the true factor(s) of the efficacy? Many Chinese doctors have tried to spread or objectify the belief that 'deqi' that is felt firstly by patients and secondly by acupuncturists. Many studies have used to secure empirical data by medical measuring devices. Those studies could persuade people that acupuncture has a medically curative or improving effect. Be that as it may, those measurements and empirical data may be different sources from deqi kinds. In other words, those measurements and empirical data are objectified and useful data for proof of medical efficacy of acupuncture, while the deqi is entirely subjective. If more studies successfully connect the two opinions, the objective and the subjective, will the efficacy of acupuncture be acknowledged?

In fact, a more fundamental thing is meridian system in the answer to the question. Almost for more than two thousand years the meridian system has been elaborated and believed in as a reality of qi inside body. For Asian people and doctors of traditional medicine, it is accepted, *a priori*, prerequisite of medicine. Based on the idea of meridian system, TCM or other Asian traditional medicine has secured the truth as coherence. However, the Western medicine has developed a very different truth that ignores such system. From the viewpoint of the Western medicine, the meridian system of qi looks to be counted as metaphysics. Therefore many TCM researchers have made efforts to verify the efficacy of acupuncture by securing empirical data.

However, the more serious task of those researchers is to convince the skeptics that the meridian system is valid. How to successfully do this is the question.

References

Colquhoun, D./Novella, S P.: "The Acupuncture is Theatrical Placebo". *Anesthesia & Analgesia*, Vol. 116, No. 6: 1360–1363, the International Anesthesia Research Society, June 2013.

Ee, C./Xue, C./Chondros, P./Myers, SP./French, SD./Teede, H./Pirotta, M.: "Acupuncture for Menopausal Hot Flashes: A Randomized Trial". *Annals of Internal Medicine*, Vol. 164, No. 3: 146–154, American College of Physicians – American Society of Internal Medicine, 2016 Feb 02.

Enblom, A./Johnsson, A./Hammar, M./Oneloev, E./Steineck, G./Boerjeson, S.: "Acupuncture Compared with Placebo Acupuncture in Radiotherapy-Induced Nausea—A Randomized Controlled Study". *Annals of Ontology* Vol. 23, No. 5: 1353–1361, 2012.

Kim, S-Y./Kim, S-W./Park, H-J.: "Different Responses to Acupuncture in Electroencephalogram According to Stress Level: A Randomized, Placebo-Controlled, Cross-Over Trial". *Korean Journal of Acupuncture*, Vol. 31, No. 3: 136–145, 2014.

Wang, S-M./Harris, RE./Lin, Y-C./Gan, T-J.: "Acupuncture in 21st Century Anesthesia: Is There a Needle in the Haystack?". *Anesthesia & Analgesia*, Vol. 116, No. 6: 1356–1359, June 2013.

Yang, X-Y./Shi, G-X./Li, Q-Q./Zhang, Z-H./Xu, Q./Liu, C-Z.: "Characterization of Deqi Sensation and Acupuncture Effect". *Evidence-Based Complementary and Alternative Medicine*, Vol. 2013, Hindawi Publishing Corporation, 2013.

Andrea-Mercedes Riegel

The Names of Acupoints in Chinese Medicine: A Mirror of Chinese Culture Misunderstood in the Western World

Abstract: In Chinese Medicine all the structures in the human body have their symbolic value, they are all representatives of Heaven or Earth. This is also true for the acupoints. 365 acupoints in the human body represent the days of a year that is Heaven in man. Their names carefully chosen represent part of Chinese culture.

1 Introduction

The classical Chinese Medicine is closely related to the cosmology and mythology of the times when it came into existence. It is based on symbolism and in a large part on the symbolism of the *Yijing*. The *Yijing* (Book of Changes) is based on line symbols originally representing the sun and the moon and in a broader sense the two opposite poles Yang and Yin. This book is extremely important for Chinese culture, we may even say it is its foundation. Its main ideas are: Heaven, Man and Earth are one entity (*tian ren he yi* 天人合一), Heaven and Earth are father and mother of all things and consequently man's main duty on Earth is procreation, nothing goes beyond the opposite poles of Yin and Yang, all things and situations are in permanent change. These ideas are represented in trigrams and hexagrams. We find references to the symbolism of the *Yjing* everywhere in Chinese medical texts, medicine is the perfect mirror of the *Yijing*'s ideas and symbols. The fact that the symbolism of the Book of Changes is the base for Chinese medicine was pointed out by several medical thinkers in the statement *yi zhe yi ye* 医者易也, "medical science is the science of symbols". Sun Simiao even stated that a man who doesn't know the *Yijing* is unable to talk about medicine and in the Ming dynasty (1368–1644) Zhang Jiebin (1563–1640) asked "Can we practice medicine without knowing the symbolism [of the changes]?"[1]

The interweaving between medicine and the *Yijing* may best become clear in Zhang Jiebin's statement about Heaven and Earth in man:

> Heaven and Earth take the number of 6 as a standard. The three potentials taken two times, make six lines, six even and six uneven, this makes 12. Heaven has 12 months,

---

1 Zhang, Jiebin: *Leijing*. Zhongguo zhongyiyao chubanshe: Beijing, p. 666.

man has 12 inner organs, Heaven has 12 houses man has the 12 channels, Heaven has 12 double hours, man has 12 main joints. Knowing this one knows that the circulation of Ying-Qi and Wei-Qi and of the 12 channels having an inner–outer relationship and the luo vessels are symbolized here.[2]

As for the channels *Lingshu* (15) mentions 28 channels "flowing up and down, left and right and front and back".[3] These channels are the twelve main channels twice, the Qiaomai[4] on the right and on the left side and Renmai and Dumai. They symbolize the 28 great star constellations in Heaven and their flow of Qi represents the interrelation between these constellations.

The channels have 365 special points which may be used for diagnosis and treatment. This number of course also has a symbolic value, the number of points represents the days of a year. For this the points – as well as the channels – represent Heaven in man.

As these points may be effectively used for the treatment of diseases and pain they exert a certain attraction on the practitioner. In Chinese medicine all the points were denominated and the names were carefully chosen. In the western world many practitioners who want to preserve the traditional doctrine try to find explanations for the effects of the points by interpreting their names. We might find hints to the effects of the points in the names but the Chinese and the Western ways may diverge and new ideas may come up which are far away from the Chinese original.

2 What Is an Acupoint?

The acupoint is a special unit in the Chinese medical system. It is part of the body which is able to manifest pathologies in the human body and to resolve them. The base for all the theories about the characteristics and the functions of the acupoints is the idea of *tian ren he yi*. So Huangdi said "I heard man has 365 acupoints as a correspondence to one year".[5] The acupoint is called *xuewei* 穴位 or *xuedao* 穴道. This means it is not a point on the surface of the skin but it is a kind of a hole or a dwelling, a space made by the removal *ba* 八 of earth. In the *Huangdi neijing* we find some synonyms like Qixue 氣穴, Qifu 氣府 or

---

2 Ibid.
3 *Lingshu yishi*. Shanghai kexue jishu chubanshe: Shanghai, 1997, p. 152.
4 For man one chooses the Yangqiao, for woman the Yinqiao.
5 *Suwen* (58); Yang, Weijie: *Huangdi neijing shijie*. Yuejun wenhua shiye gongsi: Taibei, 1990, p. 409.

shuxu 输穴. *Shu*[6] means to transport, to transmit.[7] The character may also be written with the radical for flesh (130) *rou* 月(肉) or the carriage *che* 車 (159). The radical for flesh makes obvious that this space is located somewhere in the flesh of the body, the carriage symbolizes the function of transport. So the *shuxue* denotes a hole, in which Qi may flow in or out. Their main function is to ensure the flow of Ying-Qi and Wei-Qi in order to guarantee the function of the inner organs, the sense organs and all the other tissues.

The acupoints are holes in the body which also guarantee man's contact to the cosmos. The classical literature attributes to the points a spiritual power. *Suwen* (26) states: "Qi and blood are man's *shen*, one has to nourish them."[8] *Shen* makes up the human being. So *Lingshu* (54) defines *shen*-Qi:

As soon as blood and Qi are united, Ying-Qi and Wei-Qi do have contact, the five viscera are ready, the *shen*-Qi resides in the heart, *hun* 魂 and *po* 魄 are mature, then the human being is complete.[9]

Shen-Qi may describe the power of consciousness, it is correlated with the emotions and *po* and *hun* as we read in *Lingshu* (12): "The channels do receive fluids and conduct them, the five viscera unite *shen*, *hun* and *po* and store them."[10]

Its state is reflected in the eyes. *Lingshu* (1) makes a union between the *shen*-Qi and the acupoints. It states: "The points are spaces, where *shen*-Qi streams in and out, they are not located in the skin, the flesh, the sinews or the bones."[11] So the acupoints may be seen as collecting pools where blood and Qi and *shen*-Qi are concentrated and pass by. So they do have a material and an immaterial component and one may conclude that by this they regulate both parts of man, the body and the mind. It is the *shen* 神 aspect which brings about the contact between man and his surroundings and the cosmos. And the points may be influenced by consciousness which is even required by the *Lingshu* which states, "The method of needling must first be based on *shen*."[12]

---

6 The character may also be read *yu*.
7 See Wilder, George Durand/Ingram, James Henry: *Analysis of Chinese Characters*. Caves Books Ltd.: Taibei, 1974, p. 795.
8 Yang Weijie, p. 226.
9 *Lingshu yishi*, p. 335.
10 Yang Weijie, p. 130.
11 *Lingshu* (1); *Lingshu yishi*, p. 9.
12 *Lingshu*(8); *Lingshu yishi*, p. 75.

2.1 The Denomination of Acupoints

In Chinese acupuncture all the acupoints do have names. The *Huangdi neijing* states: "Each of the acupoints (Qixue) does have its [fixed] location and a name."[13] We already find 160 names in the *Huangdi neijing* and 349 the *Zhenjiu jiayijing*.[14] This means the names were chosen very early in acupuncture history, during the Han Dynasty or shortly after. These names are composed of two or three characters and very profound as Sun Simiao stresses: "As for all the acupoints, their names were not merely fixed, the names do all have a profound meaning."[15]

The single characters are well chosen and as the Chinese Medicine is a system of imaging thinking the characters may symbolize various things at the same time. In most cases a character is chosen for the diversity of its meanings.[16] The compounds may make visible the unity of Heaven, Man and Earth or tell us stories about the point or the relationship between different points which are located in the same area or which have the same character in the compound. Each point's name reflects a part of Chinese culture.

Criteria for Denomination

There are several criteria which played an important role for denomination. And metaphors, outstanding persons and allusions to the *Yijing* are found everywhere. There may be[17]:

A reference to one of the tidal hexagrams as representative of the corresponding meridians
A reference to an anecdote or an important legendary person
A reference to heaven, i.e. a constellation of the stars
A reference to the earth, i.e. to landscapes, rivers, mountains, etc.
A reference to architecture
A reference to the body, the anatomy, and the anatomy of the part of the body where the point is located

---

13 *Suwen* (5); Yang Weijie, p. 49.
14 The *Zhenjiu jiayijing* was written by Huangfu Mi and accomplished in 282 A.C.
15 *Qianjin yifang*; see also Frühauf, https://www.classicalchinesemedicine.org.
16 In the western world up to now only two authors tried a new and correct translation of the points' names, Heiner Frühauf and A. Riegel. H. Frühauf gives an exhaustive interpretation of the meanings of the two characters in the name of the point Tianfu (Lu3). See H. Frühauf, *The Spirit of Symbols*, https://www.classicalchinesemedicine.org.
17 The following list of criteria is based on H. Frühauf.

A reference to the physiologic function of the point
A reference to pathology, i.e. the action of the point

It is not seldom that the *Yijing* which is the base for acupuncture theories occurs directly in the name in the shape of a reference to the trigrams and their symbolism or in the shape of an allusion to the numbers of the Hetu and the Luoshu.

For the translation of the points' names we must be very aware of these facts. One has to analyze each character on different levels: the character itself as a symbol, different meanings of each of the characters of the name and the relationship between the two or three characters in the name.

How are the points normally translated into western languages?

The first translations of points' names in European languages were made by Soulié de Morant who in the beginning of the 20th century lived and worked in Beijing.[18] A lot of his translations are found in later works and it seems they were just adopted without having been verified. As for the translation into the German language the first translation of the points' names was done by the Japanologist Otto Karow in 1954. It was followed by the translation by Bachmann in 1959 who widely adopted Karow's translation.[19] In 1973 Stiefvater published a textbook on acupuncture where he translated the names of 185 points. He also widely referred to Karow. In 1973 Manfred Porkert tried a latin translation and in 1985 he translated the points' names into the German language. In cooperation with Carl-Herman Hempen he published a textbook on acupuncture.[20] Hempen's atlas of acupuncture (1995)[21] gives the names in German and Latin languages. In 1982 the World Health Organization (WHO) published the "Standard Acupuncture Nomenclature" which was revised in 1993. When we have a look at all these works we see that all the authors relied on prefabricated translations. They pick out one possible meaning of each of the characters in the compound and they establish a relationship between them except the WHO nomenclature. As for the interpretations of the compounds we mostly find the relations adjective-adjective,

---

18 See his works *Précis de la vraie Acuponcture Chinoise*. Mercure de France: Paris, 1934 and *L'Acuponcture Chinoise*. Mercure de France: Paris, 1938.
19 See also Schmidt, Josef: *Die klassischen Akupunkturpunkte. Geschichte und Synopsis ihrer deutschen Übersetzungen von 1954 bis 1988*. Medizinisch literarische Verlagsgesellschaft: Uelzen, 1990, pp. 12–13.
20 All the following German translations are based on Porkert's translation. See Schmidt 1990, p. 26.
21 Hempen, Carl-Hermann: *DTV-Atlas Akupunktur*; see the references. It is the most frequently used work of reference in Germany.

verb-noun, adjective-noun or noun-noun. The WHO nomenclature however only offers one translation for each of the characters in the compounds without establishing a relation between them. Instead of giving a translation of the compounds the WHO nomenclature tries to give a short explanation for each point's name or each point's main indication.

2.1.1 Generalities

There are characters in the names which refer to the outer appearance of the location of a point. The characters of *gu* 谷, *xi* 溪, *gou* 沟 or *du* 渎 refer to small hollows in the extremities and serve as metaphors for valleys whereas the characters *shan* 山, *qiu* 丘 *ling* 陵 or *xu* 墟 serve as metaphors for peaks like in the Chenshan 承山 (Bl 57) which is located between the two parts of the gastrocnemius muscle, Daling 大陵 (Pc 7) at the wrist, Liangqiu 梁丘 (St 34) on top of the vastus lateralis muscle or Qiuxu 丘墟 (Gb 40) which is located at the end of the malleolus lateralis. The characters which refer to water accumulations are *quan* 泉, *chi* 池, *hai* 海 or *ze* 泽. As the main meridians were seen as channels nourishing the tissues with fluid and energy, the big joints as locations where this fluid could accumulate, we have a lot of points located near the elbow, the knee or the wrist which do have these characters in their names like Sidu 四渎 (TB 9), Houxi 後溪 (SI 3), Zhigou 支沟 (TB 7), Chize 尺泽 (Lu 5) Shuiquan 水泉 (Li 8), Quchi 曲池 (LI 11), Xuehai 血海 (Sp 10), Yanglingquan 阳陵泉 (Gb 34) or Yinlingquan 阴陵泉 (Sp 9). Other metaphors were chosen because of the shape of the point's area like Futu 伏兔 "The cowering rabbit" (St 32) or Dubi 犊鼻 "The calf's nose" (St 35).

The points which are located in the upper part of the body which is the heavenly part of man, may have the word *tian* 天, Heaven, in their name like Tianfu 天府 (Lu3),[22] Tianchi 天池 "The pool of Heaven" (PC 1), Tianzong 天宗 "The heavenly clan" (SI 11), Tianding 天鼎 "Celestial vessel" (LI 17), altogether they are fifteen points.[23]

As for direct references to anatomy we find names like Wangu 完骨 "Processus mastoideus" (Gb 12) or Wangu 腕骨 "The wrist bone" (SI 4), Ermen 耳门

---

22 As for Tianfu Frühauf gives an exhaustive explanation of the point's name on his website https://www.classicalchinesemedicine.org.
23 Even this number of fifteen may have a symbolic value because this number establishes the connection to the Earth: It is the magic number of the Luoshu which represents the Earth and it represents 3 times 5, the number of three symbolizing Heaven, Man and Earth and 5 the turning point between the generating and the completing numbers.

(TB 21) "Entrance to the ear" or Dazhui 大椎 "The great vertebra" (Du 14) which indicate the location of the point at a special kind of bone. As for foramina we find the character of *liao* 髎 in points' names. Actions of points are hidden in the *shu*-points' names like Shenshu 肾俞 (Bl 23), Ganshu 肝俞 (Bl 18), etc. And the action on the psychic aspects of the inner organs becomes obvious in the names of the points located laterally to the *shu* points on the lateral branch of the bladder channel like Shentang 神堂 (Bl 44) Hunmen 魂门 (Bl 47), Pohu 魄戶 (Bl 42) or Zhishi 志室 (Bl 52). The point Yingxiang 迎香 "To welcome the odor" helps for smelling, the point Tinggong 听宫 (SI 19) "The palace of hearing" is indicated for tinnitus or deafness and Xuehai 血海 (Sp 10) regulates and strengthens blood. Sanyinjiao 三阴交 (Sp 6) is the point where the three foot-Yin channels unite and we may imagine how to use this point. It is the same for the point Sanyangluo 三阳络 (TB 8). These examples are all very easy to understand. But there are names which cannot be easily interpreted (see below).[24]

2.1.2 *Manifold Meanings of Single Characters Used in the Names of Different Points*

There are several points with the character *bai* 白 in the name. Normally *bai* is translated with "white" or metaphorically with "bright". There are the points Xiabai 侠白 (Lu 4), Yinbai 隐白 (Sp 1), Taibai 太白 (Sp 3), Sibai 四白 (St 2), Yangbai 阳白 (Gb 14) and Fubai 浮白 (Gb 10).[25]

Xiabai 侠白

Hempen: Eingezwängte Weiße [The constrained white], Candor coercitus Deadman: Clasping the White

The WHO Nomenclature: "White color refers to the lung. When both arms are hanging freely, this point is precisely on both sides of the lung."[26]

In this case the white color refers to the color of the lung according to the Five phases. The character *xia* 侠 first indicates the location of the point on the border between the white and the red flesh. In this sense the main idea here is to describe the location of the point. *Xia* also denotes a knight errant in the

---

24 We want to refer to Hempen's *DTV Atlas Akupunktur* 2006, the WHO Nomenclature (second edition 1993) and to Peter Deadman's *Manual of Acupuncture* as a reference in English language.
25 We do not want to give an exhaustive explanation of the points' names but only pick out some aspects.
26 WHO Nomenclature, p. 10.

compound *xiake* 侠客. Written with the radical "hand" 挟 the character may mean "to protect". This is also an argument for the use of the character *xia* in the name, because the lung protects all the other organs and defends the organism against pathogen factors.

Yinba i 隐白

Hempen: Verborgene Weiße [The concealed white], Candor occultus
    Deadman: Hidden White
The WHO nomenclature: "the point is in a hidden region, where the colour is white."[27]

In this case the character "*bai*" makes reference to the point Ma 45, Lidui. It indicates that here the metal of Lidui 历兑[28] is absorbed. The metal's color is white. Metal is hard and it may symbolize the hardness of Yang, in this case the hardness of the Yangming channel. Here at the first point of the spleen channel the Yang passes into Yin, the Yin of the Foot-Taiyin channel. But at this point Yin is still hidden. Moreover the phase of metal here indicates that the point has a good action on the Qi of spleen and lung because the earth nourishes metal.[29] Here the character of *bai* lets us imagine the passage of the Qi from the Foot-Yangming channel into the Foot-Taiyin channel and it indicates the action of the point.

Taibai 太白

Hempen: Das größte Weiße [The biggest white], Candidum majus
    Deadman: Supreme White
The WHO nomenclature: "The point is in the white skin of the big toe, where the white skin is the widest."[30]

The two translations choose the attribute–noun relation without interpretation of the compound. The WHO nomenclature interprets the white color as locally limited to the area where the point is located.

Yinbai was the first point of the Foot-Taiyin channel, here we have the third point which is also the *yuan* point. At the first point the Yin and Qi of the channel were still hidden, now they are great *tai*. We may see in the denomination the development of the Taiyin channel and its Qi. *Bai* may be interpreted as the white color of metal. From the point of view of the Five Transport points this point

---

27 WHO Nomenclature, p. 55.
28 The trigram Dui 兑 is a symbol for metal. See below.
29 Qi, Hao: *Shiyong liujie xuewei cidian*. Beijing chubanshe: Beijing, 1994, p. 407.
30 WHO nomenclature, p. 56.

Taibai represents the earth, from the point of view of its name it also represents the phase of metal. As white is great *tai*, this point must have a significant action on the lung and its Qi. But the name reveals still another aspect: Taibai is the name of the planet Venus which is associated with metal, the West, the fall and the white tiger. The metal is hard, the tiger is brave and able to chase away the demons. The planet Venus is the most brilliant of all the planets. On the level of the organism Taibai's brilliance might be interpreted in the sense that the point must be an effective point to restore the order in the inner organs and to help the patient to recover. As the tiger is brave and able to chase away the demons the point Taibai must be effective against pathogen factors (the "demons") and it concentrates on Yin factors because the white tiger is a symbol for Yin. The action on the immune system, i.e. the Qi organs spleen and lung is indicated in the character *bai* as well in the compound *taibai* "supreme white" and in the quality of the point as "earth-point". The two elements metal and earth do work together for convalescence and strength. So in the point's name we directly see its actions and its importance for man's health.

Sibai 四白

Hempen: Rand des Wangenbeins [Margin of the cheekbone], margo zygomaticus
Deadman: Four Whites

The WHO nomenclature: "This point is below the eye and is indicated in treating diseases of the eyes. It is said to improve the vision and give one sharp eyes in all four directions."[31]

The point is located in a straight line under the pupil. The number of four *si* indicates the four directions. *Bai*, white, here does not refer to the color of metal but is means "clearness" or "bright, translucent". The name indicates the main indications of the point, to clear man's eyesight. This is what the WHO nomenclature explains. The translation could be "clear sight in all directions".

Yangbai 阳白

Hempen: Die Weiße des Yang; [The white of Yang], candor Yang
Deadman: Yang White

The WHO nomenclature: "Yang here refers to the head. The point is at the head and its function is to brighten the eye".[32]

---

31 Ibid., p. 29.
32 Ibid., p. 169.

This point is located in a straight line above Sibai (St 2) on the forehead. The head is Yang. As the point is located above Sibai, the character Yang indicates that it represents the Yang aspect of man even more than Sibai. Moreover it is a point where the Yang-channels Foot-Yangming, Shou-Yangming, Foot-Shaoyang and Shou-Shaoyang and Yangweimai join up. So the point is not only located in the Yang region, its quality is also Yang. It is able to clear heat in the region of the head and the eye. Its action on the eyes corresponds to Sibai. One might translate the compound with "Clearness in the Yang region".

Fubai 浮白

Hempen: Oberflächliche Weiße [Superficial White], candor superficialis
　　Deadman: Floating White
　　The WHO nomenclature: "The point is on the superficial layer of the body and functions in clearing the mind and brightening the eyes."[33]

Here the authors also choose the attribute-noun translation. *Fubai* here refers to a metaphor which goes back to the period of the Warring States (445–221 B.C.). The *Fudabai* 浮大白 (floating Great White) was a metaphor for an overfull cup of wine.[34] This metaphor was integrated in the everyday's language where it became a metaphor for dizziness and drunkenness. In the *Laozi dabai* is used in the sense of a certain debauchery.[35]

So the Great White *dabai* 大白 might be interpreted as a white misty cloud or the feeling of dizziness. *Bai* here is a symbol for a white cloud and a metaphor for dizziness. Combined with the character *fu* 浮 for "floating" we have the image for the feeling of floating on a white cloud. Floating on the great white cloud symbolizes the feeling of drunkenness or dizziness. In the scope of medicine symptoms like dizziness, vertigo and headache which go along with drunkenness when awaking the very next morning are associated with "phlegm". So the name of the point indicates the main actions of the point: It resolves phlegm and it is indicated for all symptoms associated with phlegm in the upper part of the body.

The character *shang* 商 is also found in several points' names. Whereas the character *bai* 白 very often symbolizes the color of metal, *shang* is used as a symbol

---

33　Ibid., p. 167.
34　See Liu, Xiang: *Shuoyuan; Shuoyuan jiaozheng*. Zhonghua shuju: Beijing, 1987, p. 276.
35　See Li, Shuhuan: *Daojiao cidian*. Juliu tushu gongsi: Taibei, 1989, p. 208 and *Laozi* (41). It states "(…) The great White looks disgraceful." *Daodejing shiyi*. Santai chubanshe: Xian, 1988, p. 102.

for the metal's sound. We find the points Shangqu 商曲 (Ki 17), Shangqiu 商丘 (Sp 5), Shaoshang 少商 (Lu 11), and Shangyang 商阳 (LI 1).

Shangqu 商曲

Hempen: Hohe Krümmung [High flexion],[36] curvatura alta
  Deadman: Shang Bend
  The WHO nomenclature: "The large intestine also pertains to metal. This point corresponds to the flexure of the intestines."[37]
  Shang here symbolizes the phase of metal and the Yangming organs stomach and large intestine. The character *qu* 曲 here indicates the flexure of stomach and large intestine where the point is located. *Shang* also implicates the hardness of metal. By this the character also indicates the indications of the point, heat and dryness in the large intestine manifested in constipation and hard stool. Moreover there is obstinate stagnation of Qi in stomach and large intestine in the scope of the point's indications. One might translate the name as "flexion of the metal-organs".

Shangqiu 商丘

Hempen: Kleiner Fersenberg [little hill of the heel], monticulustali
  Deadman: Shang Mound
  The WHO nomenclature: "This is the Jing-River point of the spleen meridian and pertains to metal. The point is below the medial malleolus, which looks like a hill".
  Shang here has the same meaning as in Shangqu. It symbolizes the hardness of metal and by this it gives a hint to the indications of the point: it resolves stagnations of Qi and dampness and strengthens weak function of the pair spleen-stomach and large intestine. From the point of view of the Five Transport points it represents the phase of metal which is also hidden in the character of *shang*. The character of *qiu* 丘 indicates the anatomic position of the points at the inner ankle. One could translate the name with "Metal-hill".

Shaoshang 少商

Hempen: Junges Shang [Young Shang], Metallum structivum
  Deadman: Lesser Shang

---

36 Hempen seems to interpret the character of *shang* 商 here as *gao* 高 high.
37 Ibid., p. 133.

The WHO nomenclature: "The lung pertains to metal in the Five Elements and to the *shang* sound in the Five Sounds. This is the last point of the lung meridian, where the Qi is less."[38]

Here *shang* once more symbolizes metal. This is the last point in the Shou-Taiyin channel of the lung. So metal begins here and is very little at this point, which is indicated in the character of *shao* 少. We may imagine that here Yang begins to grow in the Yin, the Shou-Taiyin channel passes into the Shou-Yangming channel.

Shang Yang 商阳

Hempen: Äußerstes Yang [Extreme Yang], Yang extremus
Deadman: Shang Yang
The WHO nomenclature: "The large intestine pertains to metal and is ascribed to the shang sound. Yang refers to the Yang meridian."[39]

This is the first point of the Shou-Yangming channel. Here at this point the phase of metal on the Yang side begins to grow. The last point of the Shou-Taiyin channel was called Shaoshang and it is only logic that the very first point of the Shou-Yangming channel now is called Shang Yang: At this point the Qi of the Shou-Yangming channel adopted from the Shou-Taiyin channel begins to grow. By these two names Shaoshang and Shang Yang one can imagine the transmission of the Qi from the Yin channel to the corresponding Yang channel. Hempen's translation is the opposite of what is meant here. One might translate "Yin metal passes to Yang metal".

2.2 Heaven, Man and Earth in the Points' Names

There are several points who's names indicate directly the entity of Heaven, Man and Earth.

The first example to discuss is Taiyi 太乙 (St 23). The point Taiyi (St 23) is translated by Hempen with "Das mächtige Eine" (The mighty one) and Deadman calls it "Supreme Unity". *Taiyi* has several meanings. On the human level the compound may be interpreted as a symbol for the center of life. The point is located on the level of the curvature of the stomach and the curvature of the large intestine. The character of *yi* 乙 is a symbol for this curvature, the character *tai* 太 being hint to the large intestine (*dachang*). So on the one hand the compound is a symbol for

---

38 Ibid., p. 14.
39 Ibid., p. 17.

the anatomic location of the point, on the other hand it indicates the function of the point to regulate the middle and lower burner.

But *Taiyi*, the Supreme One, on the cosmic level, has several meanings: First, it is identifiable as the Dao in the *Laozi*'s sense. It is the ultimate source of all phenomena "invisibly animating and regulating the universe".[40] The *Laozi* (42) states: "The Dao produces the One, the One makes the Two, the Two makes the Three, the Three makes the ten thousand things".[41] And the *Liji* states: "Now the Rites necessarily have their origin in the Supreme One which divides to become Heaven and Earth, revolves to become Yin and Yang and changes to become the four seasons."[42]

During the second millennium BC the Taiyi was regarded as the pole star[43] and during the Han Dynasty the Supreme One was also worshipped as the most important deity who's abode was the Pole of the Dipper. It was considered to dwell in the center as the Son of Heaven.[44] This means that Taiyi completes the correlation of the Imperial palace in Heaven with the imperial palace on Earth. On Earth the region of the Taiyi represents the imperial palace, in man this region is the most important site for metabolism in the center of the organism. The shape of the large intestine opening in the rectum resembles the shape of the Great Dipper in Heaven and the imperial palace on Earth. The Dipper is the Supreme Lord's carriage. It revolves around the center, regulating each one of the four regions. "It divides Yin and Yang, establishes the four seasons, liberates the Five Element Forces, deploys the seasonal junctures and angular measures, and determines the various periodicities – all are tied to the Dipper."[45] This statement of the *Shiji* demonstrates the unity of the Supreme One in the Dipper, the Son of Heaven in his imperial palace on Earth and the center of metabolism in man.

The point Taiyi is followed by the point Tianshu (St 25) which is located on the level of the umbilicus. First Tianshu is also a star's name. It is the first star in

---

40 Pankenier, David: *Astrology and Cosmology in Early China*. Cambridge University Press: Cambridge, 2015, p. 90. In the Warring States there existed a text called "*Taiyi sheng shui*" (The Supreme One springs from water) in which the Supreme One was interpreted as the Dao.
41 *Laozi* (42); *Daodejing shiyi* 1988, p. 104; see also Wilhelm, Richard: *Laotse. Tao Te King*. Diederichs: München, 1978, p. 85.
42 *Liji* (*Li yun*); *Liji jijie*: Wen shichechubanshe: Taibei, 1990, p. 617.
43 Needham, Joseph: *Science and Civilisation*. Vol. 3. Cambridge University Press: Cambridge, 1995, p. 260.
44 See Pankenier 2015, p. 89.
45 *Shiji* (27). Sima Qian: *Shiji*. Zhonghua shujju: Beijing, 1985, p. 1291.

the Great Dipper (Ursa major) and via another star it directly points to the pole star. During the Han it was considered the pole star[46] which was the center for orientation and a kind of a clock. In man this center is symbolized in the umbilicus. Tianshu is located on the level of the umbilicus and encircles it. Drawn as a bear the star Tianshu is directly located in the loins of the bear at the same level as Tianshu is in man. In old books the star Tianshu was also called the "killing star" (*shaxing* 杀星) and the "peach blossom star" (*taohuaxing* 桃花星) symbolizing the strength and impulsiveness of the star and its popularity among the stars. In Daoism it was also called "the spirit of Yangming" and the "greedy wolf" (*tan lang* 贪狼) because of its flexibility and qualities. On the human level this means that the point is crucial for curing all problems in the Yangming organs stomach and large intestine, it brings about a rigorous but soft regulation in the flow of Qi above and below the umbilicus. *Shu* 枢 as a single character denotes a pivot. Here in the center of the body there is the pivot from the Heaven part of man to the Earth part. In the point Tianshu this turning point is indicated by the character *tian*, Heaven. This indicates that the Heaven part in man ends here. Needling this point may resolve blockages in the flow of Qi between the two parts, Heaven and Earth, in man. In the end the name Tianshu as a whole indicates that accumulations of masses and Qi may be resolved, the metabolism in the middle and lower burner be regulated. This is also the case for blockages on the mental level, on the level of the *shen* which is stored in the heavenly part of the body.

Tianzong 天宗 (SI 11) also unites Heaven, Man and Earth. *Zong* 宗 denotes an affiliation, familiar or dynastic. The character *tian* first indicates the location of the point in the heavenly part of the body. It is located in the midst of the scapula on the same level as Shentang (Bl 44), the "Hall of *shen*". In the cosmos the three heavenly entities are the sun, the moon and the stars, they constitute the "heavenly clan". On earth the three entities are the rivers, the oceans and the mountains. We are reminded to a star constellation, a "heavenly clan" by the image of the lineage between Naoyu (SI 10), Tianzong (SI 11), Bingfeng (SI 12) and Quyuan (SI 13). The stars' constellations directly influence the oceans and – in the ancient Chinese society – man's life. The point Tianzong's association to celestial bodies demonstrates that here the contact to the cosmos may be established. Its location near Shentang (Bl 44), i.e. the heart, moreover makes clear the point's action on the soul and body of man. It may open the pores and the heart and therefore be effective for the treatment of depression or chronic nervousness as well as for (psychosomatic) pain in the back and shoulders.

---

46 See Needham ibid.

Tianfu 天府 (Lu 3),[47] the "Heavenly treasure" is another example which shows how an acupoint unites the microcosmic and macrocosmic levels of existence and the whole range of meanings of this point in its manifoldness becomes obvious "as soon as we deal with the multidimensional aspects of its symbolic code."[48] The first aspect is that Tianfu is the third point on the lung channel because this shows the threefold process of prenatal energy in postnatal energy according to the *Laozi*'s statement concerning the creation of the world.[49] Zhongfu 中府 (Lu 1) is the first point, i.e. the first state, where the mineral ore is still in the earth, Yunmen 云门 (Lu 2) introduces the change and the coming out of the heavenly Qi in the Earth, Tianfu (Lu 3) represents the Taiyin essence in its pure metal condition. At this point the pulse is first palpable on the body surface. We can imagine this image just when looking at the names of the first three points of the Lung channel. *Fu* 府 is also the term which denotes the collection of material substance in a central space and a central headquarter where the government officials meet. *Fu* in the point's name is the functional unit which serves the purpose of fulfilling the Taiyin function which is to process material essence in the microcosm of the human society and to deal with it.

In his description of the two stars' constellations called Tianfu which existed during the Han Dynasty Frühauf demonstrates the pendants on the Earth and human levels. So we see that Tianfu is an excellent example for the unity of Heaven, Man and Earth in some points' names.

The symbolism of the numbers in the points' names

In the acupoints' names the numbers of 3 and 5 occur several times and these numbers are far away from being a mere kind of measure. There are the points Shousanli 手三里 (LI 10) and Zusanli 足三里 (St 36), Wuchu 五处 (Bl 5), Wushu 五枢 (Gb 27), Diwuhui 地五会 (Gb 42), Shouwuli 手五里 (LI 13) and Zuwuli 足五里 (Li 10).

As Chinese Medicine is based on symbolism all the numbers do have a symbolic value. The number of 3 symbolizes the three potentials *San cai* 三才, Heaven, Man and Earth, we see this in the three levels for needling, the nine (3 × 3) positions for pulse diagnosis (*sanbujiuhou* 三部九候), the nine inner organs and

---

47 Tianfu is exhaustively described in all its facets by H. Frühauf. (see above).
48 Frühauf, "der Akupunkturpunkt Tianfu". https://www.classicalchinesemedicine.org/2009/04/die wurzeln-der-chinesischen-medizin.
49 *Laozi* (42), see above.

the nine orifices as they are described in the *Suwen* (9), the nine needles, the 81 (27 × 3) chapters of the *Nanjing* or the *Huangdi neijing*.

Suwen (9) states:

[…] three times three [the three potentials Heaven, Man and Earth] makes the nine, the 9 is the symbol for the 9 regions, the 9 regions make the 9 organs, that is why we have 4 material organs[50] and 5 organs which store spiritual energies,[51] altogether they are the 9 organs for storage, which correspond to this.[52]

As for the number of 5 one has to think of the central position of the number of 5 in the two circular arrangements of the trigrams, the Hetu and the Luoshu. Moreover according to the Great Appendix there are five numbers for Heaven and five numbers for the Earth, and the number of 5 is the number of the Earth. The number of Heaven and Earth is 55.[53] The Great Appendix states:

> The numbers of Heaven are five [1,3,5,7,9], the numbers of Earth are five [2,4,6,8,10]. The five places find together [1 and 2, 3 and 4, 5 and 6, 7 and 8, 9 and 20] and every [number] finds its complement [1 and 6, 2 and 7, 3 and 8, 4 and 9, 5 and 10]. The number of Heaven is 25 [1 + 3 + 5 + 7 + 9], the number of Earth is 30 [2 + 4 + 6 + 8 + 10]. The number of Heaven and Earth is 55. This is why there is a marvelous continuous run of birth and completion brought about by change.[54]

In a row of ten numbers the number of 5 is the turning point between the generating and the completing numbers. And in heaven there are 28 stars divided into 5 mansions.

Shousanli 手三里 (LI 10) and Zusanli 足三里 (St 36) are both points of the Yangming channels and they are closely related to the Earth. Zusanli is the *he* point of the Foot-Yangming channel and represents the Earth. Shousanli is located 3 *cun* distal to Zhouliao 肘髎 (LI 12) and 2 cun distal to Quchi 曲池 (LI 11) which is the *he* point of the ShouYangming channel and represents the Earth. The Zusanli is located 3 *cun* distal to the lower border of the patella. In this sense the character *li* 里 may be interpreted as a "mile". From the point of view of anatomy these two points Shousanli and Zusanlido correspond to one another and from this point of view and the equality of names of the channels they form a pair. As representatives of

---

50 Stomach, large intestine, small intestine and bladder.
51 Spleen, kidney, liver, heart and lung.
52 Yang Weijie, p. 84.
53 See *Zhouyi zhezhong*. Jiuzhou chubanshe: Beijing, 2003. The number of 55 is the result of the addition of all the numbers from 1 to 10.
54 *Zhouyi zhezhong*, p. 875.

the three potentials they are able to cure diseases which are located on every level of the human body, the region of Heaven (the region above the point Tianshu 天枢)[55] and the region of the Earth (the region below Tianshu). As for Shousanli this may also be symbolized in the anatomic position of the point Shousanli on the forearm: The forearm hanging down the point is located parallel to Tianshu. This idea concerning the indications may also be symbolized in the character *li* 里 because *li* also means "to regulate", "to restore order". Both points do have a strong effect on the large intestine and on the earth organs and by this on Qi and the immune system. This aspect also may be seen in the character of *li* 里 itself which is composed of the field *tian* 田 and the earth *tu* 土.

The point Wuchu (Bl 5) is the fifth point of the bladder channel. It occupies the place in the midst of Qucha (Bl 4), Chengguang (Bl 6), Shangxing (Du 23) and Muchuang (Gb 16). All these points do have nearly identical indications of healing eye problems, opening the orifices and clearing heat. It occupies the place number five, that is the middle position like the number of 5 in the Luoshu.

The point Wushu 五枢 (Gb 27) is located on a level three *cun* distal to Tianshu 天枢 (St 25) which also has the character *shu* 樞 (枢) in its compound; and these two points must be seen in relation to one another. The number of 5 in the compound Wushu symbolizes the Earth and the center. As the number of 5 is also the turning point in the row of the ten numbers from the generating to the completing numbers the number of 5 itself symbolizes a pivot. As the point is located somewhat distal to Tianshu this location already is part of the Earth part of the body. And it regulates disharmonies in the Middle and particularly in the Lower Burner and of the five viscera gallbladder, bladder, large intestine, small intestine and stomach. The Wushu is also a point pertaining to the girdle vessel (Daimai) which divides the body into the two parts of Heaven and Earth.

The point Wushu is also related to the stars: One may also interpret the number of 5 as the fifth place; in the Southern Dipper the fifth star is also called Tianshu. So the name Wushu may also refer to the Tianshu in the South Dipper. So there may be indicated that these two points Tianshu and Wushu are correlated.

The point Diwuhui 地五会 (Gb 42) is located on the instep that means in the earth area of the human body. This fact is indicated in the character *di* 地, "earth" and in the number of 5 which is the number of the Earth. The character of *di* also indicates that at this point the pathogens of the earth (dampness, cold, and wind) may concentrate and also be eliminated via this point. The character of hui 会 may

---

55 Tianshu (Ma 25) "The Heaven's Pivot" is the turning point between the parts of Heaven and Earth in the human body.

be associated with the characters *di* 地 and *wu* 五 and in this sense it means that the earth pathogens do gather at this point which represents "Earth five". *Hui* may also refer to Yang channels and combined with the number of 5 it indicates that all the Yang channels of the foot join up at this point.

The point Zuwuli 足五里 (Li 10) is located three *cun* distal to Qichong 气冲 (St 30). In the surroundings of five *cun* of this point Qichong there is no other point located. So here *li* must be used in the sense of "regulation". In allusion to the central position of the number of 5 in the Luoshu here the number of 5 refers to the position in the middle of the body and moreover to the five Yin organs. So this point located on the lower extremities (symbolized in the character *zu* 足) may be used not only for the regulation of the lower extremities but also for the regulation of the inner organs. There is a parallel point called Shouwuli 手五里 (LI 13). Here the number of 5 may have two meanings: on the one hand the point is located 5 *cun* above the apex of the elbow,[56] on the other hand there is the allusion to the central position of the number of 5 in the Luoshu like in the Zuwuli. This point has great effect on the inner organs which is so strong that in the classical acupuncture it was recommended not to needle this point.[57] As it is the parallel point to Zuwuli it may also be used for the regulation of eye problems of all kinds just like Zuwuli.

2.3 The Yijing Deeply Rooted in the Points' Names

As acupuncture theories are deeply rooted in the *Yijing* we also find references to this work hidden in the points' names. The most obvious examples are those where the name of a trigram occurs in the point's name.

There are three points which directly refer to one of the trigrams, the Lidui 厲兌 (St 45), the Duiduan 兌端 (Du 27) and the Duichong 兌冲 (H 7).[58]

The trigram Dui represents metal. And as for the inner organs Dui represents the small intestine and in the body structures it represents the mouth. As it is the case for the characters *bai* 白 and *shang* 商 Dui may symbolize different aspects of the phase of metal.

In the name Lidui the *dui* symbolizes the mouth or an opening in the sense that the Yangming channel opens its mouth and its Qi passes through into the Taiyin channel. *Li* 歷 also may denote the passage from Heaven to Earth and here the passage from the head to the toe. So the compound *lidui* symbolizes the fact

---

56 This corresponds to the location of the point Zhouliao (LI 12).
57 See p. ex. *Zhenjiu jiayijing jiaozhu*. Renmin Weisheng chubanshe: Beijing, 1996, p. 642.
58 Duichong is an alternative name for Shenmen (H 7).

that the Qi of the Yangming channel passed from the head to the toe and turns into the Taiyin channel via an opening. The trigram Dui is a Yin trigram symbolizing the Sea and the youngest daughter. The point is located at a very deep point of the body where Yin factors (dampness and cold) may penetrate the body. The danger of penetrating pathogen factors may also be symbolized in the character *li*, which may mean "peril, disease" or "depth". *Li* also denotes a calendar. From the point of view of the calendar Dui symbolizes autumn, harvest and metal. The direction of autumn and metal is falling, sinking. So in this point the action of drainage of pathogen factors like dampness, cold and phlegm may be indicated. From the point of view of the Five Transport points the point Lidui symbolizes metal which is also indicated in the character *dui* 兑. As a partly correct translation we might translate the name as "Passage through an opening".

In the point Duiduan 兑端 (Du 27) the name indicates the location of the point: the extreme pole of the mouth, the mouth being symbolized in the character, i.e. the trigram Dui. So Duiduan could be "The extreme pole of the mouth".[59] Shenmen's 神门 (H 7) alternative name is Duichong 兑冲. Chong 冲 denotes a strong stream or as a verb it means "to infuse" or "to dash against". *Dui* in this case symbolizes the small intestine. So one knows that here at this point the Qi of the heart channel is ready to pass or pour into the channel of the small intestine. From the point of view of the Five transport points Duichong represents the Earth. The point which represents metal is Lingdao 零道 (H 4). There is a row of four points (H 4, H 5, H 6, H 7) with special qualifications each and with partly similar indications. So a connection of the four points with one needle can be recommended. The trigram Dui also represents happiness which is symbolized in the Yin line floating on two Yang lines or the little waves dancing on the surface of the sea. One of the most important indications of Duichong – as of the other three points in the row – is to calm the spirit. So Hempen takes this aspect as the most important one and translates with "Straße zur Heiterkeit" (Road leading to happiness). Lingdao as well as Duichong –who's main name is Shenmen – are directly connected to the *shen*. So connecting Lingdao with Duichong via Tongli and Yinxi can be recommended for mental disorders.[60]

Allusions to the *Yijing* or especially to the Luoshu may also be found in the points Shenmai 申脉 (Bl 62) and Jinmen 金门 (Bl 63). In Shenmai (Streching the sinews) the character of *shen* 申 indicates the beginning of the Yangqiaomai

---

59 Hempen picks out the wrong correspondence of Dui by translating "Vorgebirge der Freude"/Promontorium laetitiae (The cape of happiness).
60 See also Hempen, p. 123.

because *shen* may mean "to stretch". On the other hand *shen* belongs to the earth branches. It represents the number of 9 and indicates the time between three and five o' clock in the afternoon, which is the active time of the bladder channel. In the Luoshu *shen* corresponds to the direction of SW, where the trigram Kun 坤 is located. The character *shen* 申 marks the second part of the character for *kun* 坤. The following point is Jinmen 金门, "The door to metal" (Bl 63). Metal *jin* 金 is represented by the Trigram Dui 兑 ☱, which in the Luoshu is located next to Kun on the position West (W). This indicates that in acupuncture practice these two points are inseparable.

3 Misleading Translations, the Base for Aberrations in Acupuncture Theories in the Western World

Each point's name has its own symbolism which may be manifold. But this symbolism which is hidden in the characters and in their combinations could not be understood by the experts in the western world because one only adopted prefabricated translations without taking into consideration the Chinese culture and without consulting any Chinese commentaries. Consequently the translations not seldom are senseless or misleading. In some cases misinterpretations of acupoints' names could become the base for new and strange theories.

3.1 The General Psychologization of Points

In the 1970s Jack Reginald Worsley (1923–2003) founded the school of the "Classical Five Element Acupuncture" (CEFA) where he wanted to teach the classical Chinese medicine. The theories and treatments should be deeply rooted in ancient wisdom and adapted for the modern world. The main pivot of the school was the strict application of the Five Elements' theories in practical treatment. Worsley's teachings were spread all over Europe and are still very popular.

In Worseley's acupuncture theories there took place what one might call a general "psychologization" of the points based on their names, that is, based on the prefabricated translations which already existed of the names. In an introduction to Worsley and his teachings in 2014 his follower Peter Borten explained some selected "spirit points" and their actions derived from the presumed names. Some examples might make the obvious aberrations from the Chinese way:

Muchuang 目窗 (Gb 16), "Eye window". This point who's alternative name is Zhirong 至荣 (Highest brilliance) is located 1 *cun* cranial to Toulinqi 头临泣 (Gb 15) and it is surrounded by several points which do have influence on the eyesight and on the *shen*. These are Benshen 本神 (Gb 13), Chengguang 承光

(Bl 6), Zhengying 正营 (Gb 17). In this sense it is a kind of "window" for the eye; and also because when man concentrates on something he turns his eyes upward toward Muchuang and by that absorbs and concentrates the essence in the eye. The point being a "window" is also an entry for wind and this explains the point's indications for wind-diseases.

Borten sees in the name the idea that this point enables man to look at problems from another point of view. He says: "(…) For a patient who is unable to see themselves (sic!) Allows them to open the eye that looks inward. For when a person seems blind to the world, wrapped up in their own frustration and struggle (…)".[61]

Qimen 期门 (Liv 14), "Gate to the cycle" is the last point of the liver channel. *Qi* as a verb means "to meet, to make an appointment". As a noun it denotes the period of one month or one year.[62] In the body the Qi of the lung channel joins the Qi of the liver channel regularly every day at the same time and a new cycle of Qi begins. It begins in the point Zhongfu (Lu 1) and ends here at the point Qimen. Qimen is the door (*men*) for the new cycle of Qi – and moreover for the regularity of the monthly cycle; because the liver regulates the menstruation and this point is a main point for irregularities in menstruation. Borten offers the translation "Gate of Hope" and he attributes to the point the function to give people hope in desperate situations. He states,

[…] people of all CFs can get blocked against this gate. When a person is banging up against this gate, they're not seeing what might lie beyond. Open up this gate and they can see the hope.

Shaoshang 少商 (Lu 11), which we translated with "Young Shang" is translated here with "Little Merchant".[63] And Borten states,

> This point is not a supermarket, not a department store. Just a little store in the neighborhood, run by a familiar merchant. The Little Merchant is available whenever you need a little something. He helps in the little things that are so important. Sometimes the spirit is so comforted by the little things. Little Merchant can be a way for a patient who is trying to bring things together to get a little help.

---

61 For Borten's statements see his presentation *"Worsley Five Element Acupuncture"*; https://peterborten.com/wp-content/uploads/2014/08/CEFA-presentation1.pdf.
62 See *Shuowen jiezi duanzhu*. Chengdou guji shudian: Sichuan, 1981, p. 332. The phonetic part *qi* 其 may be interpreted as a demonstrative, the radical is *yue* 月, "month" or "moon". In the sense of "one year" the character is an alternative character for *ji* 稘.
63 In the classical Chinese language *shangren* 商人 denoted a merchant.

Other examples may be the points Taiyi (St 23) and Tianshu (St 25) which we also already discussed as names which make obvious the unity of Heaven, Man and Earth. Borten states,

> St–23: The Great Oneness. Powerful point for a person who feels a lack of the oneness, wholeness, roundness, inclusiveness of Earth. When a person is out of touch with the wholeness, in its absence they feel a bleakness, as if they're in the dark. They can't see the light. In these cases, this point can be combined with K-21-Dark Gate (needle Dark Gate first) – for when a person (Earth CF) feels they've been under a cloud for years (sic!). [...]

St–25: Heavenly Pivot

> [...] For when a person is lost, they can't find the ground beneath them. The point connects them to what is Divine within them (of the Earth Element). Makes them grounded, nourished, secure, comforted, anchored, consistent, home.

In the first case Borton (or Worsely) introduces a new kind of needling treatment for depressive episodes, Youmen (Ki 21) and Taiyi (St 23).[64] In Tianshu he only sees a mental effect of the point.

Another follower of Worsley's way is the German psychologist Josef Viktor Müller. In 2001 he published a book on the points' names and their psychological implications called "Ben shen. Die Punktenamen als Bindestriche zur Psychosomatik" (Ben shen. The points' names as a linkage to psychosomatics).[65] He also was led astray by prefabricated translations and tries to find explanations for the actions of the points one might say by mere fantasy. Sometimes the text is not understandable. One example may demonstrate the confusion in his reasoning:

Guilai 归来 (St 29), "Returning home". This point is called "returning home" for two reasons: First it helps prolapsed organs to return to their original place by its effect of raising Qi in the abdomen. In a second sense the name refers to the wife who proved to be sterile, to be unable to bear children. As descendants was extremely important in Confucian China a woman unable to bear children was sent back home to her parents. In this sense the name indicates the point's positive effect on the ovaries and the uterus and its main indications for irregularities of menstruation, sterility and infertility in particular of women.

Müller states,

> When the earth cannot bear fruits because it is dried up there cannot be any harvest. Undernourishment in our society is scarcely a social problem of distribution of ailment but rather a question of mental attitudes as it is the case in anorexia. The absence of

---

64 There are no evidences of the effect of this point combination.
65 It was followed by a second volume in 2012.

menstruation caused by undernourishment is the most evident manifestation of sterility. Giving up these concepts of making sterility impossible in this respect is the most important aspect of the point St 29.[66]

These examples might demonstrate how far the way of this school – and also of others as one might expect – became detached and even alienated from the Chinese way of acupuncture; because these ideas about the meanings of the points' names led to new needling concepts which do not exist in the original acupuncture practice.[67]

3.2 The Points of Ancestors

It maybe in the eighties that a new concept was founded in the CEFA, the concept of the "points of the ancestors". As is indicated in some publications about the points and the points' names,[68] one assumed that these points could help to see problems in another way, to get the help of the ancestors, to call ancestral energies and to make use of the ancestors' wise insight.

The Ancestors

The most important precondition for the coming into existence of this theory probably is a misunderstanding of the word "ancestor". Who are the ancestors? Are these the ancestors of the patient, of the individual? We do have the ancestral Qi (*zong* Qi) which comes into existence in the breast by melting the air which was absorbed from outside (*kong* Qi 空气) and the *gu* Qi 谷气, the Qi which is the result of a changing process of the essence selected by the spleen. The air, the Qi from outside, the cosmos, bears the spirit of the primary ancestors of man which are Heaven and Earth. On Earth the most important ancestors are those of the emperor who do have their own temple where they are worshipped. They are protected by a courtyard and by the stars in heaven and their spirit protects the emperor who protects his people. The ancestors were human beings who have become a kind of dieties. In former times they were regarded as a means

---

66 Müller, Josef Viktor: *Den Geist verwurzeln. Die Namen der Akupunkturpunkte als Bindestriche der Psycho-Somatik*. Müller & Steinicke: München, 2001, p. 79 (transl. by the author). The last sentence seems to be incomprehensible.
67 As Müller's book is called "the golden book" in the most renowned German Association of Traditional Chinese Medicine one can imagine how widely these ideas might spread.
68 There are no special publications on these points of ancestors and their actions. The concept is taught in the scope of seminaries.

of connection to the supreme power of Heaven Tian or of the supreme ruler in Heaven, Shangdi. In an abstract sense they are the reproductive forces on Earth and by this the forces which do preserve the creative order of Heaven. In Confucianism the respect and the veneration of the ancestors is one of the most important rules, it is the most important part of filial piety.

Confucianism in the points' names

It is a matter of fact that Confucianism largely influenced Chinese medicine. So one presumption for the birth of the theory in question might be that Confucian values must be hidden in the names. The character *xu* 墟 and in some cases *ling* 陵 in the names of the points of ancestors are interpreted and translated as "ancestral tombs". The character *zong* 宗 is generally interpreted as "ancestor". Among the points of ancestors there are points like Wailing (St 26), Qiuxu (Gb 40), Tianzong (SI 11), Huizong (TB 7), Lingxu (Ki 24); and the point Gongsun (Sp 4) is also included into this group of points.

Müller translates the points' names as follows:

> Wailing 外陵 (St 26) Äußerer Grabhügel (Outer grave mound)
> Qiuxu 丘墟 (Gb 40) Ahnengrabhügel in der Wildnis (Ancestral grave mound in the wilderness)
> Tianzong 天宗 (SI 11) Himmlischer Vorfahr (Heavenly ancestor)
> Huizong 会宗 (TB 7) Ahnenversammlung (Assembly of the ancestors)
> Lingxu 零墟 (Ki 24) Grabstätte des Ling (The ling's tomb)
> Gongsun 公孙 (Sp 4) Vorfahr und Abkömmling (The ancestor and the descendent)[69]

In Müller's analysis of Tianzong[70] 天宗 we directly see his idea of Confucianism influencing medicine. He states,

> The heavenly principle Tian combined with another principle, which was of extreme importance in China, the worshipping of the ancestors, helps the small intestine which too strictly differentiates between the pure and the impure to adopt a less polarizing attitude. [...][71]

In Huizong 会宗 the character *zong* 宗 may have the denotation of "ancestor", "root" and also of "assembly". *Hui* also means "to gather". The ancestor is the father of descendants. Before there are descendants there must be a father. As

---

69 It is not clear whether this list is complete.
70 As for the analysis of Tianzong see above Section 2.2.
71 Müller, p. 131.

for this point it is the father of Sanyangluo (TB 8), the point of confluence of the three Yang channels of the hand. The assembly of the Yang channels has its roots in Huizong. According to the location of the point one *cun* laterally to Zhigou (TB 6) and the translation "Ahnenversammlung" (Reunion of the ancestors) for Huizong Müller draws a strange conclusion,

> The assembly of the ancestors leaves the normal tract of the channel and takes a special seat from where one can develop new sights. As all the points of ancestors […] do this point helps man to have a look at his problems from another angle and here in particular the problems of adaptation, integration and immunity […].[72]

The most interesting point in this group of the points of ancestors is the Gongsun 公孙 (Sp 4). Hempen translates with "Enkel des Fürsten" (The lord's grandson), Deadman calls it "Grandfather/Grandson". Accepting this interpretation of a special relation between the grandfather and his grandson Müller states,

> Translated literally with Grandfather/Grandmother Grandson/Granddaughter this must be seen in the context of the traditional Chinese family structure, in which only the grandchildren could enjoy the care of the grandparents because the grandparents' own children were seen to be responsible for the care for the parents. In a broader sense the point Sp 4 may be helpful for psychic problems which are caused by lacking care of the parents (and in particular the mother as the incorporation of the Earth) for the child. Instead of longing for the lacking care and in most cases hoping vainly the mentally undernourished child can mentally get into contact to the archetype of the great mother. […] Ancestor/descendant may refer energetically to the *luo*-vessel to the stomach channel but also to the point's function as opening point to the Chongmai which in this case is the ancestor of the spleen channel in its quality as the sea of blood.[73]

Here the author falls into the trap of a senseless translation. Of course *gong* 公 may denote the feudal lord or the ruler of a state. And *sun* 孙 may denote the grandson (*sunzi* 孙子). But the characters and the compound were chosen for other reasons. Qi Hao points out that *Sun* means that the point is the *luo* point of the spleen channel to the stomach channel and it does have connections to all the tertiary vessels *sunluo* 孙络 and to all the *luo* vessels in the body. From this starting point one reaches all the networks to the inner organs. *Gong* mays also mean "center". So here also the location of the point in the central position (*gong zheng* 公正) of the inner side of the foot is indicated. The point is located in the center of the foot and this location is comparable to the location of the spleen in the center of the body. The point is as important for the spleen as the spleen

---

72 Ibid., p. 218.
73 Ibid., p. 95; translation by the author.

is for the whole process of metabolism. And the spleen is as important for the metabolism as the earth is for man. This idea indicates that this point which is the *luo* point of the spleen channel is the most important point on the spleen channel and one of the most important points in the body. As there is a special relationship between the spleen and the heart[74] this point may establish this connection between these two organs. This may be the explanation for the fact that Gongsun is an excellent point against nausea which in Chinese language is *e xin* 恶心, the "evil heart". *Gongsun* as a compound is also the name of the Yellow Emperor, Huangdi. So once more the importance of the point for the human body is indicated: it is as important for the middle burner as the center of the human body as Huangdi was for the Chinese culture.

As for Qiuxu 丘墟 (Gb 40) the name is a metaphor for the location of the point in a deep valley which is surrounded by mountains.

Müller interprets the "ancestral tomb in the wilderness" in a psychic way which is hard to understand. He states,

> Gb 40 which is the ancestral tomb in the wilderness, extends our comprehension by connecting us with the serenity of the ancestors. The decisions made from this point of view do not have the etiquette of undecidedness, nor of obstinate dogmatism. The wilderness is also a symbol of integrity. Far from any kind of conditioning by civilization one accepts oneself as a member in the chain of the life which follows a plan dominated by necessity.[75]

One can clearly see that this concept of the points of ancestors is a theory which is based on a misunderstanding of the role of Confucianism in medicine and a misunderstanding resulting from wrong translations of the points' names. One must only think about the real situation and ask questions which do emerge when looking at this concept: Does this concept refer to the ancestors of the individual? Were all the ancestors really wise? What can we do when an ancestor of the patient was a murderer or a thief? Worshipping is one thing and it was an absolute duty for every person in ancient China. But in this case – seen from the point of view of the Westerner – the application of the points of ancestors – if they existed – would not really be a good idea.

4 Conclusion

The points' names are meaningful and they do reflect Chinese culture. To find the right translation is not easy and requires a lot of research work including the

---

74 One branch of the spleen channel connects with the heart.
75 Ibid., p. 250.

consultation of etymological dictionaries, classical works and commentaries because it is impossible to make out the basic ideas hidden in the names when just looking at them from the surface. The concept of the points of ancestors is just one example for strange theories coming into existence on the base of misunderstandings of Chinese culture and literature in the western world. Worsley, Borten or Müller, who is a psychologist by profession, make several mistakes which are nevertheless typical for Westerners: They trust in prefabricated translations, they ignore the Chinese cultural background and they provide their own interpretation from the point of view of a Westerner educated in Western disciplines. By this these experts create theories which seem to be more Chinese than the original Chinese theories by getting more and more detached from the original.

References

Borten, Peter: *Worsley Five Element Acupuncture.* peterborten.com/wp-content/uploads/2014/08/CEFA-presentation1.pdf.

Deadman, Peter: *A Manual of Acupuncture.* Journal of Chinese Medicine Publications: Sussex, 1998.

Duan, Yucai: *Shuowen jiezi duanzhu.* (Explanation of Simple Characters and Analysis of Compounds). Chengdou guji shudian: Sichuan, 1981.

Frühauf, Heiner: *The Spirit of Symbolism.* https://ClassicalChineseMedicine.org.

Hempen, Carl-Hermann: *DTV-Atlas der Akupunktur.* Deutscher Taschenbuch Verlag: München, 2006.

(*Huangdi neijing*) *Lingshu yishi.* (Modern Translated and Annotated Edition of the Huangdi neijing Lingshu) Shanghai kexue jishu chubanshe: Shanghai, 1997.

Jia, Xiaoqian: *Yi yi tan wei* (Searching the Secrets in the Relations Between the Yijing and Medicine). Shanxi kexue jishu chubanshe: Taiyuan, 2009.

Kubiena, Gertrude: *Bestzeitakupunktur–Chronopunktur. Akupunktur der Meister nach der energetischen Zeit.* Maudrich: Wien, 2002.

Li, Guangdi: *Zhouyi zhezhong.* (The Analysis of the Book of Changes). Jiuzhou chubanshe: Beijing, 2003.

Li, Shuhuan: *Daojiaodacidian* (The Great Dictionary about Daoism). Juliu tushu gongsi: Taibei, 1989.

Liu, Xiang: *Shuoyuan jiaozheng.* (Revised Edition of the Shuoyuan). Zhonghua shuju: Beijing, 1987.

Müller, Josef Viktor: *Den Geist verwurzeln. Die Namen der Akupunktur-Punkte als Bindestriche der Psycho-Somatik.* Müller & Steinicke: München, 2001.

Needham, Joseph: *Science and Civilisation.* Vol. 3. Cambridge University Press: Cambridge, 1995 (orig. 1959).

Pankenier, David W.: *Astrology and Cosmology in Early China.* Cambridge University Press: Cambridge, 2015.

Qi, Hao: *Shiyong liujie xueweicidian.* (Practical Dictionary of the Acupoints Analyzed in Six Categories). Beijing chubanshe: Beijing, 1994.

Ren, Farong: *Daodejing shiyi.* (Explanations of Dao De Jing). Santai chubanshe: Xian, 1988.

Riegel, Andrea-Mercedes: *Die klassischen Akupunkturpunkte. Wesen, Wirkung, Indikationen.* Elsevier: München, 2012.

Schmidt, Josef M.: *Die klassischen Akupunkturpunkte. Geschichte und Synopsis ihrer deutschen Übersetzungen von 1954 bis 1988.* Medizinisch literarische Verlagsgesellschaft: Uelzen, 1990.

Sima, Qian: *Shiji.* (The Records of the Grand Historian Sima Qian). 10 vols. Zhonghua shuju: Beijing, 1985.

Soulié de Morant, George: *Précis de la Vraie Acuponcture.* Mercure de France: Paris, 1934.

Soulié de Morant, George: *L'Acuponcture Chinoise.* Vol. 1. Mercure de France: Paris, 1938.

Sun, Simiao: (*Beiji*) *Qianjin yaofang* (Recipes Worth One Thousand Gold pieces for Emergency). Renmin Weisheng chubanshe: Beijing, 1983 (orig. ca. 652).

Sun, Xidian: *Liji jijie.* (Explanations of the Book of Rites). Wen shichechubanshe: Taibei, 1990.

Unschuld, Paul-Ulrich: *Nan-Ching. The Classic of Difficult Issues.* Caves Books Ltd.: Taibei, 1986.

Wang, Deshen: *Zhenjiu xueming guoji biaozhunhua shouce.* (Manual of the International Standardization of the Names of the Acupoints). Renmin Weisheng chubanshe: Beijing, 1988.

Wilder, George Durand/Ingram, James Henry: *Analysis of Chinese Characters.* Caves Books Ltd.: Taibei, 1974 (orig. 1922).

Wilhelm, Richard: *Laotse. Tao Te King.* Diederichs: München, 1978.

World Health Organisation: *Standard Acupuncture Nomenclature. A Brief Explanation of 361 Classical Acupuncture Point Names and their Multilingual Comparative List.* 2nd edition. Regional Office for the Western Pacific: Manila, 1993.

Xu, Guoqian: *Zhenjiu jiayijing jiaozhu.* (Corrected and Annotated Edition of the Systematic Classic of Acupuncture).

Yang, Weijie: *Huangdi neijing Suwen yijie*. (An Annotated Modern Translation of the Simple Questions of the Classic of Inner Medicine of the Yellow Emperor). Wenhua shuye gongsi: Taibei, 1990.

Zhang, Jiebin: *Leijing*. (The Classic of Internal Medicine of the Yellow Emperor Divided in Categories). Renmin Weisheng chubanshe: Beijing, 2000 (orig. ca. 1624).

Zhang, Qicheng: *Yixue yu Zhongyi. Dongfang shengming huayuan*. (The Science of the Book of Changes and Chinese Medicine. The Eastern Garden of Life). Zhiyuan shuju: Taibei, 2002.

Ephraim Ferreira Medeiros, Andrea-Mercedes Riegel,
Mildred Ferreira Medeiros, and Fengli Lan

Understanding Baomai 胞脉 and Baoluo 胞絡: A Multidisciplinary Approach

Abstract: Combining traditional Chinese and Western medicine perspectives, we found prenatal neurocognitive development to be influenced by the Bao Mai and Bao Luo channels. We propose that, to help us better understand the mutual interactions between pregnant and fetus, the function of these channels should be expanded to include these mechanisms.

1 Etymologycal Aspects of Baomai/Baoluo

1.1 Bāo 胞

The *Shuowen*, the original Han dynasty dictionary by Xu Shen define Bāo (胞) as "Uterus, place inside the mother from which a baby is born. The character is created using Moon/Meat (月肉) for the meaning part and the use of 包/ "package" as phonetic part."[1]

The character *bao* 胞 represents a "wrapper" bao and is written with the radical for flesh (肉 (月 ↔ 月) Radical 130 in Kangxi Dictionary 康熙字典). Therefore, *bao* is part of the human body. As for the female body "*bao*" is often translated as "uterus". But the *bao* may just be a kind of muscular wrapper in the body as *Lingshu*, chapter 63, states[2]:

> when [the sour taste] resides in the stomach, the inner of the stomach is harmonized and warm, it flows down to the bladder, the bladder's bao being thin and weak shrinks when accepting the sour taste [...]
> (*Lingshu*, chapter 63)[3]

---

1 《说文解字》胞，婴儿生在其中的娘胎。字形采用"肉（月）"作边旁，采用"包"作声旁。
2 Bao here is interpreted as the wrapper around the bladder but the bladder itself may also be seen as a kind of bao.
3 *Lingshu yishi*. In: Nanjing TCM University (eds.): *Annotated and Translated Edition of the Spiritual Pivot of the Classic of Internal Medicine of the Yellow Emperor*. Shanghai kexue jishu chubanshe: Shanghai, 1997.

Fig. 1: Bāo 胞 in Seal Script 篆書 (zhuànshū). From meat 月肉 and phonetic 包. Meaning womb. 包 is also related to womb ("Etymology", Chineseetymology.Org, accessed in April 2, 2017)[4].

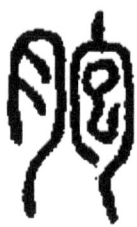

1.2 Mai 脉 and Luo 絡

"Xue mai 血脈", "jing 經" and "luo 絡" appeared together in the *Han Shu·Yi Wen Zhi* or *Treatise on Literature of The History of The Former Han Dynasty* 汉书·艺文志, "Medical classics explore the origins of blood vessels 血脈, jing-luo 經絡, bone marrow, yin-yang, exterior and interior in order to treat various diseases from the root", where seemingly differentiated blood vessels from Jing Luo.

Jing Luo 經絡 functions to carry and move qi and blood in the body. *Guan Tzu. Water and Earth* states that "Water is the qi and blood of the earth, running on the earth which is just like qi and blood flowing in the vessels". Judged from the cognizing order, the flow of qi and blood in man is analogized and inferred from the natural phenomenon of water flow in the rivers under the earth. The extensions from "vessel 脈" to "jing-luo 經絡" and from "blood" to "qi and blood" are also closely related to the application of acupuncture, moxibustion, tuina, qigong, etc, which explore the phenomenon of Qi and blood flowing in the body, thus enriching the understanding on the "vessels".

Seeing that "jing 經" and "luo 絡" are subdivisions of "Mai 脉" or Vessel, i.e. Jing Vessel and Luo Vessel, Jing-Luo system is surely the "Vessel system" – being mainly composed of Jing Vessels and Luo Vessels.

The standardized translation for "经脉" approved by the World Health Organization (WHO) is *meridian*, which implies a two-dimensional grid. Seeing that "*Jing Mai* 经脉" can carry and move qi and blood and so must be a three-dimensional tube, and that "Channel" – another popular translation in the West, indicating a three-dimensional tube – is a polysemant, whose meaning is not clear and definite, and that "*Jing Mai*" and "*Luo Mai*" are further divisions of "*Mai* or Vessel", "Vessel" can refer to a three-dimensional tube of the human being and

---

4 "Etymology." Retrieved on April 2, 2017 from http://www.chineseetymology.org/.

therefore is a strict and proper translation for *jing mai* worth to be popularized in the future (Lan, 2012, p. 214)[5].

2 Important Actors in the Prenatal Development: Uterus, Bao Mai and Bao Luo, Hearth, and Kidneys

Traditional Chinese medicine (TCM) describes all the aspects of female reproduction – the organs, the glands and their secretions, and the psyche – in terms of kidney function, heart function and the uterus. TCM texts say: "the Uterus, the Heart and Kidney form the core of reproductive activity." The uterus describes the arena where all of this happens[6]. When we use the term uterus in a Chinese medicine context it is a translation of the term Bao Gong (胞宮), which includes all the reproductive organs: uterus, ovaries, fallopian tubes and cervix. Judging by the number of times bao appears as the uterus (13 times in 9 chapters) in *Suwen*, women's reproductive health formed an important aspect of Han medicine. This is not surprising given the Confucian environment with its family-centered ethics, ancestor worship, and a strong emphasis on healthy offspring (Leo, 2011, p. 126)[7].

Bao, seen as the uterus, pertains to the so-called "extraordinary organs" (qi hang zhifu 奇恒之腑) and chapter 11 of *Suwen* calls it *nüzibao* 女子胞. The pathways or channels, Bao Mai (Uterus vessel 胞脉) and Bao Luo (Uterus channel 胞絡), provide the means of communication between heart, uterus and kidneys (Lyttleton, 2013, p. 10)[8], with Renmai, Chongmai and Dumai also playing important roles. Wiseman translates the Baoluo as "uterine network vessels" and Baomai as "uterine vessels" (1996, p. 401)[9] and suggests that there are more than one Baoluo or Baomai. In the same sense Unschuld and Tessenow translate

---

5   Lan, F.: *Culture, Philosophy, and Chinese Medicine: Viennese Lectures (Culture and Knowledge)*. Peter Lang Publishing Group, 2012, p. 214. Similar discussions also appear in op. cit. pp. 290, 329–332.
6   The process of understanding the importance and roles of the uterus took place around differing opinions and points of view. For a view about the history of this process, see Wu, Y-L.: *Reproducing Women: Medicine, Metaphor, and Childbirth in Late Imperial China*. University of California Press: Berkeley, 2010, pp. 92–97.
7   Leo, J.: *Sex in the Yellow Emperor's Basic Questions*. Three Pines Press: Dunedin, 2011, p. 126.
8   Lyttleton, J.: *Treatment of Infertility With Chinese Medicine*. Elsevier Health Sciences: London, 2013, p. 10.
9   Wiseman, N.: *English-Chinese Chinese-English Dictionary of Chinese Medicine*. Hunan kexue jishu chubanshe: Changsha, 1996, p. 401.

Baoluo as the "network vessel of the uterus" and Baomai as "uterus vessel" (2008, p. 20)[10,11].

Suwen, in chapter 33, makes these two vessels responsible for a regular menstruation and pregnancy and considers them very sensitive to emotional disturbances. In chapter 47, Su Wen says "[t]he Uterus Channel extends to the Kidneys."[12] Also, the Uterus is physiologically related to the Heart via a channel called the Uterus Vessel (Bao Mai).

Chapter 33 of the *Suwen* or *Simple Questions* says: "When the period does not come it means that the Uterus Vessel is obstructed. The Uterus Vessel pertains to the Heart and extends to the Uterus."[13]

The *Selected Historical Theories of Chinese Medicine* (《中医历代医话选》) says:

> The Pericardium (Xin Bao) is a membrane wrapping the Heart on the outside [...] the Uterus connects downwards with the Kidneys and upwards with the Heart where it receives the name of Connecting Channel of the Envelope of the Heart' (Xin Bao Luo) (Maciocia, 2015. p. 168.)[14]

In TCM it is said that Kidney jing dominates reproduction. Kidney jing plays a key role in feminine physiology at all stages from puberty to pregnancy to menopause. Aspects of the kidney also influence libido and sexual function (Lyttleton, 2013, p. 9).

We also can see that of the eight extraordinary vessels in Chinese medicine, Ren Mai and Chong Mai are greatly involved in reproduction and fertility. Both vessels originate in the kidneys and flow through the uterus. These two vessels are critical in female reproductive function and exert strong influence on the organs of the abdomen as the vessels pass through them (*ibid.* p. 21).

After the woman has conceived, the uterus vessel has to stay healthy to bring the pregnancy to completion. If it does not function properly, it can play havoc with her health.

---

10 Unschuld, P./Tessenow, H.: *A Dictionary of the Huang Di Nei Jing Su Wen*. University of California Press: Berkeley, 2008, p. 20.
11 They offer a literal translation of *mai* and *luo* in order to maintain the difference that is made in the original text. They do not explain the difference between the two vessels or of the meaning of the vessels.
12 《素问·奇病论第四十七》 胞络者，系于肾.
13 《素问·坪热病论第三十三》月事不来者胞脉闭也，胞脉者属心而络于胞中.
14 Maciocia, G.: *The Foundations of Chinese Medicine*. Elsevier Health Sciences: London, 2015. p. 168.

While the kidneys and the heart control the processes necessary for female fertility, they are not the only organs or systems involved. The spleen and liver also contribute in less direct ways to aspects of reproduction and fertility. The spleen produces blood through transforming food and nutrients and the liver stores and moves the blood. Therefore, these two organs contribute to nourishing the uterus. The spleen also controls the circulation of blood in the vessels. The liver is responsible for the smooth movement of Qi and therefore plays a critical role in events surrounding ovulation and menstruation. The lungs are less involved in this process but also influence Qi circulation (*ibid.* p. 9).

2.1 Baozhong: The Place of Activity of Baomai and Baoluo

The main pathology of Baomai and Baoluo vessels is disruption *jue* 绝 resulting in an undernourishment of the *baozhong* which, in women, leads to missing menstruation or even sterility and abortion. As there are no anatomical descriptions of these two kinds of vessels, we can only hypothesize that Baomai is (are) nourished by the heart's blood – needed in the whole genital apparatus – and whether the Baoluo takes essence from the kidneys to nourish the *baozhong*[15,16] (Flaws, 2005, p. 9).

Baozhong is introduced in *Suwen*, chapter 33 as the structure to which the Baomai connects. We can attempt to understand it as the "center of the uterus", but attention must be drawn to the fact that this area or structure must also exist in the male organism. Rochat de la Vallee states that here the *baozhong* does not exactly represent the uterus, but, "the center of what is wrapped and protected and thus designates the protection of the origin of life." (Rochat de la Vallee/Larre, p. 165)[17] Indeed a new life does come into existence in the uterus, but also by the action of the female and male gonads.

Both Huang Fumi in his *Zhenjiu jiayijing jiaozhu* 《针灸甲乙经》 and Li Shizhen in his *Bencao gangmu.* 《本草纲目》 (Outline of the materia medica) state that the *Baozhong* is also the origin of Renmai, Dumai and Chongmai and several classics mention the term without strictly defining it.

---

15 See also *Lingshu*, chapter 65.
16 Flaws, B.: *A Compendium of Chinese Medical Menstrual Diseases*. Blue Poppy Press: Boulder, 2005, p. 9.
17 Rochat de la Vallee, E./Larre, C.: *The Extraordinary Fu*. Monkey Press: London, 2003, p. 165.

In other texts, *Baozhong* is associated with several structures like the Mingmen (Riegel, 2010; Unschuld, 1986, p. 320; ibid. p. 399; Lingshu, p. 369)[18,19], the uterus and the palace of sperm[20] (*Lingshu*, 393f), the extraordinary vessels (Riegel, 2016)[21] and the classic book *Leijing* 《类经》 correlates it with the Lower Dantian.

2.2 *Bao* and the Palace of *jing*

The palace of *jing* may be seen as the testes and the epididymis, the reservoir for sperm. The same palace of *jing* exists in the female organism as the ovaries, where the female *jing* is stored. Both structures do emerge from the primordial kidney, making the kidney responsible for the gonads. When *Lingshu*, chapter 44, states that Chongmai is the Great *luo* of the Shao Yin channel and originates under the kidney we may assume that this is the primordial kidney and thus the kidney channel is also associated with it.

But all the structures described here do meet at a place which in the female organism becomes the uterus. Seen from both genders this place is only the center of the urogenital system and the center of the "origin of life". The Baomai has contact with this region but we do not know when Baomai comes into existence. As it is only active in the adult female organism, we may see *baozhong* as this origin of life or the whole of uterus, ovarian tubes, and ovaries. In the male organism we may understand the *baozhong* as the region of the testes including the epididymis, the "palace of *jing*" and the penis, which is needed to bring the fertile sperm to the "entrance" of *bao* in the female.

---

18 Riegel, A.M.: *Die Niere shen. Klassische Konzepte der traditionellen chinesischen Medizin im Lichte der modernen Schulmedizin*. Bacopa: Schiedlberg, 2010.
19 Unschuld, P.U./ Bian, Q.: *Nan-ching the Classic of Difficult Issues*. University of California Press: Berkeley, 1986.
20 Bao or baozhong does exist in man and woman. In women, the baozhong may refer to the uterus, in man the "palace of sperm" may be interpreted as the testes with the reservoir that is the epididymis. See also *Lingshu*, chapter 65, which deals with the question why women do not have a beard.
21 Riegel, A.M.: "Qijing bamai – The eight extraordinary vessels. A concept of Chinese medicine based on the Yijing". In: Wallner, F. G./Kluenger, G. Nordhausen (eds.), *Constructive Realism – Philosophy, Science and Medicine (libri nigri 53)*. Verlag Traugott Bautz, 2016.

2.3 Baomai, Baoluo, Renmai and Chongmai, the Vessels Which Are Responsible for Blood

The sexual potentials of man and woman are bound to the kidney and have their origin in the primordial kidney. We also find the origin of the Renmai and Chongmai there. Moreover, these two vessels are responsible for blood, particularly so in the female organism, where they provide the menstrual blood. That Renmai and Chongmai can be called the "sea of blood" might also be seen in the embryonic development. In the embryonic tissue, we find the AGM – aorta-gonad-mesonephros – region, located close to the urogenital system, generating the gonads and the metanephros. Pietilä and Vainio (2005 p. 805)[22,23] found that this region produces hematopoietic stem cells and that "[t]he AGM region is the first intra-embryonic area where hematopoietic stem cells (HSCs) capable of colonizing adult bone marrow have been detected" (*ibid*. p. 804). As this area pertains to *baozhong* in the embryo this could be an explanation for the responsibility of the two extravessels for blood.

Suwen, chapter 33, makes clear that the Baomai is (are) necessary to provide blood for the *baozhong*. It assumes that Baomai is active in the female organism but this does not necessarily mean that man doesn't have Baomai. The character *mai* is used for channels and for blood vessels. As blood vessels the Baomai may be interpreted – at least in part – as coming from the aorta, originating in the heart and running downward, and dividing in numerous branches. In the female *baozhong*, Baomai might then be the arteria uterine, the arteria ovarica, and their branches. These are branches of the aorta iliaca anterior, itself a branch of the aorta abdominalis. In the male *baozhong*, Baomai on the other hand might represent the corresponding vessels in the male organs (e.g. the arteria testicularis and the arteria deferentis) which are branches of the aorta iliaca interna, all being – in terms of Chinese medicine – the sun-luo 孫絡 of the aorta abdominalis.

2.4 Baomai and Baoluo as a Circuit

In this sense Baomai and Baoluo prescribe a circuit, although Bob Flaws sees quite another circuit, summarized in the following way:

> [...] the baomai is the pathway by which heart blood is transported down to the uterus. Whereas, the bao luo is the pathway by which yin essence is transported to the uterus

---

22 Pietilä, I./Vainio, S.: "The embryonic aorta-gonad-mesonephros region as a generator of haematopoietic stem cells", *Journal Compilation APMIS*, 12(113), pp. 804–812.
23 They can be found there since the eleventh day of pregnancy. (ibid. p. 805).

but also from thence upward via the chong mai/bao mai to the heart and upper body.
The uterus is the juncture between the bao mai and bao luo, and, therefore, also between
the heart and kidneys or the upper and lower burners.
(Flaws, *2005*. p. 10)

First, he sees Baoluo as a plural, the "network vessels distributed over the *bao gong* which supply and fill the *bao gong* with kidney essence" (*ibid.*, p. 9). Therefore, Flaws interprets the character luo as small connecting vessels whereas the *Suwen* commentary by Yang Weijie interprets the character as the "xinbao luo", an indication that this vessel(s) pertain to the pericardium.

As for Baomai, he associates this vessel with the pericardium and states that it is "the vessel by which the heart sends blood down to the uterus" (*ibid.*, p. 9). In the end he interprets Baomai as a synonym for Chongmai. "Baomai" then is "a term used in theoretical and introductory discussions" (*ibid.*) This metaphor does not hold logically: the Baomai transports blood downward whereas the Chongmai transports Qi and blood upward, and a vessel or channel can only flow in one direction.

3 Prenatal Cognitive Development: Classical Chinese Medicine and Western Medicine Perspectives

3.1 Modern Science Perspectives on Prenatal Cognitive Development

Pregnant women can attest that the fetus responds and even communicates to stimuli. But since "of all the measures available for examining cognition in infants, only Heart Rate is available presently for use in the fetus" (Kisilevsky/Hains, 2010, p. 60–75)[24], western science is starved of data. It has been taking steps though, by using, e.g. "exposure learning, classical conditioning and habituation" (Hepper, 1996)[25] and "focusing on audition and olfaction/taste, [it] has shown that the fetus is capable of learning and that some reflexive behaviour of the fetus allows simple communicative acts" (Huotilainen, 2004)[26]. It is easier to assess the newborn, even if the methodologies are not necessary so, and researchers have found

---

24 Kisilevsky, B.S./Hains, S.M.J.: "Exploring the relationship between fetal heart rate and cognition". *Infant & Child Developoment*, 19, 2010, pp. 60–75. doi:10.1002/icd.655.
25 Hepper, P.G: "Fetal memory: Does it exist? What does it do?". *Acta Paediatrica Supplement*, 416, 1996, pp. 16–20.
26 Huotilainen, M.: "Foetal learning – a bridge over birth". Retrieved on April 27, 2017 from https://www.edu.helsinki.fi/lapsetkertovat/lapset/In_English/Huotilainen.pdf.

that "the neonate even prefers the smells and tastes that he/she was exposed to during pregnancy" (Liley, 1972)[27] and "prenatal music exposure alters the fetal behavioral state and is carried forward to the newborn period." (James/Spencer/Stepsis, 2002, pp. 431–438)[28].

It is interesting to point that auditory, acoustics and cognition remind us about the relation between Kidneys (Ear/hearing) and cognitive development. Fetal Heart Rate and Cognition highlights the relationship between Heart and Mind (Shen 神) in early stages of human life.

3.2 Ancient Chinese Perspectives on Prenatal Cognitive Development

Taijiao (Fetal Education)

> Taijiao is a series of purposive preparations during gestation that exert direct or indirect influences on physical and psychological aspects of pregnant women for the sake of positive fetal development regarding physiological and mental health. Taijiao inception is recommended as early as the second month of pregnancy. Its benefits comprise better embryonic growth of sensory, neurological, and physical functions, along with infantile development in language learning and psychological well-being, thus indicating an extended impact on progression from the fetus and adolescent stages to the whole life span. (Cheng, 2016)[29].

The concept of *taijiao* (fetal education) is different from 'prenatal education'. The current Western notion of prenatal education encompasses ideas of proper nutrition and health for the pregnant woman, and hence the fetus. The concept of *taijiao* also includes the idea that the mind, body, and spirit of the fetus can be molded by the outside world while it is still in the womb.

> Later exhortations to avoid frog and rabbit meat were to prevent a colicky baby or one born with a harelip, respectively. Poetry and music, on the other hand, could engender peaceful and intelligent offspring.
> (Cheng, *op. cit.*)

---

27 Liley, A.W.: "The foetus as a personality". *Australian and New Zealand Journal of Psychiatry*, 6, 1972, p. 99.
28 James, D.K./Spencer, C.J./ Stepsis, B.W.: "Fetal learning: A prospective randomized controlled study". *Ultrasound in Obstetrics and Gynecology*, 20(5), 2002, pp. 431–438. See also prenatal maternal speech influences newborns' perception of speech sounds.
29 Cheng, F-K.: "Taijiao: A traditional Chinese approach to enhancing fetal growth through maternal physical and mental health". *Chinese Nursing Research*, 3(2), 2016, pp. 49–53.

Fetal education instructed pregnant women to discipline their emotions, behavior, and environment to nurture the physical and moral development of the impressionable fetus (Richardson, 2015)[30].

To use a more modern metaphor found in a 1915 issue of the *The Ladies' Journal*: "When taking photographs, if there is a smile, then after developing the image, there is the same smile. If there is anger, then after developing, there is the same anger." (Lackner and Vittinghoff, 2004, p. 671)[31] These quotes emphasize that the impressionable fetus can be influenced by the signs and sounds experienced by the pregnant woman, as well as the woman's own emotional state during pregnancy – her smiles or anger.

The blocked passage of Baomai and Baoluo during pregnancy may cause disturbance of the education of the fetus, but it is also the psychic situation which determines the success of all the efforts of prenatal education. This is because the heart blood directly influences the fetus via the Baomai vessels. Heart blood stores the shen. In case of blood deficiency, the shen cannot be stored. Disturbances of shen are the result. And disturbances of the shen directly influence the fetus and impairs his development, from the mental and physical point of view.

3.3 Some Fetal Cognitive and Behavioral Effects Due to Exposure to Maternal Psychosocial Experiences

A review by Monk, Spicer and Champagne remarks that recent data suggests children gestated under significant stress, anxiety or depression are more likely to display characteristics considered precursors to psychopathologies, evidence that "fetal exposure to maternal psychosocial experiences contributes to the determination of children's neurodevelopmental trajectories" (Monk et al., 2012)[32]. That's particularly harmful, they argue, due to the "important role of epigenetic mechanisms in regulating gene activity, neurobiology, and behavior and the potential role of environmentally-induced epigenetic variation in linking early life exposures to long-term biobehavioral outcomes" (ibid.).

---

30 Richardson, N.C.: *A Nation in Utero: Pregnancy and Fetal Education in Early Republican China, 1912–1937*. PhD Dissertation, University of California: Davis, 2015.
31 Lackner, M./Vittinghoff, N.: *Mapping Meanings. The Field of New Learning in Late Qing China*. Sinica Leidensia, Vol. LXIV. BRILL: 2004, p. 671.
32 Monk, C./Spicer, J./Champagne, F.A.: "Linking prenatal maternal adversity to developmental outcomes in infants: The role of epigenetic pathways". *Development and Psychopathology*, 24 (04): 2012, pp. 1361–1376.

Cecil Reynolds, expands on that, noting that "in view of the complexity of the cortex and its prolonged development" (Reynolds, 2014)[33] it's unreasonable to blame cortical developmental issues only on genetic defects, for a multitude of other factors, including "psychoactive drugs (e.g., nicotine, antidepressants), toxic substances, or brain trauma, and nutritional or other environmental circumstances (e.g., maternal stress)" (ibid) could play a similarly important role.

On a different direction, a previous study by Jarrett Barnhill reminds us that "the impact of abnormal brain development plays a pivotal role in the lives of many people with intellectual disabilities, [...] influenc[ing] not only brain function but also sensitivity to environmental stress, deficits in adaptive skills, affect regulation, impulse control, and communication skills." (Barnhill, 2004)[34], a sentiment amalgamated by Callander and Travis – founders of Wellness Associates, a resource center for healthcare and well-being practitioners:

> [S]cores of studies in recent years have documented the potential for increased risk of lifelong problems for prenates exposed to excessive maternal stress, anxiety, and depression. [...] Parents – and hence their unborn – do better when living in a calm, addiction-free environment, supported by family and friends.
> (Callander/Travis, web)[35]

3.4 Some Fetal Cognitive and Behavioral Effects Due to Exposure of Alcohol and Drugs during Pregnancy

Cognition is the act or process of acquiring knowledge through perception, attention, association, memory, reasoning, judgment, imagination, thought and language. The teratogenic and cognitive development effects caused by antenatal exposure to alcohol, cocaine and cannabis have been investigated worldwide by different researchers that aimed to evaluate if maternal drug use was related to cognitive and behavioral disorders in infants (Huizink/Mulder, 2006)[36].

---

33 Reynolds, C.: *Handbook of Clinical Child Neuropsychology*. Springer, 2014, p. 29.
34 Barnhill, J.: "Developmental neuropsychiatry: Embryology and psychopathology". *NADD Bulletin*, VII (5), Article 3: 2004.
35 Callander, M.G./Travis, J.W.: "Myth: The fetus' brain and personality development are independent of their womb experience." Retrieved on April 27, 2017 from http://www.thewellspring.com/flex/pregnancy/2388/myth-the-fetus-brain-and-personality-development-are-independent-of-their-womb-experience.cfm.
36 Huizink, A.C./Mulder, E.J.: "Maternal smoking, drinking or cannabis use during pregnancy and neurobehavioral and cognitive functioning in human offspring". *Neuroscience & Biobehaviral Review*, *30*(1), 2006, pp. 24–41.

Many researchers have identified that a routine antenatal exposure to any of these chemical substances is responsible for promoting many adverse child behavioral and cognitive outcomes including Attention Deficit Hyperactivity Disorder, increased externalizing behavior and decreased cognitive function (Passeya et al., 2014)[37].

3.4.1 Prenatal Alcohol Exposure

The negative influence of maternal alcohol intake during pregnancy was previously analyzed and an adverse alcohol effect on cognitive development was not detected in children without Fetal Alcohol Syndrome (FAS) diagnosed. FAS refers to a pattern of anomalies that include craniofacial, central nervous system (CNS), body growth, and various sensory anomalies due to moderate to intense mother alcohol ingestion during pregnancy (Bailey et al., 2004; Bhutta et al., 2002; Kelly et al., 2009; da Silva-Lopes et al., 2016.)[38,39,40,41].

Michael Church and James Kaltenbach, classify the hearing disorders associated with FAS into four types: "developmentally delayed auditory function, sensorineural hearing loss, intermittent conductive hearing loss owing to recurrent serous otitis media, and central hearing loss" (Church/Kaltenbach, 1997)[42] and that, improvements to the children functional levels are possible with "early identification and intervention to treat hearing, language, and speech problems." (ibid).

---

37 Passeya, M.E./Sanson-Fisher, R.W./D'Este, C.A./Stirlinga, J.M. & Stirlinga, J.M.: "Tobacco, alcohol and cannabis use during pregnancy: Clustering of risks." *Drug and Alcohol Dependence, 134,* 2014, pp. 44–50.
38 Bailey, B.N./Delaney-Black, V./Covington, C.Y./Ager, J./Janisse, J./Hannigan, J.H., et al.: "Prenatal exposure to binge drinking and cognitive and behavioural outcomes at age 7 years." *American Journal of Obstetrics and Gynecology, 191,* 2004, pp. 1037–1043.
39 Bhutta, A.T./Cleves, M.A./Casey, P.H./Cradock, M.M./Anand, K.J.S.: "Cognitive and behavioural outcomes of school-aged children who were born preterm: A meta-analysis." *JAMA, 288,* 2002, pp. 728–737.
40 Kelly, Y./Sacker, A./Gray, R./Kelly, J./Wolke, D./Quigley, M.A.: "Light drinking in pregnancy, a risk for behavioural problems and cognitive deficits at 3 years of age?". *International Journal of Epidemiology, 38,* 2009, pp. 129–140.
41 da Silva-Lopes, L./Amelio, P.A./Ferraz, P.R./Silva, S.M.G./Rodrigues, M.R./Ferreira Medeiros, M.: "Sistematização De Cuidados De Enfermagem Para Gestantes Usuárias De Crack Baseada Em Estudo Bibliográfico". *Revista Eletrônica Estácio Saúde,* 5, 2016, pp. 123–137.
42 Church, M.W./Abel, E.L.: "Fetal alcohol syndrome. Hearing, speech, language, and vestibular disorders". *Obstetrics & Gynecology Clinics of North America, 25*(1), 1998 (March), pp. 85–97.

Martin and Dombrowsky's review examines studies that collectively show negative effects on higher-level cognitive functioning, including "cognitive flexibility, response inhibition, and planning and concept formation/reasoning" (Martin/Dombrowsky, 2008, p. 156)[43], impairment of "memory, recall and recognition of verbal information, memory for stories or designs, and spatial memory" (loc. cit.). They also remark that "[a]ttention deficits and hyperactive behavior are considered a hallmark of prenatal alcohol exposure and may be as sensitive an indicator of prenatal alcohol (and dose dependent) exposure as physical features" (ibid. p. 157).

3.4.2 Prenatal Marijuana Exposure

The Martin and Dombrowsky book also indicate that marijuana exposure during pregnancy may also have deleterious effects, and that it "has been associated with increased tremors, exaggerated and prolonged startle response, visuospatial reasoning capacity, short term memory, sustained attention and attentional deficits, altered sleep patterns and reduced habituation to visual stimuli." (ibid., p. 156)

3.4.3 Prenatal Crack Cocaine Exposure

Ross points out that the "vast majority of drugs of abuse do cross the placenta and, then it can directly act on its molecular target in the fetus" (Ross et al., 2015)[44] and, unsurprisingly, cocaine exposure also leads to "language deficits, behavior defects, and executive functioning abnormalities. [...] [and also] abnormalities related to lower arousal, poorer quality of movement and self-regulation, higher excitability, jitteriness, and more non-optimal reflexes". A previous work by Hurt found problems in "language, attention and perceptual reasoning skills" (Hurt et al., 2009)[45] and another by Singer reported that "cocaine-exposed children had significant cognitive deficits and a doubling of the rate of developmental delay during the first 2 years of life [...] it is possible that these children will

---

43 Martin, R.P./Dombrowski, S.C.: *Prenatal Exposures/Psychological and Educational Consequences for Children*. Springer: New York, 2008.
44 Ross, E.J. et al.: "Developmental consequences of fetal exposure to drugs: What we know and what we still must learn." *Neuropsychopharmacology*, 40(1), 2015, pp. 61–87. Doi: 10.1038/npp.2014.147. Epub 2014 Jun 18. Accessed on 23 April 2017.
45 Hurt, H./Betancourt, L.M./Malmud, E.K./Shera, D.M./Giannetta, J.M./Brodsky, N.L./Farah, M.J.: "Children with and without gestational cocaine exposure: a neurocognitive systems analysis". *Neurotoxicology and Teratology*, 31(6), 2009 Nov–Dec, pp. 334–341. doi: 10.1016/j.ntt.2009.08.002. Epub 2009 (August 15).

continue to have learning difficulties at school age." (Singer et al., 2002)[46] This more worrisome conclusion is reflected also in Ross' work: "behavioral outcomes observed at birth due to the cocaine exposure continue and sometimes worsen after 12 months of age" (Ross, 2015). These children display behaviors that can be "associated with less sociability, more withdrawn behavioral problems, more anxious/depressed behaviors and symptoms" (ibid.), all commonly considered to be "precursors of later psychiatric problems" (ibid), e.g. "disruptive behaviors including aggression and delinquent behavior at 9 years of age" (ibid) where reported in literature.

Trying to elicit causes, Lamy argues that some of these problems might result from misdiagnosed withdrawal syndrome then echoes the already listed consequences and adds "attention deficit disorders with impulsivity or with hyperactivity (ADHD), and memory disorders" (Lamy et al., 2015)[47] to the list, reinforcing that "the prevalence of depressive or anxiety disorders may also be increased in these children." (ibid.), and Martin and Dombrowsky state that, "[conceptually] cocaine's effect on the monoaminergic system [...] was thought to presage later difficulties with attention, aggression, impulsivity and mood lability." (Martin/Dombrowsky, p. 169).

3.5 The Chinese Medicine Perspective

Chinese medicine describes a central role of the Heart when it is dealing with emotional imbalance. The Heart is said to be the house of the spirit and when it is damaged there can be many psychological manifestations – some of them deep in the subconscious, some of them manifesting in high levels of anxiety and a number of other clinical symptoms. The Heart also has a direct link to the uterus and in fact is of key importance in controlling the 'opening and closing' of the uterus. Disturbed Heart Qi during pregnancy can lead to inappropriate opening of the uterus and miscarriage.

---

46 Singer, L.T./Arendt, R./Minnes, S./Farkas, K./Salvator, A./Kirchner, H.L./Kliegman, R.: "Cognitive and motor outcomes of cocaine-exposed infants". *JAMA*, *287*(15): 2002, pp. 1952–1960.

47 Lamy, S./Laqueille, X./Thibaut, F.: "Consequences of tobacco, cocaine and cannabis consumption during pregnancy on the pregnancy itself, on the newborn and on child development: A review." Retrieved on October 9, 2017 from https://www.ncbi.nlm.nih. gov/pubmed/25439854, translated from: *Encephale*. 2015 Jun; 41 Suppl 1: S13–S20. doi: 10.1016/j.encep.2014.08.012.

Treatment to prevent miscarriage should always be mindful of the heart and be settling or calming to the mind. Addressing the heart Qi is recognized as a very important part of TCM infertility treatment. (Lyttleton *op. cit.*, p. 311)

A basic therapeutic principle of pregnancy diseases is to "calm the fetus" (prevent miscarriage) while treating the disease. If the mother's disease causes the fetus to be restless, the emphasis is on treating the mother's disease, the dispelling of which will allow the fetus to calm itself. If the mother's disease is secondary and caused by the threat of miscarriage, measures should be taken to calm the fetus. When the fetus is calm, the mother's disease will be cured automatically. Calming the fetus is done by reinforcing the kidney, strengthening the spleen and soothing the liver in order to reinforce the foundation of the fetus, boost the source of blood and regulate qi movement. (Zhaoling 2015, pp. 366–367)[48].

As we can see, TCM describes the importance of communication between the heart and the uterus via the Bao vessel. After experiencing shock or great stress, the heart and kidney can be practically traumatized. This often leads to heart heat, which causes Heart *qi* to stagnate and, if the uterus opens suddenly, can cause a miscarriage or intermenstrual bleeding (Hemm, 2017)[49].

Alcohol or drug abuse, if extreme, can create such toxic conditions for the fetus that it cannot survive. Or they damage the mother's health sufficiently that her body is unable to sustain the pregnancy. In TCM such agents are usually said to create internal Heat, which at a certain level damages the endometrium and, as we discussed above, increases the risk of miscarriage due to disharmony in the Heart–Uterus connection via the Bao vessel (affected by toxic or internal Heat) (Lyttleton *op. cit.*, p. 278).

Sudden upset, shock, emotional trauma or more chronic agitation or anxiety are often symptoms of Heart Qi stagnation. The patient may complain of palpitations, insomnia, and diagnosed psychosis. The treatment principle in this pathology would be to calm the shen and circulate the Heart Qi (ibid., p. 285).

If the Heat affects the Heart, then there is a high risk of miscarriage because the Heart–Uterus connection via the Bao vessel can be disturbed. TCM theory posits that the Heart Qi has much to do with 'opening' of the Uterus and, when its Qi is disturbed (for example by Liver-Fire), the disruption in the Bao vessel may precipitate an untimely opening of the Uterus. For this reason, the cautious

---

48 Zhaoling, Y.: *Gynecology in Chinese Medicine*. PMPH-USA, 2015, pp. 366–367.
49 Hemm, D.: "Physiology and pathology of fertility and reproduction from the TCM perspective", *Musculoskeletal Key*, last modified 2017, retrieved on April 27, 2017, http://musculoskeletalkey.com/physiology-and-pathology-of-fertility-and-reproduction-from-the-tcm-perspective/.

doctor is ever mindful of the Heart and Kidney relationship in early pregnancy. What this means is that the mental and emotional state of the newly pregnant woman can influence the pregnancy and a skillful doctor will take measures to safeguard the fetus by using acupuncture or herbs to calm the woman's mind if she is excessively anxious or agitated (ibid.).

Women, are cautioned to control their emotions, especially during pregnancy. Suwen's explains, in chapter 44, how emotions such as sadness can disharmonize the flow of Qi[50], thus affecting the uterus. According to Suwen, this can manifest itself clinically as bloody urine, but it also follows that internal agitation of Yang will adversely affect fetal health, possibly leading to an abortion:[51]

> When sadness and grief are excessive, then the network [vessels] of the uterus rupture. When the network [vessels] of the uterus rupture, then the yang qi is agitated internally. When it is effused, then a collapse occurs below the heart. [Patients] frequently pass urine with blood[52].

Yang Shangshan in Chapter 44 of Taisu. adds: "When there is excessive sorrow, the collateral network vessel of the uterus is severed. When this is the case, yang qi cannot move internally"[53] (Leo 2011, pp. 126–127).

---

50 *Suwen* in Chapter 39 《举痛论》 explains how the sorrow produces disharmony in the Qi flow: "When one is sad, then the heart connection is tense. The lobes of the lung spread open and rise and the upper burner is impassable. The camp [qi] and the guard [qi] do not disperse. Heat qi is in the center. Hence, the qi dissipates." (悲则心系急，肺布叶举，而上焦不通，荣卫不散，热气在中，故气消矣).

51 The text mentions bloody urine but illustrates what could happen to other Lower Burner organs – as the uterus. For a pregnant woman, this could cause vaginal bleeding that might indicate high abortion risk (or an actual abortion). We find similar passages in another text as *Tài sù* by Yáng shàngshàn 《太素·五脏凄》卷二十五，杨上善注 e Zhòng guǎng bǔ zhù huángdì nèijīng sù wèn by Wáng bīng 《重广补注黄帝内经素问·痞论》卷十二，王冰注.

52 《痿论》悲哀太甚，则胞络绝，胞络绝则阳气内动;发则心下崩，数溲血也

53 Also in *Taisu*: 《太素·五脏凄》卷二十五，杨上善注[悲哀大甚胞络绝，绝则阳气内动，发则心下崩，数溲血。]胞络者，心上胞络之脉。心悲太甚，则令心上胞络脉绝，手少阳气內动有伤，心下崩损，血循手少阳脉下，尿血，致令脉虚为脉痹，传为脉痿。

3.6 Pathologies of Baomai and Baoluo

The *Suwen* lists some pathologies of the two vessels Baomai and Baoluo which are based on disruption, i.e. an impaired flow of Qi and blood due either to mental disturbances or mechanical obstruction[54].

In Western medicine, it is a well-known phenomenon that a long-term grief, sorrow and mental pressure result in menstrual disorders, either in mid-cycle bleedings or in amenorrhea. If this severe impairment of *shen*, i.e. the psyche occurs during pregnancy this might be a reason for abortion. Chinese medicine explains this by undernourishment of the *bao* by stagnation of Heart Qi in the upper part of the body, in Western medicine the mechanism is not clear.

The other pathology that concerns pregnancy is the syndrome which we may identify as the compression syndrome of the caval vein[55]. The Suwen Chapter 47 states:

> When a woman is pregnant and in the ninth month she loses speech what is the reason for this? Qibo said: <This is because the luo and mai of the bao are disrupted.> Huangdi: <What does this mean?> Qibo: <the Baoluo is bound to the kidney; the shaoyin channel pertains to the kidney and is bound to the tongue, therefor she cannot speak. (Yang 1990, p. 356)

In late pregnancy the unborn fetus becomes heavy and presses not only on the vessels and channels, i.e. on Baomai and Baoluo but also on the kidney channel. The Qi of the kidney channel cannot rise upward to nourish the tongue.

This passage shows the close affiliation between the two shaoyin channels of heart and kidney. Both channels do have contact to the root of the tongue. The pressure on Baomai, Baoluo and shaoyin channels in this case might be interpreted as a compression of the caval vein during late pregnancy (see above) which goes along with temporary loss of consciousness, dyspnea and hypotonus; or on the other hand a precursor of a preeclampsia which goes along with hypertension edema and proteinuria (EPH). These symptoms all make visible the stagnation of Qi in the heart and kidney channels and a disruption of the flow of Qi between the upper and the lower part.

3.7 The Significance of Baomai and Baoluo for Treatment

Baomai and Baoluo are two different kinds of vessels. On the one hand we may interpret Baomai as arteries, branches of the aorta abdominalis which provide

---

54 *Suwen*, chapters 33 and 44.
55 Y. Weijie (1990) p. 356.

blood to the uterus and the ovarian tubes or in man to the gonads (testes) and the penis. The Baoluo in this context may be interpreted as the caval vein. On the other hand, both vessels are close to the channels of heart and pericardium, the Baomai being close to the heart channel, the Baoluo to the channel of pericardium on the one hand and to the kidney channel on the other hand. According to the statement of *Suwen* (47) the Baoluo seems to be a branch of the kidney channel or at least to have a direct contact to this channel.

The statements of the *Suwen* (33) and (44) make clear that one could observe the influence of the psyche on the menstrual behavior and in a broader scope of pregnancy. The descriptions based on the theory of the channels attribute the impairment of the menstrual cycle or abortion to a lack of heart blood in the uterus. This becomes plausible when one attributes the production or the circulation of gonadotropines and gonadal hormones to the circulation of blood *xue*. And one might imagine that sterility, infertility and abortion may be due to undernourishment of the endometrium with blood. But there is also the shen aspect which may be impaired by the disruption of Baomai or Baoluo. Impairment of the *shen* may also result in menstrual disorders, sterility and even abortion or delayed development of the fetus.

The preeclampsia, which may be described in Suwen (44), really goes along with alterations in the mother's blood along with hypertension, which may be understood, in Chinese medicine as a disharmony between heart and kidney – or Baomai/Baoluo and kidney – or as a stagnation of the heart-Qi and -blood in the upper part. Hypotony in the late pregnancy is said to be due to a blockage of both, Baomai and Baoluo. And in particular the Baoluo – interpreted as the vessels leading to the caval vein – may be seen as responsible for the lack of blood in the upper part which makes hypotension, vertigo and dyspnea.

Therefore, we see that Baomai and Baoluo were mixed concepts of anatomy and channel theory that particularly served to explain certain pathologies in menstrual behavior and pregnancy. As for the male organism, the two vessels and their pathologies were no subject of discussion. However, we might imagine that erectile dysfunction due to nervousness and stress might have its source in undernourishment of the male genitals due to the disruption of Baomai or Baoluo. So in this case instead of only soothing the liver one has to calm the spirit, clear the heat of the heart and activate the blood circulation downward. In acupuncture, there are several points on the Shaoyin- and Jueyin-channels that are useful: Pc 6, Pc 7, H 7, Ren 14, Ren 17, Liv 3, Ki 3 and Yingtang. The points Pc 6, Pc 7, H 7 and Yingtang are also apt for pregnancy.

4 Conclusions

The concept of Baomai and Baoluo is discussed in different ways.

There are experts who see a connection between Baomai and Baoluo and the vessels of Renmai and Chongmai. An argument for this idea is the fact that in the specialized literature following the *Huangdi neijing* there is a little mention of the two vessels and problems of menstruation and pregnancy are mainly discussed in relation to Renmai and Chongmai. It seems nevertheless more plausible that Baomai and Baoluo be different from Renmai and Chongmai. The two vessels are described as nourishing vessels, especially for the genitals that means their scope of activity is rather restricted. Moreover, there is no question about their origin in the *baozhong*.

The concept of Baomai and Baoluo may have its source partly in anatomic findings and it seems to be a mixed concept between anatomy and channel theory. As part of the channels they may be understood as branches of the heart channel and the pericardium channel, respectively. The characters of *mai* and *bao* in their names may also be a hint to the location of the vessels: the Baomai might nourish the deeper layers of the corresponding tissues, and the *luo* might nourish the superficial layers of the tissues, as it is the case for the rest of the channels and luo vessels. As anatomically visible vessels they may represent the small arteries and veins which are branches of the aorta abdominalis (Baomai) and the caval vein (Baoluo).

Baomai and Baoluo can also be placed as possibly important actors for pre-natal psycho/neurocognitive processes. As a relatively new field of study for Western medicine, Chinese Medicine's views about the physiology of the channels and organs involved in a pregnancy can provide enriching insights and Strangifications (Greiner/Wallner/Gostentschnig, 2006) for further research and discussions.

During pregnancy, Bao Mai and Bao Luo are responsible for the flow of Qi, Blood and Essence (Jing) in the uterus, nourishing and supporting the development of the fetus. We can understand this dynamic as a bi-directional information flow between pregnant and fetus. The fetus exhibits cognitive capacities since early gestation stages and various factors (stress, substance abuse, and environment) can affect its development.

As shown above, heart and kidneys play key roles on processes involved in fertility and gestation. We have also shown that heart and kidneys are involved on the pre-natal psycho/neurological development, as one of heart's function is to house the Mind/Shen, and the kidneys are also linked to the brain and related with the development of the nervous system (Maciocia op. cit., pp. 156–157).

For these reasons, we can't neglect the importance of the Bao Mai and Bao Luo channels when studying pre-natal psycho/neurocognitive processes, for it's through these channels that heart and kidney communicate with the uterus, and when analyzing the citations to the Bao Mai and Bao Luo channels in ancient texts we can ascribe to them a central role on the interaction dynamics between environment, pregnant and fetus.

Heart and kidneys use the Bao Mai and Bao Luo channels not only to support the physical development of the fetus, but also serve as information exchange pathways between pregnant and the fetus[56].

During pregnancy, Bao Mai and Bao Luo are responsible for the flow of Qi, blood and essence (Jing) in the uterus, nourishing and supporting the development of the fetus.

Current research shows that the fetus, since its first weeks, already develops cognitive capacities essential to further post-natal developments and that those capabilities can be harmed by the pregnant exposure to stress, malnutrition, abuse of toxic substances, polluted environment, and others. The ancient Chinese belief is that the fetus was highly impressionable by outside forces which aligns with modern observations of the development of cognitive abilities in the fetus from external stimuli.

The ancient Chinese believed that pregnant and fetus exchanged information, and prescribed that the gestation happened in a harmonically balanced environment, stress-free, with the pregnant following a strict diet and avoiding exposure to factors detrimental to fetal development.

What astonishes is the fact that the concept of Bao Mai and Bao Luo seems to have fallen into oblivion during Chinese medical history. But it can explain several phenomena which we know in Western medicine and its understanding opens new ways in diagnosis and treatment of menstrual disorders, sterility, infertility, the female psyche, and the erectile dysfunction and impotence of man.

We propose to extend the Bao Mai/Bao Luo functions to include their possible connection to the dynamics of pre-natal psycho/neurocognitive development in addition to their already known roles on ovulation, menstruation and fertility. By doing this we are not trying to diminish or ignore the importance of other

---

56 Here we consider "information" to be all stimuli (e.g. sounds, hormonal changes) that can be directly (or indirectly) physiologically sensed by pregnant and fetus.

channels as Dumai, Ren Mai and Chong Mai[57] (or all the 5 Zang organs)[58] for fetal development but, instead we believe that this could help understand how, and through which specific pathways, the mutual interactions between pregnant and fetus happen on processes related to neurocognition. Further reflections and a deeper understanding of the role of heart and kidneys on the pregnant–fetus relationship might allow a reframing of ancient practices as the Taijiao, removing them from mere folk beliefs or traditional culture, positioning fetal education as a practice with support on fundamental Chinese medicine theories, and opening a dialog with modern scientific observations.

A deeper understanding will also foster the development of preventive and follow-up strategies, focused on the pre-natal psycho/neurocognitive processes, with the aim to enrich the gestation process since the first weeks for better fetal cognitive development. It also allows for new reasoning to support initiatives that advocate for the gestation to happen in a tranquil environment, facilitating lifestyle changes for all those involved. We have shown that both Chinese tradition and modern science agree that while pregnant and fetus are the main actors, the whole family (father, family relations and friends) and multiple societal aspects can also have persistent, long-term influences (positively or adversely) on how the children – and future adult – will perceive and relate to the world.

References

Bailey, B.N./Delaney-Black, V./Covington, C.Y./Ager, J./Janisse, J./Hannigan, J.H., et al.: "Prenatal exposure to binge drinking and cognitive and behavioural outcomes at age 7 years." *American Journal of Obstetrics and Gynecology, 191*, 2004, pp. 1037–1043.

Barnhill, J.: "Developmental neuropsychiatry: Embryology and psychopathology". *NADD Bulletin*, Vol. VII(5), Article 3, 2004.

Bhutta, A.T./Cleves, M.A./Casey, P.H./Cradock, M.M./Anand, K.J.S.: "Cognitive and behavioural outcomes of school-aged children who were born preterm: A meta-analysis." *JAMA, 288*, 2002, pp. 728–737.

---

57 Late imperial authors stated that the womb vessels were in fact the thoroughfare and controller vessels, two circulation tracts that had a special relationship with the womb. See Y-L. Wu *op. cit.*, p. 91.

58 See Theoretical Research of Five Organs Regulating the Female Reproduction in Traditional Chinese Medicine 中医五脏调控女性生殖的理论研究 《河北医科大学》 2015 年班光国.

Callander, M.G./Travis, J.W.: "Myth: The fetus' brain and personality development are independent of their womb experience", 2015, Retrieved on April 27, 2017 from http://www.thewellspring.com/flex/pregnancy/2388/myth-the-fetus-brain-and-personality-development-are-independent-of-their-womb-experience.cfm.

Cheng, F-K.: "Taijiao: A traditional Chinese approach to enhancing fetal growth through maternal physical and mental health". *Chinese Nursing Research*, 3(2), 2016, pp. 49–53.

Church, M.W./Abel, E.L.: "Fetal alcohol syndrome. Hearing, speech, language, and vestibular disorders". *Obstetrics and Gynecology Clinics of North America*, 25(1), 1998 (March), pp. 85–97.

Church, M.W./Kaltenbach, J.A.: "Hearing, speech, language, and vestibular disorders in the fetal alcohol syndrome: A literature review". *Alcoholism: Clinical and Experimental Research*, 21(3), 1997, pp. 495–512.

da Silva-Lopes, L./Amelio, P.A./Ferraz, P.R./Silva, S.M.G./Rodrigues, M.R./Ferreira Medeiros, M.: "Sistematização De Cuidados De Enfermagem Para Gestantes Usuárias De Crack Baseada Em Estudo Bibliográfico". *Revista Eletrônica Estácio Saúde*, 5, 2016, pp. 123–137.

"Etymology." Retrieved on April 27, 2017, from http://www.chineseetymology.org/.

Flaws, B.: *A Compendium of Chinese Medical Menstrual Diseases*. Blue Poppy Press: Boulder, 2005.

Greiner, K./Wallner, F.G./Gostentschnig, M.: *Verfremdung*. Peter Lang: Frankfurt am Main, 2006.

Hemm, D.: "Physiology and pathology of fertility and reproduction from the TCM perspective", *Musculoskeletal Key*, last modified 2017, retrieved on April 27, 2017, http://musculoskeletalkey.com/physiology-and-pathology-of-fertility-and-reproduction-from-the-tcm-perspective/.

Hepper, P.G.: "Fetal memory: Does it exist? What does it do?" *Acta Paeditrica Supplement*, 416, 1996, pp. 16–20.

Huotilainen, M.: "Foetal learning – a bridge over birth". Retrieved on April 27, 2017 from https://www.edu.helsinki.fi/lapsetkertovat/lapset/In_English/Huotilainen.pdf.

Huizink, A.C./Mulder, E.J.: "Maternal smoking, drinking or cannabis use during pregnancy and neurobehavioral and cognitive functioning in human offspring". *Neuroscience & Biobehavioral Reviews*, 30(1), 2006, pp. 24–41.

Hurt, H./Betancourt, L.M./Malmud, E.K./Shera, D.M./Giannetta, J.M./Brodsky, N.L./Farah, M.J.: "Children with and without gestational cocaine exposure:

A neurocognitive systems analysis". *Neurotoxicology and Teratology, 31*(6), 2009 Nov-Dec, pp. 334-341. doi: 10.1016/j.ntt.2009.08.002. Epub 2009 (August 15).

James, D.K./Spencer, C.J./Stepsis, B.W.: "Fetal learning: A prospective randomized controlled study". *Ultrasound in Obstetrics and Gynecology, 20*(5), 2002, pp. 431-438.

Kelly, Y./Sacker, A./Gray, R./Kelly, J./Wolke, D./Quigley, M.A.: "Light drinking in pregnancy, a risk for behavioural problems and cognitive deficits at 3 years of age?". *International Journal of Epidemiology,* 38, 2009, pp. 129-140.

Kisilevsky, B.S./Hains, S.M.J.: "Exploring the relationship between fetal heart rate and cognition". *Infant and Child Development,* 19, 2010, pp. 60-75. doi:10.1002/icd.655.

Lackner, M./Vittinghoff, N.: *Mapping Meanings: The Field of New Learning in Late Qing China.* Sinica Leidensia, Vol. LXIV. Brill: Leiden & Boston, 2004.

Lamy, S./Laqueille, X./Thibaut, F.: "Consequences of tobacco, cocaine and cannabis consumption during pregnancy on the pregnancy itself, on the newborn and on child development: A review." Retrieved on October 9, 2017 from https://www.ncbi.nlm.nih.gov/pubmed/25439854, translated from: Encephale. 2015 June; 41(Suppl. 1): S13-S20. doi: 10.1016/j.encep.2014.08.012.

Lan, F.: *Culture, Philosophy, and Chinese Medicine: Viennese Lectures (Culture And Knowledge).* Peter Lang Publishing Group: Frankfurt am Main; New York, 1st edition, 2012.

Leo, J.: *Sex in the Yellow Emperor's Basic Questions.* Three Pines Press: Dunedin, 2011.

Liley, A.W.: "The foetus as a personality". *Australian and New Zealand Journal of Psychiatry,* 6, 1972, p. 99.

Lyttleton, J.: *Treatment of Infertility with Chinese Medicine.* Elsevier Health Sciences: London, 2013.

Nanjing Zhong yi xue yuan. Zhong yi xi: *Lingshu yishi.* In: Nanjing TCM University (eds.): *Annotated and Translated edition of the Spiritual Pivot of the Classic of Internal Medicine of the Yellow Emperor.* Shanghai kexue jishu chubanshe: Shanghai, 1997.

Maciocia, G.: *The Foundations of Chinese Medicine.* Elsevier Health Sciences UK: London, 2015.

Martin, R.P./Dombrowski, S.C.: *Prenatal Exposures/Psychological and Educational Consequences for Children.* Springer: New York, 2008.

Monk, C./Spicer, J./Champagne, F.A.: "Linking prenatal maternal adversity to developmental outcomes in infants: The role of epigenetic pathways". *Development and Psychopathology, 24*(04), 2012, pp. 1361-1376.

Passeya, M.E./Sanson-Fisher, R.W./D'Este, C.A./Stirlinga, J.M./Stirlinga, J.M.: "Tobacco, alcohol and cannabis use during pregnancy: Clustering of risks.". *Drug and Alcohol Dependence, 134*, 2014, pp. 44–50.

Pietilä, I./Vainio, S.: "The embryonic aorta-gonad-mesonephros region as a generator of haematopoietic stem cells", *Journal Compilation APMIS, 12*(113), 2005, pp. 804–812.

Reynolds, C.: *Handbook of Clinical Child Neuropsychology.* Springer: New York, 2014.

Richardson, N.C.: *A Nation in Utero: Pregnancy and Fetal Education in Early Republican China, 1912-1937.* PhD Dissertation: University of California: Davis, 2015.

Riegel, A.M.: *Die Niere shen. Klassische Konzepte der traditionellen chinesischen Medizin im Lichte der modernen Schulmedizin.* Bacopa: Schiedlberg, 2010.

Riegel, A.M.: "Qijing bamai – The eight extraordinary vessels. A concept of Chinese Medicine based on the Yijing". In: Wallner, F.G./Kluenger, G. (eds.), *Constructive Realism – Philosophy, science and Medicine (libri nigri 53).* Verlag Traugott Bautz: Nordhausen, 2016.

Rochat de la Vallee, E./Larre, C.: *The Extraordinary Fu.* Monkey Press: London, 2003.

Ross, E.J., et al: "Developmental consequences of fetal exposure to drugs: What we know and what we still must learn." *Neuropsychopharmacology, 40* (1), 2015, pp. 61–87. Accessed on 23 April, 2017. doi: 10.1038/npp.2014.147. Epub 2014 Jun 18.

Singer, L.T./Arendt, R./Minnes, S./Farkas, K./Salvator, A./Kirchner, H.L./Kliegman, R.: "Cognitive and motor outcomes of cocaine-exposed infants". *JAMA 287*(15): 2002, pp. 1952–1960.

Unschuld, P.U./Bian, Q.: *Nan-ching the Classic of Difficult Issues.* University of California Press: Berkeley, 1986.

Unschuld, P./Tessenow, H.: *A Dictionary of the Huang Di Nei Jing Su Wen.* University of California Press: Berkeley, 2008.

Wiseman, N.: *English-Chinese Chinese-English Dictionary of Chinese Medicine.* Hunan kexue jishu chubanshe: Changsha, 1996.

Wu, Y-L.: *Reproducing Women: Medicine, Metaphor, and Childbirth in Late Imperial China.* University of California Press: Berkeley, 2010.

Yang, W.: *Huangdi neijing Suwen shijie (Modern Translation and Expanations to the Simple Questions of the Classic of Internal Medicine of the Yellow Emperor).* Yuejun shuju: Taipei, 1990.

Zhaoling, Y.: *Gynecology in Chinese Medicine.* PMPH-USA, 2015.

Andrea-Mercedes Riegel
Baomai and *Baoluo*: Two Vessels of Importance Not Only for Female Health

Abstract: Baomai and Baoluo are not well defined in Chinese medical literature. The comparison between the development of the extraordinary vessels in the embryo and the development of the germ layers helps us to understand and define these structures called Baomai and Baoluo as a mixed concept between anatomy and channel theory.

1 Introduction

Baomai and Baoluo are not very well-known vessels or even networks and the concept of these vessels seems rather obscure. There are only a few chapters in the *Huangdi neijing* which mention these two vessels and they do not explain exactly what they are or how one should imagine them from an anatomic point of view. The *Suwen* (33) makes these two vessels responsible for regular menstruation and pregnancy and considers them very sensitive to emotional disturbances. The main pathology of these two vessels is disruption of *jue* 绝 which results in an undernourishment of the *baozhong*, causing women to miss menstruation, become sterile or suffer miscarriage.

Suwen (33) states, "If the monthly affair doesn't flow, this is due to an obstruction of Baomai. Baomai pertains to the heart and connects to *baozhong*." And *Suwen* (47) states, "The Baoluo is bound to the kidney; the Shaoyin channel extends to the kidney (...)"[1]

Baomai is mentioned here – as one might interpret – as a branch of the heart channel; and it is mentioned in relation to the female uterus. One might therefore draw the conclusion that Baomai, being connected to the heart, transports heart-blood to the uterus.

For the nourishment of the uterus it seems that both vessels, Baomai and Baoluo, are responsible in this respect; and both therefore seem to be complements to Renmai and Chongmai.[2] Baomai transports heart blood to the uterus

---

1 Yang, Weijie: *Huangdi neijing Suwen shijie* 1990, p. 356.
2 Bob Flaws sees Baomai as being a synonym to Chongmai because there are no disharmony patterns mentioned in the classic literature referring to Baomai but only to Chongmai. See Flaws, Bob: *A Compendium of Chinese Medical Menstrual Diseases*. Blue Poppy Press: Boulder, 2005, p. 9.

and Baoluo, being bound to the kidney, provides essence. Wiseman suggests there are several Baomai and Baoluo. He translates the Baoluo with "uterine network vessels" and Baomai with "uterine vessels".[3] Unschuld/Tessenow however translate Baoluo with "network vessel of the uterus" and Baomai with "uterus vessel".[4] Some practitioners interpret the Baomai as the vessels nourishing the deeper layers of the uterus and Baoluo as vessels supplying the superficial layers according to the concept of *mai* 脉 and *luo* 络 in the *jingluo*-system.

We want to make clear what these two vessels Baomai and Baoluo are and define their place of activity.

2 The Place of Activity of Baomai and Baoluo: Baozhong

Right here we are faced with a new concept, which is the concept of *baozhong*. We must first take a closer look at the character *bao* and ask what kind of connotations this word has. Originally the character *bao* 胞 just denoted the female womb where the fetus could develop.[5] The character follows the radical no. 130 *rou* 肉 (flesh), the phonetic part *bao* 包 originally shows a person bending over to enfold an object. The primitive meaning of *bao* 包 being gestation[6] the whole character has to do with the development of new life. New life always develops in the female womb. But may we accept the idea that *bao* 胞 as a "muscular wrapper" also exists in the male body? There is evidence that in a broader sense the character *bao* indeed may just denote a muscular wrapper in general. The *Lingshu* (63) states,

> when [the sour taste] resides in the stomach, the inner of the stomach is harmonized and warm, it flows down to the bladder; the bladder's *bao*, being thin and weak when accepting the sour taste, shrinks […][7]

---

3 See Wiseman, Nigel: *English-Chinese Chinese-English Dictionary of Chinese Medicine*. Hunan kexue chubanshe: Changsha, 1996, p. 401.
4 Unschuld, Paul/Tessenow, Herrmann: *A Dictionary of the Huang Di Nei Jing Su Wen*. University of California Press: Berkeley, 2008, p. 20. They offer a literal translation of *mai* and *luo* in order to maintain the difference which is made in the original text. They do not give an explanation of the difference between the two vessels or of the meaning of the vessels.
5 See *Zhongwen dacidian*. Zhongguo wenhua daxue chubanshe: Taibei, 1982 vol. 7, p. 999.
6 See Wilder, George D./Ingram, James H. *Analysis of Chinese Characters*. Caves Books Ltd.: Taibei, 1974.
7 *Lingshu yishi*, p. 372. Bao here is interpreted as the wrapper around the bladder but the bladder itself may also be seen as a kind of *bao*.

Seen as the uterus, the *bao* pertains to the so-called "extraordinary organs".[8] The *Suwen* (11) calls it *nüzibao* 女子胞.[9]

The concept of *baozhong* is introduced in *Suwen* (33).[10] It is the structure to which the Baomai connects. At a first glance this seems easy to understand as the "center of the uterus". But we need to pay attention to this term because this area or structure must also exist in the male organism. Regarding this, Rochat de la Vallee states that the *baozhong* does not exactly represent the uterus here. She states it is, "the center of what is wrapped and protected and thus designates the protection of the origin of life."[11] Indeed new life comes into existence in the uterus but also by the action of the female and male gonads.

Baozhong is the origin of Renmai, Dumai and Chongmai[12] and the Baomai connects to it. The term is mentioned in several classics without being strictly defined. It seems associated with several structures. What is *baozhong*?

Baozhong and the Mingmen

Rochat's translation establishes a connection between *baozhong* and the *mingmen*, the gate of life, and the gate of life is bound to the kidney. The theories about the *mingmen* are manifold in Chinese medical history,[13] it is first mentioned in the *Nanjing*. *Nanjing* (36) states,

[...] It is like this: the kidneys are not both kidneys. The one on the left is the kidney, the one on the right is the gate of life (*mingmen*). The gate of life is the place where the spirit essence (*shenjing*) lodges; it is the place to which the original influences (Yuan Qi) are tied. Hence in males it stores the essence, in females it holds the womb. Hence one knows that there is only one kidney.[14]

---

8   See *Suwen* (11). The extraordinary organs are the brain, the marrow, the bones, the vessels, the gallbladder and the uterus. Yang Weijie, p. 100.
9   See Yang Weijie, p. 100.
10 See also *Lingshu* (65).
11 Rochat de la Vallee/Larre, Claude: *The Extraordinary Fu*. Monkey Press: London, 2003, p. 165.
12 See Huangfu, Mi: *Zhenjiu jiayijing jiaozhu*. Renmin Weisheng chubanshe: Beijing, 1998, p. 385 and Li, Shizhen (*Qijing bamai kao*); *Li Shizhen yixue quanshu*. Zhongguo zhongyiyao chubanshe: Beijing, 2007, p. 1636 and 1639.
13 For further information see Riegel, Andrea-Mercedes: *Die Niere shen. Klassische Konzepte der chinesischen Medizin im Lichte der modernen Schulmedizin*. (Doctoral thesis) Bacopa: Schiedberg, 2010.
14 Unschuld, Paul: *Nan-Ching. The Classic of Difficult Issues*. University Press Group Ltd.: Dhaka, 1986, p. 382.

Nanjing (39) repeats this statement and adds the words, "The influences of the gate of life are identical with [those of] the kidney."[15] This might be confirmed by the statement of *Lingshu* (62), "Chongmai is the great network of the shaoyin channel, it originates from under the kidney."[16]

One idea about the *mingmen* was that the *mingmen* might be the right kidney, or this might be the space between the two kidneys; and Huangfu Mi (215-282) called the point Du 4 Mingmen, maybe because he identified the *mingmen* with the lower *dantian*, "the center of breath and the body energy [...] the place from where the Qi of Dumai originates."[17] From this point of view the *mingmen* would be the place *baozhong*.

Baozhong and the Lower Dantian

Zhang Jiebin (1563-1640), the most famous physician of the Ming Dynasty (1368-1644) raised doubts about the statement of the *Nanjing* that the *mingmen*, the place for reproduction, is associated with one kidney. Based on the trigram Kan ☵ he stated,

> The two kidneys correspond to the two Yin lines in the trigram Kan. The *mingmen* is represented in the Yang-line in the middle of the two Yin lines [...] This means that the *mingmen* dominates both kidneys and both kidneys pertain to the *mingmen*. Therefore the *mingmen* is the palace for fire and water the safefor Yin and Yang, the ocean for essence and Qi, the reservate for life and death. When the *mingmen* is exhausted the five viscera do not have any sustain.[18]

He saw the *mingmen* as being located in the region between the points Guanyuan (Ren 4) and Qihai (Ren 6) that is, in the "lower *dantian*", the space where the original Qi (Yuan Qi) is stored. He saw this as the place where the human being begins his life, where he absorbs the mother's Qi. In a narrow sense he considered the cervix as the entrance "*men*" [門] for the fertile sperm to the uterus, the entrance where the uterus absorbs the sperm and where the human being at birth leaves the motherly womb.

Although Zhang Jiebin identified *baozhong*, uterus and the *mingmen*; on the other hand or in a broader sense, he saw the lower *dantian* as the location of the *mingmen*. The medical compendium of the Qing Dynasty (1644-1911), the

---

15 Ibid., p. 399.
16 *Lingshu yishi*, p. 369.
17 Riegel, Andrea-Mercedes: *Die klassischen Akupunkturpunkte. Bedeutung, Indikation, Wirkung*. Elsevier: München, 2012, p. 40.
18 Zhang, Jiebin: *Leijing*. Zhongguo zhongyiyao chubanshe: Beijing, 2000, p. 683.

Baomai and *Baoluo*: Two Vessels of Importance 243

Yizong jinjian,[19] (The Golden Mirror of Medical Doctrine), which summarizes the medical knowledge throughout the medical history, also gives an interesting explanation of the character *bao*, identifying it also with the *dantian*. It states,

> The Dumai arises within the lower abdomen, externally in the abdomen, internally in the *bao*, also called *dantian* in both men and women, In women it is the uterus; in men it is the room of sperm.[20]

The Baozhong – Uterus and Palace of Sperm

This statement of the *Yizongjinjian* confirms the idea that *bao* or *baozhong* does exist in man and woman. We may draw the same conclusion from the text of *Lingshu* (65) which deals with the question why women do not have a beard:

> Huangdi said: <That women do not have a beard is it that they do not have [enough] blood and Qi?>Qibo said:<Chongmai and Renmai do arise from the *baozhong*, they run upward in the interior of the back, they are the ocean of the channels and networks. When they come to the surface they run upward along the abdomen, at the throat they come together. Here one branch separates and runs around the mouth and lips; when Qi and blood are abundant they moisten the skin and warm up the flesh. When only blood is abundant it penetrates the skin and makes hairs grow. The characteristics of women is that they are rich in Qi and poor in blood because they often lose blood; Chongmai and Renmai do not nourish the mouth and lips, for this the beard does not grow. [...]
> Huangdi said: <The Daoist priests are injured in their genitals, their Yin-Qi is disrupted and doesn't rise upward, the genitals lost their function but their beard didn't disappear, what is the reason for this? It is only in the eunuchs of the imperial palace that [their beard] disappeared. I would like to hear the reason for this.>Qibo said: <The eunuchs removed the whole of their genital sinews, they injured their Chongmai, the blood was discharged and did not recover the skin is knotted in the interior, the mouth and lips are not nourished [by Renmai and Chongmai], for this the beard-hair doesn't grow.>
> Huangdi said: <There are eunuchs by birth, whose genitals were not injured and who not [regularly] lose blood but their beard hair doesn't grow neither. What is the reason for this? > Qibo said: <This is an innate deficiency, their Renmai and Chongmai are not filled up, their whole genitals are not complete, there is Qi but no blood, for this their beard hair doesn't grow.[21]

In women the *baozhong* may refer to the uterus; in men the "palace of sperm" may be interpreted as the testes with the reservoir which is the epididymis. Dumai,

---

19 The work was published in 1742.
20 *Yizongjinjian* (44) *siyun men*; Wu, Qian: *Yizong jinjian*. Liaoning kexuejishu chubanshe: Chenyang, 1999, p. 431.
21 *Lingshu yishi*, p. 393f.

Renmai and Chongmai arise from the *baozhong*. All of them are responsible for the nourishment of the uterus with blood, but they are also present in the male organism. As the extraordinary vessels come into existence in an early embryonal state and as they precede the coming into existence of the regular channels and the inner organs, one might expect that this location of *baozhong* also comes into existence in an early embryonic stadium; and it also exists in the male embryo.

2.1 Baozhong and the Extraordinary Vessels

The Eight extraordinary vessels are the vessels which do control the regular channels and the network vessels *luomai*. They do not have the inner–outer relationship like the twelve main channels and they do not transport Qi and blood in an endless circle. That's why they are called "extraordinary".[22] In the body they do represent Heaven and Earth by being directly associated with the eight trigrams of the *Yijing*. In the body the development of the eight extraordinary vessels precedes the development of the regular channels. They build up the framework of the unborn fetus and are involved in the development process of the embryo. As they are still active in the living being, they are a linking part between pre-Heaven and post-Heaven.

The *Yiyixiangjie* 医易相结 (Medicine and the Changes are correlated), a book on the relationship between medicine and the *Yijing* which was written during the Ming Dynasty, describes the development of the eight extraordinary vessels in the embryo. It states,

> In the beginning the fetus isn't but little Yang-Qi, this is the origin of the process of Qian ☰, which corresponds to Chongmai. In the second month Qi changes into fluid which corresponds to Dui ☱ and Dumai. During the third month Qi and fluid mix up and develop heat which corresponds to Li ☲ and Renmai. In the fourth month the fetus begins to move in correspondence to Zhen, the thunder, and Daimai. [...]

The development begins with Chongmai and the Trigram Qian. In man, Qian represents the head which is the palace of *shen* 神 (consciousness). It also represents the original Yang and Heaven. Movement of Heaven brings about the two poles Yang and Yin which are represented in the embryo by Dumai and Renmai. These two poles are already mixed poles (Dumai symbolized by Dui is Yin in the Yang, Renmai, represented by Li, is Yang in the Yin.) With Dumai and Renmai, the body's Yang and Yin sides are completed and the flow of energy between the front and the back side may begin. In the following process, the Yin and Yang

---

22 See Li Shizhen: *Bencao gangmu*; *Li Shizhen yixue quanshu*. Zhongguozhongyiyaochubanshe: Beijing, 2007, p. 1631.

poles above and below the waist must develop. Daimaitherefore develops. These four vessels are called the vessels of the "first generation". All the other extraordinary vessels are those of the "second generation". They are responsible for the nourishment of all tissues.[23]

According to this statement, the development of the first three vessels takes place during the first three months of pregnancy and in the chronology Chongmai, Dumai, and Renmai. During this time, the embryo's gender cannot yet be determined; the sexual organs are still indifferent.[24]

These three vessels are said to have their origin in the *baozhong*. In the embryo in the state of cell accumulation, it seems strange that these three vessels should arise from a muscle (uterus) or male testes. Perhaps taking a look at the embryonic development could bring some enlightenment:

2.2 The Extraordinary Vessels and the Germ Layers

In Chinese medicine, the three vessels Chongmai, Dumai and Renmai have the following main functions which may be derived from the symbolism of the trigrams which they represent:

Chongmai: Chongmai, though it is a Yin-vessel from the point of view of its trigram, represents highest Yang. And it represents the head, the lung but also the lower abdomen. As it is associated with Heaven, it is also responsible for fertility of man.

Dumai: Dumai is already a representative of Yang and of Yin, it symbolizes flexibility and strength at the same time. It is responsible for the small intestine and the whole lower burner. According to its trigram (Dui, the Sea), it regulates problems which are related to water. As one branch has contact to the brain, Dumai regulates the central nervous system and the sense organs.

---

23 See also Riegel, Andrea-Mercedes: "Qijing bamai – The Eight Extraordinary Vessels. A Concept of Chinese Medicine based on the Yijing". In: Friedrich Wallner/Gerhard Klünger (eds.). Traugott Bautz (librinigri 53): Nordhausen, 2015.
24 See below. In Chinese Medicine one believed that during the first three months of pregnancy it would be still possible to change the sex of the embryo, to change a female into a male embryo. In ancient medical literature we find statements on how to change the sex of the unborn child. Mostly they are entitled "*Zhuan nü wei nan*", "How to change a female fetus into a male one." For further information see Riegel, Andrea-Mercedes: *Das Streben nach dem Sohn. Fruchtbarkeit und Empfängnis in den medizinischen Texten Chinas von der Hanzeit bis zur Mingzeit.* (Doctoral thesis) Herbert Utz: München, 1999, pp. 139–141.

Renmai: With Renmai, fire comes into the developing process. The trigram Li is the symbol for the eye and the heart. As the trigram Li is the representative of Heaven at the human level, Renmai is responsible for reproduction, it regulates the genital organs. It is also responsible for the production of blood, being the "sea of blood". As one branch runs along the spine, Renmai also nourishes the spine. In the body it strengthens Yin and Yang.

The development of the embryo

After having developed to the state of the blastula, the implantation of the fertilized egg (zygote) in the endometrium takes place. First the entoderm develops, followed by the ectoderm and mesoderm. This might find its parallel in the development of the three vessels Chongmai, Dumai and Renmai. Chongmai can represent the entoderm, Dumai the ectoderm and Renmai the mesoderm. When we take a look at the structures which develop under the primordial involvement of the three layers, we find astonishing parallels between western medicine and Chinese medicine, i.e. between the anatomical structures and the responsibilities of the vessels:

Entoderm: Pharynx, oesophagus, the respiratory tract, large intestine, urinary bladder, thyroid gland which is interpreted as part of the neck, vesiculaseminalis, prostate, thymus gland

Chongmai: organs of the upper part that is head, neck and breast (respiratory tract), and lower abdomen including the urogenital tract

As it is the "sea of the twelve channels" and the "sea of the *wuzangliufu*"[25] (五藏六腑之海) it is the base for the development of all the body structures.

Ektoderm: Skin, anus, central nervous system, glial cells, hypophysis, urethra in man, lips of the vulva, tooth enamel, sense cells of the nose and ear

Dumai: central nervous system, sense organs, urinary system

Mesoderm: Renal tubuli, renal pelvis, urethra, tubaeuterinae, uterus, vagina, pleura, pericardium, adrenal gland, skeletal muscles, spine

Renmai: heart and genital organs, spine

From the 13th day of pregnancy the mesoderm develops and from the mesoderm, the urogenital system develops. The final kidney is preceded by two kidneys which do exist temporarily. The pro-nephros which comes into existence during the third week of pregnancy in the region of the neck remains without function and only creates the pro-nephrotic ductus which is the origin of the next kidney, the mesonephros or primordial kidney. The pro-nephrotic ductus is here called

---

25 See *Lingshu* (38); *Lingshu yishi*, p. 257.

the Wolffian duct and serves as a primitive ureter. The final kidneys, the metanephros, develop out of the Wolffian ducts during the 6th week of pregnancy.

During the first eight weeks of pregnancy the gonads of the embryo are still undifferentiated.[26] The Wolffian ductus reaches the cloaca. The Mullerian ductus develops parallel to the Wolffian ductus. In the little pelvis, the Mullerian ducts pass the Wolffian ducts ventrally and they unite to form one utero-vaginal channel. In the female fetus, the Mullerian ducts further develop becoming the ovarian tubes and the utero-vaginal channel whereas the Wolffian ducts become obliterate. The distal parts of the Mullerian ducts merge and the uterus as well as the upper part of the vagina develops from this. In the male fetus by the action of the anti-Mullerian hormone in the eighth week of pregnancy the Mullerian ducts shrink whereas the Wolffian ducts develop into the epididymis, the ductus deferens, the vesicular seminalis and the ductus ejaculatorius. When the fetus is eight weeks old the urogenital system consists of primitive gonads, the mesonephros (primordial kidney) and the (mesonephric) Wolffian ducts, and the (paramesonephric) Mullerian ducts.

What does this mean for the interpretation of *bao* and the palace of *jing*? The palace of *jing* may be seen as the testes and the epididymis, which is the reservoir for sperm. The same palace of *jing* exists in the female organism in the shape of the ovaries. The female *jing*, the ovocytes, is stored here. Both structures emerge from the primordial kidney. This fact also shows that the kidney is responsible for the gonads. One may even see the primordial kidney as the treasure for the primordial *jing*, the Yuan *jing*, because from here the male and female *jing*, i.e. the sperm and eggs develop. It is plausible to assume that in this primordial kidney we find the *bao* and the origin of the three extraordinary vessels Renmai, Chongmai and Dumai. They develop at a stage when this primordial kidney exists. When the *Lingshu* (44) states that Chongmai is the Great *luo* of the shaoyin channel and originates under the kidney we may assume that, originally, it is this primordial kidney and that the kidney channel is also associated with it.

But all the structures described here do meet at a place which becomes the uterus in the female organism. In both genders, this place is solely the center of the urogenital system and the center of the "origin of life".

The Baomai has contact to this region but we do not know when Baomai comes into existence. In the adult female organism we may see *baozhong* as representing this origin of life or the whole of uterus, ovarian tubes and ovaries. In the male organism we may understand the *baozhong* as the region of the testes including

---

26 See below.

the epididymis, the "palace of *jing*" and the penis, the organ, which is needed to bring the fertile sperm to the "entrance" *men* 门 of *bao* 胞 in woman.

3 Baomai, Baoluo, Renmai and Chongmai, the Vessels Which Are Responsible for Blood

The sexual potentials of man and woman are bound to the kidney and have their origin in the primordial kidney. We also find the origin of the Renmai and Chongmai there. And these two vessels are responsible for blood, in particular in the female organism where they have to provide the menstrual blood. That Renmai and Chongmai can be called the "sea of blood" might also be seen in the embryonic development. In the embryonic tissue we find the so-called aorta-gonad-mesonephros (AGM) region which is located in close proximity to the urogenital system generating the gonads and the metanephros. This is the region which is able to produce hematopoietic stem cells[27] as Pietila and Vainio state:

> The AGM region is the first intra-embryonic are where hematopoietic stem cells (HSCs) capable of colonizing adult bone marrow have been detected.[28]

As this area pertains to *baozhong* in the embryo, it could explain the responsibility of the two extra vessels for blood. The *Suwen* (33) makes clear that the Baomai are also necessary for blood provision for the *baozhong*. It assumes that Baomai are active in the female organism but this does not necessarily mean that males do not have Baomai. It's just that we cannot see the result of obstruction of the Baomai because a man doesn't menstruate. The character *mai* 脉 is used for the channels as well as for the blood vessels. The Baomai may be interpreted – at least in part – as blood vessels coming from the aorta which originate in the heart and run downward dividing into numerous branches. In the female *baozhong*, Baomai might then be the arteria uterina and the arteria ovarica and their branches, all being branches of the aorta iliaca anterior being itself a branch of the aorta abdominalis. In the male *baozhong* the Baomai, on the other hand, might represent the corresponding vessels in the male organs (such as the arteria testicularis, the arteria deferentis) which are branches of the aorta iliacainterna, all being – in terms of Chinese medicine – the *sun-luo* 孙络 of the aorta abdominalis.

---

27 They can be found there from the eleventh day of pregnancy onwards. See Pietilä, Ilka/Vainio, Seppo: "The Embryonic Aorta-mesonephros Region as a Generator of Haematopoietic stem Cells". *Journal Compilation APMIS* 12(113), 2005, p. 805.
28 Ibid.

As for Baoluo, we find statements in the *Suwen* which may help us to understand this structure. *Suwen* (44) states,

> If there is too much grief, the baoluo will be disrupted; if the baoluo is disrupted the Yang-Qi moves in the interior [and does not reach the surface]; if it moves in the interior the heart [blood] falls downward and there is frequent blood soakage [...][29]

In the first case Yang Weijie interprets the Baoluo as "*zigong de luomai*" (子宫的络脉), the "connecting vessels of the uterus", in the second case he interprets Baoluo as the channel of the pericardium.[30]

The whole statement of *Suwen* (47) reads,

> When a woman is pregnant and in the ninth month she loses speech, what is the reason for this? Qibo said: <This is because the *luo* [and] *mai* of the *bao* are disrupted. (...) Qibo: <The Baoluo is bound to the kidney [...][31]

The first part of this statement seems to describe what might be part of the compression syndrome of the caval vein.[32] From the point of view of anatomy, the veins do transport blood from the periphery to the heart; the path goes from the small veins in the genital organs onward to vena iliacacommunis which becomes the caval vein. One side branch is the vena renalis. The vena cava accumulates the blood of the inner organs except the digestive organs and transports it to the heart.

Seen from this point of view, the Baomai can describe the arteries supplying the organs of the little pelvis whereas the Baoluo describes the veins in this region re-transporting blood to the heart.

Baomai and Baoluo as a Circuit

In this sense Baomai and Baoluo describe a circuit. Bob Flaws sees quite another circuit. First of all he also sees Baoluo as being plural. As for Baomai he associates this vessel with the pericardium and states it is, "the vessel by which the heart sends blood down to the uterus".[33] In the end he interprets Baomai as a synonym for Chongmai; he states that the term "Baomai" should be "a term used in theoretical and introductory discussions".[34] As for Baoluo he sees the "network

---

29 Yang Weijie, p. 339.
30 Ibid. Flaws relies on the translation of the *Suwen* "The Baoluo connect the kidneys to the uterus" and draws the conclusion that the Baoluo supply the uterus with kidney essence.
31 *Suwen* (47); Yang Weijie, p. 356.
32 See below.
33 Flaws, p. 9.
34 Ibid.

vessels distributed over the *bao gong* which supply and fill the *bao gong* with kidney essence."[35]

He describes the circuit between the uterus, the kidneys and the heart via Baomai and Baoluo as follows,

> [...] the baomai is the pathway by which heart blood is transported down to the uterus. Whereas, the bao luo is the pathway by which yin essence is transported to the uterus but also from thence upward via the chongmai/bao mai to the heart and upper body. The uterus is the juncture between the bao mai and bao luo, and, therefore, also between the heart and kidneys or the upper and lower burners.[36]

Flaws interprets the character *luo* 絡 as small connecting vessels, whereas the *Suwen* commentary by Yang Weijie – as has been already stated – interprets the character as the "*xinbaoluo*", as an indication, that this vessel pertains to the pericardium.

The idea that Baoluo is a branch of the pericardium channel is confirmed by the statements of Xu Feng and Li Gao. Xu Feng (1439) states,

> [...] the remaining two channels are those of the Triple Burner and of the Baoluo. The Triple Burner is the father of Yang-Qi, the Baoluo is the other of Yin-Blood.[37]

And Li Gao made the following statement in his *Piweilun* (Treatise on the Spleen and the Stomach):

> Heart-fire is Yin-fire. It rises from the loser burner upward and has contact to the heart. The heart is no more the ruler-fire, the minister-fire has to replace it; the minister-fire is the fire of the *baoluo* in the lower burner [...][38]

4 Pathologies of Baomai and Baoluo

The *Suwen* lists some pathologies of the two vessels Baomai and Baoluo which are based on disruption, i.e. an impaired flow of Qi and blood, due either to mental disturbances or mechanical obstruction.

Following Yang Weijie in his comment to *Suwen* (44), the Baoluo means the Shou Jueyin pericardium channel; but the passage also makes allusion to the Baomai nourishing the *baozhong* in order to indicate the close relationship between the two vessels. The term "*xiabeng*" 下崩 makes clear that here it is a question of the menstrual blood, because menorrhagia or metrorrhagia is called *benglou* 崩漏

---

35 Ibid.
36 Ibid.
37 Xu, Feng: *Zhenjiu Daquan*. Renmin Weisheng chubanshe: Beijing, 1988, p. 203.
38 Li, Dongyuan: *Dongyuan yiji*. Renmin Weisheng chubanshe: Beijing, 1993, p. 58.

(rushing down – dripping). It is question here of the influence of the psyche on the menstrual discharge and the idea is that an impairment of the *shen*, which is the emotional part of the heart, or long-term stagnation of liver-Qi – the liver also being a Jueyin organ – may result in heat, and heat causes frequent menstruation or at least results in mid-cycle bleeding. Grief, sorrow and mental stress might have negative effects on the male organism too, which may manifest itself in problems of erection or lack of libido.[39]

Suwen (33) states,
> If the monthly affair doesn't flow this is due to an obstruction of Baomai. Baomai pertains to the heart and connects to *baozhong*. When the Qi in the upper part presses the lung the heart Qi doesn't descend, for this the menstruation doesn't come.[40]

Here two interpretations are possible: from the point of view of channel theory, Baomai may be a synonym for the heart channel as Baoluo in *Suwen* (44) represents the pericardium channel. This would be plausible, on the one hand, because heart blood is needed in the genitals, i.e. in the uterus, for the menstruation and in the penis for erection. On the other hand, the heart channel does not connect to *baozhong*, some may suggest it is the Baomai which is being described above. It is dominated by the heart and this means impairment of the *shen* may bring about an impairment of menstruation, in this case the lack of menstruation because the heart-Qi stagnates in the upper part of the body and the *baozhong* loses its source. In the sense of Western medicine one might interpret this phenomenon as the lack of menstruation (amenorrhoea) caused by mental disturbances. In the sense of Chinese medicine, this represents a dislocation of the pivot heart-kidney, a disruption between the linkage of fire and water. One may also say the kidney doesn't receive the blood of the heart and cannot produce *tiangui*, i.e. – in terms of western medicine – hormonal disturbances occur because of mental disturbances or psychological problems. Either the hypophysis doesn't produce the gonadotropins or the ovaries do not react so that there is no ovulation.

In Western medicine it is a well-known fact that long-term grief, sorrow and mental pressure result in menstrual disorders, either in mid-cycle bleeding or in amenorrhea. If this severe impairment of *shen*, i.e. the psyche occurs during pregnancy this might cause miscarriage. Chinese medicine explains this as being

---

39 This statement may be the reason why the pericardium or the pericardium channel is often erroneously translated with "circulation – sexus".
40 *Suwen* (33); Yang Weijie, p. 266.

undernourishment of the *bao* through stagnation of heart-Qi in the upper part of the body; in Western medicine, the mechanism is not clear.

The other pathology concerns pregnancy and the syndrome which we may identify as the compression syndrome of the caval vein:[41]

> When a woman is pregnant and in the ninth month she loses speech what is the reason for this? Qibo said: <This is because the luo and mai of the bao are disrupted.> Huangdi: <What does this mean?> Qibo: <the Baoluo is bound to the kidney; the Shaoyin channel pertains to the kidney and is bound to the tongue, therefore she cannot speak.[42]

In late pregnancy the unborn fetus becomes heavy and presses on the vessels and channels, i.e. on Baomai and Baoluo but also on the kidney channel. The Qi of the kidney channel cannot rise upward to nourish the tongue.

This passage shows the close affiliation between the two Shaoyin channels of heart and kidney. Both channels have contact to the root of the tongue. The pressure on Baomai, Baoluo and the Shaoyin channels could, in this case, be interpreted as a compression of the caval vein during late pregnancy (see above) which is associated with momentary loss of consciousness, dyspnea and hypotonus; or we may see a precursor of eclampsia which is associated with symptoms like impaired vision, headache and disturbances of consciousness and with hypertension, edema and proteinuria (EPH). These symptoms all reveal the stagnation of Qi in the heart and kidney channels and a disruption of the flow of Qi between the upper and the lower part.

The blocked passage of Baomai and Baoluo during pregnancy may cause yet another pathology: the disturbance of the education of the fetus. From the Zhou Dynasty onward, it was of extraordinary importance, for aristocratic women at least, to start educating the fetus when it was still in the womb. The practice of the so-called *taijiao* 胎教 (the education of the fetus) should not lose its importance in Chinese medical history. During pregnancy the mother took care of her nourishment and her behavior to an extraordinary extent. And the servants took care of her and prevented her from becoming over-stressed. In the *Lienü zhuan* (Biographies of important women) we read,

> In Antiquity it was like this: when a woman was pregnant, she did not sleep on the side, she did not sit or stand in an oblique position, she did not eat inadequate spices, when the meals were not prepared in an adequate way she did not eat them, when the sitting mat was not straight she did not sit down, her eyes did not look at harmful colors, her ears did not listen to exciting music. In the evening one had blinds to recite poems and stories

---

41 See above (2).
42 *Suwen* (47); Yang Weijie, p. 356.

dealing with virtue and righteousness. In this way the newborn child was extremely well-shaped and endowed with extraordinary skills.[43]

But the psychological condition also determines the success of all the efforts of prenatal education. This is because the heart-blood directly influences the fetus via the Baomai vessels. Heart-blood stores the *shen*. In cases of blood deficiency, the *shen* cannot be stored. Disturbances of *shen* are the result. And disturbances of the *shen* directly influence the fetus and impair its development from a mental and physical point of view. We do not have any reports in classical literature about the negative impacts of *shen* disturbances on the development of the fetus or the child, but we may imagine the consequences: behavioral disturbances, difficulties in learning, and nervousness.

5 The Relationship between the Uterus and Psyche in Western Medicine

We have seen that a disruption of Baomai or Baoluo may produce heat in the interior or in particular heat in the heart by creating a backlog of blood and Qi. The heat which develops may impair the *shen*. Impairment of *shen* may manifest itself in loss of self control, crying because of cramp, uncontrolled movements, or even loss of clear sight because the state of *shen* is reflected in the eyes. As the blocked Qi presses on the lung we may have difficulty in breathing. These symptoms remind us of those of "hysteria". Though hysteria was a discovery of Western medicine in the 19th century, symptoms such as paralysis, sudden blindness, cramps and breathing difficulties were already described in the old Egyptian papyri (1900–1500 BC).[44] One assumed that in these women unable to speak or suffering from dyspnea, the uterus had left its place and was wandering about in the body. So as therapy, one tried to tempt the uterus to go back down to its place introducing fine smells into the vagina or eating bad tasting ailments. One main cause of this disease was assumed to be mental instability, menstrual obstruction and unsatisfied sexuality. The concept of cramps and dyspnea being caused by the female genitals was adopted by Greek medicine where the above-mentioned

---

43 *Lienü zhuan* (1); *Lienü zhuan jiaozhu*. Zhonghua shuju: Taibei, 1967, p. 4b–5a.
44 For further information concerning hysteria in western medicine see Schaps, Regina: *Hysterie und Weiblichkeit. Wissenschaftsmythen über die Frau.* Campus: Frankfurt, 1992; Loges, Bernhard: *Heiliger Wahnsinn auf der Bühne. Die Figur der Hysterika in der Belcanto-Oper.* Epodium: München, 2010, pp. 26–59; Mentzos, Stavros: *Hysterie. Zur Psychodynamik unbewusster Inszenierungen.* Vandenhoeck & Ruprecht: Göttingen, 2004, chaps. I–III.

symptoms were given the name of "hysteria" based on the name of the uterus *hystera*. Hippocrates postulated that the uterus was nourished with blood by a network of "channels"[45] leading to the womb from all over the body. It should be connected to all parts of the body by phlebes and phlebia which, if an episode occurred, could widen in order to prevent excessive menstruation and to give space for the wandering of the uterus.[46] Hippocrates interpreted the uterus as able to leave its place and attach itself to other organs; it preferred the heart, liver, brain and stomach.[47] He regarded the uterus that was able to leave its place as being like an animal. This idea was adopted by Platon who interpreted the uterus as an "irrational animal"[48] seeking sexual satisfaction and craving for children. Being infertile for a long time after puberty, it should become angry and wander about in the body, obstructing the respiratory passages and causing danger for the body. Galen (2nd century BC) also was convinced that the symptoms of hysteria were caused by a liquid kind of vapor, a kind of uterus-sperm wandering through the body. During the entire Greek-Roman period of antiquity, hysteria was considered an organic disease which was caused by the uterus. Experience taught medical practitioners that these symptoms of hysteria were mostly seen in virgins or widows and so Hippocrates assumed that the best therapy would be marriage or pregnancy in order to moisten the uterus and to draw it back to its place.

During the Christian Middle Ages, another idea developed, that hysteria symptoms were related to the Devil and were known as *Stigmata diaboli*. Consequently women who showed the symptoms of hysteria were often accused of being witches. But the idea of secular medicine, that the uterus and unsatisfied sexuality were responsible for hysteria still existed. In the following centuries up to the age of enlightenment, hysteria remained primarily a female pathology and only rarely became an issue in men. A French doctor, Charles Le Pois, discovered hysteria in men and children in 1618, but his discovery did not attract the attention of his contemporaries.[49]

At the end of the 18th century and during the early 19th century, hysteria was considered to be a neurological disease. Although Charcot, the famous 19th-century neurologist, postulated that the only cause for hysteria was hereditary factors, other experts interpreted the disease as being a symptom of society. One considered this

---

45 Dean-Jones, Lesley: *Women's Bodies in Classical Greek Science*. Clarendon Press: Oxford, 1994, p. 69.
46 See Dean-Jones, p. 72.
47 Ibid.
48 Ibid.
49 See also S. Mentzos p. 33.

pathology as a possible manifestation of female dissatisfaction with the situation of the woman in society, the suppression of the female in a paternalistic society.[50] In the sense of Chinese medicine, one could say long-term liver-Qi stagnation developed heat, the heat was transported into the heart and impaired the *shen*. If psychic factors were accompanied by menstrual disorders, one could imagine an impairment of Baomai and Baoluo, resulting in menstrual disorders.

6 The Significance of Baomai and Baoluo for the Treatment

Baomai and Baoluo are two different kinds of vessels. On the one hand we may interpret Baomai as being arteries, branches of the aorta abdominalis which provide blood to the uterus and the ovarian tubes, or to the gonads (testes) and the penis in men. In this context, the Baoluo may be interpreted as veins attached to the caval vein. On the other hand both vessels are close to the channels of the heart and pericardium, the Baomai being close to the heart channel, the Baoluo to the channel of pericardium on the one hand and to the kidney channel on the other hand. According to the statement of *Suwen* (47), the Baoluo seems to be a branch of the kidney channel or at least to have a direct contact to this channel.

The statements of the *Suwen* (33) and (44) make it clear that one could observe the influence of the psyche on menstrual behavior and, in a wider context, on pregnancy. The descriptions are based on the theory of the channels and attribute the impairment of the menstrual cycle or a miscarriage to a lack of heart-blood in the uterus. This becomes plausible when one attributes the production or the circulation of gonadotropines and gonadal hormones to the circulation of blood *xue*. And one might imagine that sterility, infertility and miscarriage may be due to an undernourishment of the endometrium with blood. But there is also the *shen* aspect which may be impaired by disruption of Baomai or Baoluo. Impairment of the *shen* also may result in menstrual disorders, sterility and even miscarriage or delayed development of the fetus. In Western medicine we are aware of the phenomenon that mental stress and depression may cause amenorrhea or on the contrary overflowing bleeding or mid-cycle bleeding. And even miscarriage may be due to psychological disorders because the psyche has a great influence not only on menstrual behavior but also on regular blood circulation in the endometrium. The psyche might also be responsible for the formation of myoma. There is an expression, "The uterus is crying" – the myoma being seen as the tears of the uterus.

---

50 See Schaps p. 114ff.

Preeclampsia is definitely related to alterations in the maternal blood as well as with hypertension which may be understood in Chinese medicine as a disharmony between heart and kidney – or Baomai/Baoluoand kidney – or as a stagnation of the heart-Qi and blood in the upper part. Hypotony in late pregnancy is said to be caused by a blockage of both Baomai and Baoluo. The Baoluo in particular – interpreted as the vessels leading to the caval vein – may be seen as being responsible for the lack of blood in the upper part which creates hypotension, vertigo and dyspnea.

So we see that Baomai and Baoluo were mixed concepts of anatomy and channel theory which served particularly to explain certain pathologies in menstrual behavior and pregnancy. As for the male organism, the two vessels and their pathologies were not a subject for discussion. But we might imagine that erectile dysfunction due to nervousness and stress might also have its source in undernourishment of the male genitals due to disruption of Baomai or Baoluo. So in this case instead of only soothing the liver, one has to calm the spirit, clear the heat of the heart and activate the blood circulation downward. In acupuncture there are several points on the Shaoyin- and Jueyin-channels which are useful:

Neiguan (Pc 6) and Daling (Pc 7): these are points which calm the spirit and Neiguan also strengthens Yin-blood being the confluence point of Yinweimai.

Shenmen (H 7) calms the spirit and strengthens heart-blood. Yinxi (H 6) strengthens Yin and being the *xi*-point of the heart channel it soothes the flow of Qi in the heart channel.

Yintang (Ex 1) calms the spirit.

Juque (Ren 14) and Danzhong (Ren 17) are points strengthening the heart and pericardium being the *mu*-points of the two organs. Shentang (Bl 44) and Gaohuang (Bl 43) may be their complements.

Taichong (Liv 3) activates the liver-Qi, the liver being the complement of the pericardium as a Jueyin organ. It is an ideal complement for Neiguan (Pc 6).

Taixi (Ki 3) and Fuliu (Ki 7) are important for the nourishment of the kidney and the kidney essence which is needed for Baoluo. Shenshu (Bl 23) may be an adequate complement. Jiaoxin (Ki 8), which establishes a contact to the spleen, strengthens the essence and being the *xi*-point of the kidney channel, it soothes the flow of Qi in the kidney channel.

Taixi (Ki 3) and Shenmen (He 7) as a combination strengthen the Shaoyin-pivot heart-kidney.[51]

---

51 Cave: Taixi, Fuliu and Taichong may not be used during pregnancy.

7 Conclusion

The concept of Baomai and Baoluo is discussed in different ways. Some Western experts interpret Baomai and Baoluo as being the vessels of Renmai and Chongmai. One argument in favor of this idea is the fact that in the medical literature throughout history there is little mention of the two vessels and problems of menstruation and pregnancy are mainly discussed via Renmai and Chongmai. It seems nevertheless more plausible that Baomai and Baoluo are different to Renmai and Chongmai. The two vessels are described as nourishing vessels especially for the genitals meaning that their scope of activity is rather restricted.

The concept of Baomai and Baoluo may have its source partly in anatomic findings and it seems to be a mixed concept between anatomy and channel theory. Being part of the channels, Baomai and Baoluo may be understood as being branches of the heart channel and the pericardium channel respectively. The names of the characters *mai* and *luo* may also give a hint to the location of the vessels; as mentioned above, this is the interpretation of some experts: the Baomai might nourish the deeper layers of the corresponding tissues, and the *luo* might nourish the superficial layers of the tissues as it is the case for the rest of the channels and networkvessels. As anatomically visible vessels, they may represent the small arteries and veins which are branches of the aorta abdominalis (Baomai) and the caval vein (Baoluo).

The fact that the concept seems to have fallen into oblivion during Chinese medical history is astonishing. But it can explain several phenomena which we are familiar with in western medicine, and its understanding opens new paths in the diagnosis and treatment of menstrual disorders, sterility, infertility, the female psyche, and the erectile dysfunction and impotence of men.

References

Dean-Jones, Lesley: *Women's Bodies in Classical Greek Science*. Clarendon Press: Oxford, 1994.

Flaws, Bob: *A Compendium of Chinese Medical Menstrual Diseases*. Blue Poppy Press: Boulder, 2005.

Huangfu, Mi: *Zhenjiu jiayijing jiaozhu*. Renmin Weisheng chubanshe: Beijing, 1998, p. 385.

Li Dongyuan: *Dongyuan yiji*. (The Collected Works by Li Dongyuan). Renmin Weisheng chubanshe: Beijing, 1993.

Li, Shizhen: *Li Shizhenyixuequanshu* (The Complete Medical Writings by Li Shizhen). Zhongguo zhongyiyao chubanshe: Beijing, 2007 (orig. 1578).

Lingshu yishi. (Annotated and Translated Edition of the Spiritual Pivot of the Classic of Internal Medicine of the Yellow Emperor). Shanghai kexue jishu chubanshe: Shanghai, 1997.

Liu Xiang: *Lienü zhuan jiaozhu*. (Corrected and Annotated Edition of the Biographies of Important Women). Zhonghua shuju: Taibei, 1967 (orig. ca. 60 BC).

Loges, Bernhard F.: *Heiliger Wahnsinn auf der Bühne. Die Figur der Hysterika in der Belcanto-Oper*. Epodium: München, 2010.

Mentzos, Stavros: *Hysterie. Zur Psychodynamik unbewusster Inszenierungen*. Vandenhoeck & Ruprecht: Göttingen, 2015.

Pietilä, Ilkk/Seppo Vainio: "The Embryonic Aorta-gonad-mesonephros Region as a Generator of Haematopoietic Stem Cells". *Journal Compilation APMIS* 12(113), 2005, pp. 804–812.

Riegel, Andrea-Mercedes: *Das Streben nach dem Sohn. Fruchtbarkeit und Empfängnis in den medizinischen Texten Chinas von der Hanzeit bis zur Mingzeit*. Herbert Utz: München, 1999.

Riegel, Andrea-Mercedes: *Die Niere shen. Klassische Konzepte der traditionellen chinesischen Medizin im Lichte der modernen Schulmedizin*. Bacopa: Schiedlberg, 2010.

Riegel, Andrea-Mercedes: *Die klassischen Akupunkturpunkte. Bedeutung – Indikation – Wirkung*. Elsevier: München, 2012.

Riegel, Andrea-Mercedes: "*Qijing bamai – The Eight Extraordinary Vessels. A concept of Chinese Medicine based on the Yijing*". In: Friedrich Wallner/Gerhard Kluenger (eds.): *Constructive Realism – Philosophy, Science and Medicine*. Traugott Bautz (librinigri 53): Nordhausen, 2015, pp. 177–198.

Rochat de la Vallee/Larre, Claude: *The Extraordinary Fu*. Monkey Press: London, 2003.

Schaps, Regina: *Hysterie und Weiblichkeit. Wissenschaftsmythen über die Frau*. Campus Verlag: Frankfurt, 1992.

Schulze, Susanne: *Kurzlehrbuch Embryologie*. Elsevier: München, 2006.

Unschuld, Paul: *Nan-Ching: The Classic of Difficult Issues*. University Press Group Ltd.: Dhaka, 1986.

Unschuld, Paul/Tessenow, Herrmann: *A Dictionary of the Huang Di Nei Jing Su Wen*. University of California Press: Berkeley, 2008.

Unschuld, Paul/Tessenow, Herrmann: *Huang Di Nei Jing Su Wen. An Annotated Translation of Huang Di's Inner Classic – Basic Questions*. 2 vols. University of California Press: Berkeley, 2011.

Wilder, George Durand/Ingram, James Henry: *Analysis of Chinese Characters*. Caves Books Ltd.: Taibei, 1974.

Wiseman, Nigel. *English-Chinese Chinese-English Dictionary of Chinese Medicine*. Hunan kexue jishu chubanshe: Changsha, 1996.

Wu, Qian. *Yizong jinjian*. (The Golden Mirror of Medical Doctrine). Liaoning kexue jishu chubanshe: Liaoning, 1999 (orig. 1739).

Xu, Feng: *Zhenjiu Daquan* (The Great Compendium of Acupuncture and Moxibustion). Renmin weishengchubanshe: Beijing, 1987 (orig. 1439).

Yang, Weijie: *Huangdi neijing Suwen shijie* (Modern Translation and Explanations to the Simple Questions of the Classic of Internal Medicine of the Yellow Emperor). Yuejunshuju: Taibei, 1990.

Zhang, Jiebin: *Leijing*. (The Classic of Internal Medicine of the Yellow Emperor in Categories). Zhongguozhongyiyaochubanshe: Beijing, 2000 (orig. 1624).

Culture and Knowledge

Edited by Friedrich G. Wallner

Vol. 1   Friedrich G. Wallner: Structure and Relativity. 2005.

Vol. 2   Kurt Greiner: Therapie der Wissenschaft. Eine Einführung in die Methodik des Konstruktiven Realismus. 2005.

Vol. 3   Daniël Francois Malherbe Strauss: Paradigmen in Mathematik, Physik und Biologie und ihre philosophischen Wurzeln. Ins Deutsche übertragen von Martin J. Jandl. 2005.

Vol. 4   Friedrich G. Wallner: What Practitioners of TCM Should Know. A Philosophical Introduction for Medical Doctors. With a Supplement by *Kelvin Chan*. 2006.

Vol. 5   Kurt Greiner / Friedrich G. Wallner / Martin Gostentschnig (Hrsg.): Verfremdung – Strangification. Multidisziplinäre Beispiele der Anwendung und Fruchtbarkeit einer epistemologischen Methode. 2006.

Vol. 6   Kurt Greiner: Psychoanalytik als Wissenschaft des 21. Jahrhunderts. Ein konstruktivistischer Blick auf Struktur und Reflexionspotential einer polymorphen Kontextualisations-Technik. 2007.

Vol. 7   Kambiz Badie / Maryam Tayefeh Mahmoudi: Strangification: A New Paradigm in Knowledge Processing and Creation. 2007.

Vol. 8   Friedrich G. Wallner: Systemanalyse als Wissenschaftstheorie I: Von der Sprachlichkeit zur Kulturalität. Redigiert von Florian Schmidsberger und Kurt Greiner. 2008.

Vol. 9   Friedrich G. Wallner: Five Lectures on the Foundations of Chinese Medicine. Copyedited by Florian Schmidsberger. 2009.

Vol. 10   Friedrich G. Wallner / Gertrude Kubiena / Martin J. Jandl (eds.): Understanding Traditional Chinese Medicine. Consultant: Lena Springer. 2009.

Vol. 11   Fritz G. Wallner / Florian Schmidsberger / Franz Martin Wimmer (eds.): Intercultural Philosophy. New Aspects and Methods. 2010.

Vol. 12   Friedrich G. Wallner: Systemanalyse als Wissenschaftstheorie II: Kulturalismus als Perspektive der Philosophie im 21. Jahrhundert. 2010.

Vol. 13   Friedrich G. Wallner / Fengli Lan / Martin J. Jandl (eds.): The Way of Thinking in Chinese Medicine. Theory, Methodology and Structure of Chinese Medicine. 2010.

Vol. 14   Kurt Greiner / Martin J. Jandl / Friedrich G. Wallner (eds.): Aus dem Umfeld des Konstruktiven Realismus. Studien zu Psychotherapiewissenschaft, Neurokritik und Philosophie. 2010.

Vol. 15   Martin J. Jandl: Praxeologische Funktionalontologie. Eine Theorie des Wissens als Synthese von H. Dooyeweerd und R.B. Brandon. 2010.

Vol. 16   Friedrich G. Wallner: Systemanalyse als Wissenschaftstheorie III: Das Vorhaben einer kulturorientierten Wissenschaftstheorie in der Gegenwart. 2011.

Vol. 17   Friedrich G. Wallner / Fengli Lan / Martin J. Jandl (eds.): Chinese Medicine and Intercultural Philosophy. Theory, Methodology and Structure of Chinese Medicine. 2011.

Vol. 18   Gerhard Klünger (Hrsg.): Wörterbuch des Konstruktiven Realismus. Aus Vorlesungen, Seminaren und Werken von Friedrich G. Wallner. 2011.

Vol. 19   Fengli Lan / Friedrich G. Wallner / Claudia Wobovnik (eds.): Shen, Psychotherapy, and Acupuncture. Theory, Methodology and Structure of Chinese Medicine. 2011.

Vol. 20   Gerhard Klünger: Freiheit im Kontext der Wissenschaftskritik. 2012.

Vol. 21 Friedrich G. Wallner / Fengli Lan / Andreas Schulz (Hrsg.): Aspekte des Konstruktiven Realismus. 2012.

Vol. 22 Fengli Lan: Culture, Philosophy, and Chinese Medicine. Viennese Lectures. 2012.

Vol. 23 Fengli Lan / Friedrich G. Wallner / Andreas Schulz (eds.): Concepts of a Culturally Guided Philosophy of Science. Contributions from Philosophy, Medicine and Science of Psychotherapy. 2013.

Vol. 24 Friedrich G. Wallner / Fengli Lan (eds.). Evaluation of Acupuncture. An Intercultural and Interdisciplinary Approach. 2018.

www.peterlang.de

www.ingramcontent.com/pod-product-compliance
Ingram Content Group UK Ltd.
Pitfield, Milton Keynes, MK11 3LW, UK
UKHW041924210426
5322IPUK00002B/35